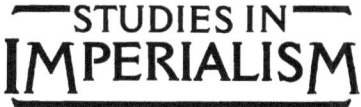
STUDIES IN IMPERIALISM

General editor: Andrew S. Thompson
Founding editor: John M. MacKenzie

When the 'Studies in Imperialism' series was founded more than thirty years ago, emphasis was laid upon the conviction that 'imperialism as a cultural phenomenon had as significant an effect on the dominant as on the subordinate societies'. With well over a hundred titles now published, this remains the prime concern of the series. Cross-disciplinary work has indeed appeared covering the full spectrum of cultural phenomena, as well as examining aspects of gender and sex, frontiers and law, science and the environment, language and literature, migration and patriotic societies, and much else. Moreover, the series has always wished to present comparative work on European and American imperialism, and particularly welcomes the submission of books in these areas. The fascination with imperialism, in all its aspects, shows no sign of abating, and this series will continue to lead the way in encouraging the widest possible range of studies in the field. 'Studies in Imperialism' is fully organic in its development, always seeking to be at the cutting edge, responding to the latest interests of scholars and the needs of this ever-expanding area of scholarship.

Insanity, identity and empire

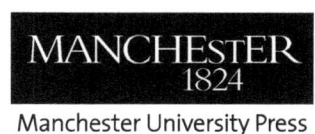
Manchester University Press

SELECTED TITLES AVAILABLE IN THE SERIES

WRITING IMPERIAL HISTORIES
ed. Andrew S. Thompson

MUSEUMS AND EMPIRE
Natural history, human cultures and colonial identities
John M. MacKenzie

MISSIONARY FAMILIES
Race, gender and generation on the spiritual frontier
Emily J. Manktelow

THE COLONISATION OF TIME
Ritual, routine and resistance in the British Empire
Giordano Nanni

BRITISH CULTURE AND THE END OF EMPIRE
ed. Stuart Ward

SCIENCE, RACE RELATIONS AND RESISTANCE
Britain, 1870–1914
Douglas A. Lorimer

GENTEEL WOMEN
Empire and domestic material culture, 1840–1910
Dianne Lawrence

EUROPEAN EMPIRES AND THE PEOPLE
Popular responses to imperialism in France, Britain, the Netherlands, Belgium, Germany and Italy
ed. John M. MacKenzie

SCIENCE AND SOCIETY IN SOUTHERN AFRICA
ed. Saul Dubow

Insanity, identity and empire

IMMIGRANTS AND INSTITUTIONAL
CONFINEMENT IN AUSTRALIA AND
NEW ZEALAND, 1873–1910

Catharine Coleborne

MANCHESTER
UNIVERSITY PRESS

Copyright © Catharine Coleborne 2015

The right of Catharine Coleborne to be identified as the author of this work has been asserted by her in accordance with the Copyright, Designs and Patents Act 1988.

Published by MANCHESTER UNIVERSITY PRESS
ALTRINCHAM STREET, MANCHESTER M1 7JA
www.manchesteruniversitypress.co.uk

British Library Cataloguing-in-Publication Data
A catalogue record for this book is available from the British Library

Library of Congress Cataloging-in-Publication Data applied for

ISBN   978 0 7190 8724 0   hardback

First published 2015

The publisher has no responsibility for the persistence or accuracy of URLs for any external or third-party internet websites referred to in this book, and does not guarantee that any content on such websites is, or will remain, accurate or appropriate.

Typeset by
Servis Filmsetting Ltd, Stockport Cheshire
Printed in Great Britain by
Lightning Source

CONTENTS

List of illustrations—vi
Founding Editor's Introduction—ix
Acknowledgements—xii

Introduction: Insanity, identity and empire	1
1 Insanity in the 'age of mobility': Melbourne and Auckland, 1850s–1880s	20
2 Immigrants, mental health and social institutions: Melbourne and Auckland, 1850s–1890s	51
3 Passing through: narrating patient identities in the colonial hospitals for the insane, 1873–1910	84
4 White men and weak masculinity: men in the public asylums, 1860s–1900s	114
5 Insanity and white femininity: women in the public asylums, 1860s–1900s	139
6 The 'Others': inscribing difference in colonial institutional settings	164
Conclusion	183

Bibliography—190
Index—218

ILLUSTRATIONS

Figures

1.1	'Emigrants landing at the Queen's Wharf, Melbourne', from a Sketch by N. Chevalier, Esq., State Library of Victoria	22
1.2	'Queen Street, Auckland', 3 October 1883, State Library of Victoria	23
1.3	'Canvas Town in 1853', from a Sketch by S. T. Gill, State Library of Victoria	35
2.1	'Night refuge at the Immigrants Home', W. H. Harrison, Melbourne 1873, Wood Engraving, reproduced with the permission of the National Library of Australia	59
2.2	'Australian Sketches: The Melbourne Immigrants' Home', London, 1872, Wood engraving by William Ralston, reproduced with the permission of the National Library of Australia	63
2.3	'Casuals at the Immigrants' Home', 19 June 1880, *Australasian Sketcher*, State Library of Victoria	66
2.4	'The Ne'er-Do-Well in the Colonies', *Illustrated Australian News*, 1 October 1890, State Library of Victoria	67
2.5	An interior view of the Costley Home New Infirmary Ward, Auckland, 9 December 1906, Sir George Grey Special Collections, Auckland Libraries	72

Map

1.1	Map of south-eastern Australia and New Zealand, showing major places mentioned in the text, created by Max Oulton, Cartographer, Geography, Tourism and Environmental Planning Programme, University of Waikato	24

LIST OF ILLUSTRATIONS

Tables

2.1	Overview of patient sample	56
2.2	Length of time in the Australian colonies from IAS report	62
3.1	Marital status of inmates in the sampled data	92
3.2	Birthplaces	93
3.3	Religious affiliations	95
3.4	Occupations	99
3.5	Medical diagnoses	104
3.6	Patient outcomes	105

FOUNDING EDITOR'S INTRODUCTION

Famously, Louisa Geoghegan, who arrived in Victoria in the 1860s, considered Australia to be an 'out of the world place'. But she persevered and coped with these distant and difficult characteristics. Others found it much more difficult and this induced them to feel, in a sense, not only 'out of the world', but be reduced to a condition where they were, in the view of some observers, 'out of their minds' and consequently needing to be placed 'out of society'. In many respects, the themes of this book are about constructions of these various forms of pushing outward, in geographical and meteorological terms, in respect of white colonial society's expectations of 'normal' behaviour, and with regard to concepts of respectability and appropriate conformity. But Catharine Coleborne explores all these issues within a much more sophisticated web of concepts of gender, class, race and ethnicity in specific settler colonial settings, comparing Victoria in Australia with the northern part of the North Island of New Zealand where both similar and contrasting white settlements were established, with some differences in economic conditions, but with many comparable developments in urban growth together with social and cultural transformations.

It is often said that the British Empire was essentially about hierarchies, layerings of class, of functions and roles, of occupations, of gender, of ethnicity and of race. But as well as thinking in terms of pyramidal structures, we should perhaps also think in terms of circles of power and social influence. Settlements established new circles, centred on rapidly growing urban spaces, on rural settlement, and mining communities, circles of authority that were carefully protected and policed, with indigenous peoples often pushed towards the edges in their confinement to specific areas, and with the outcasts of white society marginalised in other ways, notably into institutions where, as far as possible, they could be 'out of sight'. Just as indigenous peoples were spatially marginalised in order to reduce their capacity to resist, so problematic whites were institutionally marginalised in order to reduce their moral threat to what were seen as the central meanings and ambitions of colonial society.

Such colonial societies of settlement were, as Coleborne points out, essentially about aspects of mobility, the mobility of settlers to new lands, the dramatic shifts in the economic fortunes and productive capacities (in agriculture, mining, urban growth, and infrastructural developments) of the new societies, the movement also of ideas and institutions, as well as the setting up of pressures towards mobility on the part of indigenous people having to cope with revolutionary change. Such colonies invariably saw the global extension of the white bourgeois norms which emerged in the early nineteenth century and came centre stage by its second half. Colonial bourgeoisies set out to reproduce the central aspects of the social conditions, the cultural contexts, the educational and religious values, and their own constructions of the moral norms which they considered crucial to a well-ordered and secure society. All of these were to be underpinned by the institutions which upheld this complex of culturally specific ideals. These institutions included Christian churches, schools, benevolent societies, sporting bodies, libraries, museums, and art galleries as promoters of moral and intellectual well-being, together with hospitals and asylums for the maintenance of physical and mental health. Settlement colonies were particularly crucial here. As wholly new and burgeoning societies, they presented both great opportunities for the extension of bourgeois values and considerable threats to their survival. They were also to create zones of transformation and hybridity in the extension of such values. Colonial societies were to prove different in all sorts of ways, in helping to form new concepts of masculinity and femininity, fresh identities, and hybridities in terms of ideas about class, ethnicity and race.

Mental health institutions were key locations in the formation and defining of such new concepts. Colonial society soon had its own notions of what were considered to be appropriate forms of masculinity and femininity, of the articulation of ethnicity in terms of religion, 'whiteness', class and cultural difference, of coping with non-British ethnicities, both immigrant and indigenous. It is true, as Coleborne demonstrates, that asylums saw the collapse of distinctions of class and even race since all social classes, if to varying degrees, were prone to what was conceived to be mental illness, while asylums in Victoria and New Zealand could embrace Chinese, as well as other non-British groups, and Maori inmates. Nevertheless, the medical and mental health discourses of these institutions strove for what were seen as new scientific advances through the observation of patients in unique settings, as well as framing them in terms of these very bourgeois norms. Since colonial societies were new, it was hoped that they would present fresh opportunities for the advancement of ideals framed elsewhere, but it also made them vulnerable to anxieties about factors that would potentially destabilise them. This led doctors and others who worked in the mental health sector to survey aspects of difference, in class, ethnicity, heredity, social conditions, and personality to attempt to frame analyses of mental health issues in terms of mobile immigrants and then in respect of the formation of colonial-born societies. Using a considerable range of primary sources as well as building on an extensive number of works already published in the field, Coleborne has produced a strikingly original and sophisticated book that will advance these significant studies in migrant, settler and indigenous mental health issues.

John M. MacKenzie

ACKNOWLEDGEMENTS

This book emerges from a joint Royal Society of New Zealand Marsden Funded project with my co-principal investigator, Professor Angela McCarthy, at the University of Otago (2009–2011). I am grateful to the terrific team of Angela and our two postgraduate students, Dr Maree Dawson and Masters student Elspeth Knewstubb, as well as our Research Assistant, Dr Christopher Burke, for their wisdom, companionship and intellectual interest in the project for the duration: thank you. Managing the large amount of data generated by the research was difficult and time consuming for me, and I was assisted in this task by Christopher Burke, Dr Debra Powell and Dr John Armstrong: I thank you all most sincerely. Maree also provided the team with data collected at the Auckland Branch of National Archives, New Zealand. Debra helpfully contributed editorial assistance in the latter stages of my manuscript process. Dr Fiona Martin has also contributed a huge amount to the final polishing of references for this book: thank you for your attention to detail. Special thanks go to the editorial team at Manchester University Press who have supported this project, and to the anonymous reader of the manuscript, for a very helpful critique and set of suggestions about the book.

I consulted a number of libraries, repositories and archives for this study, and the staff at all of these institutions were very helpful. The Public Record Office of Victoria (PROV), and the State Library of Victoria, again proved to be lovely places to work and to conduct research. Particular thanks go to Gabriele Haveaux, the Archivist at the Royal Melbourne Hospital, Royal Park, Melbourne for access to the physical and digital records of the former Immigrants' Home at Royal Park. For permission to examine the records of the Melbourne Citymission, and for gifting me other published materials, I thank Willa Longmuir, the Senior Project Worker and Coordinator, Heritage Service, Melbourne Citymission, Children and Disability Services. In New Zealand, National Archives Auckland Branch, and the Auckland War Memorial Museum Library, provided terrific sources of material; closer to home for me, working in the University of Waikato Library's New Zealand Collection was a joy, especially since so many significant published materials relating to both colonial New Zealand and Australia are held in the collection and in the library.

Institutional support for research is fundamental to the process of pursuing ideas and publishing and the University of Waikato has pro-

ACKNOWLEDGEMENTS

vided generously over the course of this work with time, additional funds in the form of conference leave, small research grants from the Faculty of Arts and Social Sciences, as well as a period of Study Leave from late 2011 to the middle of 2012 so that I could spend some time writing portions of this book.

During the tenure of this project between 2009 and 2012 I also attended some terrific conferences where very preliminary ideas for this book were aired and feedback was generously shared: from Palmerston North, Dunedin and Wellington in New Zealand, and Sydney in Australia, to Durham in the UK and Utrecht in the Netherlands. More than one research institution generously provided space and intellectual stimulation as this book has been produced. My three weeks at the Centre for Colonialism and its Aftermath, University of Tasmania, Hobart, in 2012, enabled me to make significant progress on the work because I had space and time. Thanks to Ralph Crane, Anna Johnston and others for their help and support, as well as members of the work-in-progress seminar held that month which provided me with a very useful forum to share and extend my ideas about colonial forms of mobility. Colleagues in Canada also provided a much needed space to articulate ideas in a new setting late in 2013: I want to express particular appreciation to Professor David Wright, at the Institute for Health and Social Policy, McGill University in Montreal, for hosting my visit and hearing some of the ideas presented here in Chapter 6.

My colleagues in New Zealand have been once again interested and supportive and always ready to suggest ways forward. I wish to acknowledge, in particular, those people who have always been supportive, knowledgeable and ready with critiques and suggestions, including: James Beattie and Kirstine Moffat, both at the University of Waikato; and Katie Pickles, at the University of Canterbury, all of whom read some draft material of this book. I offer special thanks to Peter Gibbons for reading drafts, commenting, offering references and being a generally positive presence during the long process of research and writing. Lynda Johnston and Robyn Longhurst also hosted events for the Women's and Gender Research Network at the University of Waikato, a useful space in which to articulate ideas. For encouraging words at crucial moments, I thank Richard Bedford, Tracy Bowell, Anna Green, Robert Hannah, Richard Hill, Tahu Kukutai, Bronwyn Labrum, Charlotte Macdonald and Nan Seuffert. In particular, Tony Ballantyne (University of Otago) offered very useful ideas about my work as part of his commentary at the Australian Historical Association Conference plenary panel about mobility and history in July 2014 at University of Wollongong. His well-articulated insights into my work have hopefully made it better.

Research travel to Melbourne was the primary focus of time away and I value the friendships which sustain me across the Tasman as I continue to work across archives and places: in particular, I offer gratitude to Diane Kirkby, Christina Twomey, Andrew May, Katie Holmes, Kate Ryan and her family, Hans Pols, Kathleen Troup and Kai Jensen. Thanks must also go to Deborah Rechter for reminding me of the complex ethnic identities in colonial Victoria, and for pointing me to her own curatorial work about the Jewish peoples of colonial Melbourne for the Jewish Museum of Australia in Melbourne. In Hobart in 2012, Julia Hickey and family were warm and welcoming during this visit and looked after me when I needed some company. Back in New Zealand, Professor Margaret Tennant also helpfully provided me with access to her own research materials and images.

Parts of this book have appeared in an earlier form in refereed articles, and were also first presented to audiences at conferences. I acknowledge specific published articles here: Catharine Coleborne, 'Insanity, gender and empire: Women living a "loose kind of life" on the colonial institutional margins, 1870–1910', *Health and History*, 14:1 (2012), pp. 77–99; Catharine Coleborne, 'Regulating "mobility" and masculinity through institutions in colonial Victoria, 1870s–1890s', *Law, Text, Culture*, 15 (December 2011), pp. 45–71; and Catharine Coleborne, 'White men and weak masculinity: Men in the public asylums in Victoria and New Zealand, 1860s–1900s', *History of Psychiatry*, 25:4 (2014), pp. 468–76; Catharine Coleborne, 'Mobility stopped in its tracks: Institutional narratives and the failures of the mobile in the trans-Tasman world of the nineteenth century', *Transfers: Interdisciplinary Journal of Mobility Studies*, forthcoming. The patient case records accessed for the historical period examined in this study are open to the public. Given that full archival citations are made in accordance with archival research practices, the surnames of institutionalised people are used here to preserve, rather than obscure, their identities.

All of my friends and family have contributed to my work in some way – by listening, supporting and providing outlets for fun and relaxing times: I really appreciate all of you, and your own precious time. Finally, my family has now endured another long book project: so I express my very deep gratitude to Craig and Cassidy Hight for their love and patience.

INTRODUCTION

Insanity, identity and empire

In 1879, John Hayes was taken to the Yarra Bend Asylum by the police and his friends, said to be experiencing delusions. He announced that he was turned 'degenerate in colonial society'. Although his age was not known, he was single, Catholic, a cabinet maker and lived in the inner urban area of Melbourne in Little Lonsdale street. His attack of insanity was said to be caused by 'pollution of mind'.[1] Little Lonsdale Street was in the heart of the city and not far from Chinatown, a part of the city known to be frequented by opium smokers, 'shady' characters and prostitutes. Young John Hayes had perhaps strayed from his expected path as a new immigrant, and had lost his mind in the process. Advice to new immigrants warned of such misadventure and its risks, and went so far as to suggest rather sternly that the colonies were no place for men with weaknesses. It was relatively early in the colony's history for the outright mention of degeneracy in the asylum records, showing that developing imperial ideas about 'race' and heredity circulated with the migrants who arrived in the colonies.

Almost two decades later, in 1894, William Rentle, a sailor, also found his way inside the institution at the Yarra Bend. He did not know where he was, nor from where he had come. He said, his notes reported, 'he came in a ship but does not know its name nor can he tell the name of the captain, mate or any one on board'. Rentle, aged forty-five, had been drinking, but was in good physical shape.[2] Like many of the men housed in both welfare and medical institutions in the colonies, Rentle's excessive drinking was a sign of the times for colonial masculinity. His case history reaches back, too, to the imperial world, where he started his long adventure to the colony of Victoria.

These two necessarily brief stories of male inmates at the public asylum in Melbourne remind us of the varied journeys of immigrants to the colonies, and of how and where they stopped, for different reasons, inside social institutions of the period. As fragments of the patient case records of mental hospitals, known earlier as hospitals for the insane, these stories need to be read against the historical backdrop of societies in formation. This book is about their stories, how these were told and produced inside institutions for the insane, and through welfare provisions, and how, in the telling, colonial identities were asserted and formed. They are vignettes because the records on which this study rests are full of such short episodes, a fact which, as this book also demonstrates, allows us to assemble sometimes only limited narratives of colonial men and women as they came into contact with social institutions.

This history examines insanity in the context of migration to the colonies by focusing on two urban, public hospitals for the insane in the colonies of Victoria, Australia, and the province of Auckland, New Zealand, in the period 1873 to 1910. In doing so, it engages with two important scholarly projects, and the connections between them: the examination of gendered and 'raced' bodies in the imperial world of the nineteenth century on the one hand, and on the other, a consideration of the imperial discourses of insanity and the formation of colonial institutional knowledge and practice. This was a period of migration from Britain and other parts of the world for both places – part of a widespread Anglo-settler 'explosion' or 'revolution'[3] – and it was also the period during which social institutional networks were developed across the Australasian colonies. These 'social institutions' included health, medical and welfare institutions, all of which were modelled on British imperial institutional spaces and with imperial sensibilities. In particular, this book examines the creation of an institutional language of gender, class and race in two nineteenth-century colonial institutional sites formed through imperial processes.

The book contends that the populations and processes of social institutions can tell us a good deal about the processes of the shaping of colonial identities. It is in their copious records that we might examine the interplay between mobile lives and institutional fixity: institutions were places where normative expectations of a 'settling' population were formed. The peoples who passed through these institutions allow us to think about the movement of ideas, paper case files and the dynamics of settler dislocation and failure. The archival contents produced in the moments of institutional confinement are sometimes uneven, but with 'dense' pockets of detail, and it is in their 'uneven density' that meanings about specific social groups were made.[4] The major contribution of this book, then, is to draw attention to the vast records of the hospitals for the insane as sites that produced 'social categories' with meanings behind words, words that exhibited practices and forms of knowledge about colonial populations. What

INTRODUCTION

these institutional records can and do tell historians about their wider social context, including the themes of migration, poverty, social class, gender formation and the articulation of ideas about the state and ethnicity, is rarely examined in such detail or depth.

At the same time, interpreting a large sample of patients in two institutional sites also sheds new light on patterns of insanity and confinement of the insane in the Australasian colonies, enhancing historical awareness of the mental health of migrants and settlers who were unsettled by mental breakdown. This is also the first study to embed these institutions inside a much wider social context, because it also draws upon the records of other social institutions, notably the Immigrants' Aid Society of Melbourne, and the Costley Home in Auckland, as well as the official reports of welfare institutions. It surveys official parliamentary inquiries into charitable aid and welfare, as well as the Annual Reports of the Inspectors of Asylums in Victoria and New Zealand, and numerous newspapers and pamphlets. In addition, relevant medical journals of the period, the *Transactions and Proceedings of the New Zealand Institute* (later the Royal Society of New Zealand), the Intercolonial Medical Congresses of Australasia, and published accounts of migrants, travellers and colonists, all serve to form an impression of the collective wisdom about insanity and colonial populations. In this way, the book forges new and important historical connections between medical and welfare practices in the colonial communities described, rather than viewing the hospitals for the insane and their patient case records in relative isolation.

Seeking to bring the social welfare institutions and hospitals for the insane into a shared analytical framework for understanding colonial society is also a deliberate way of thinking afresh about welfare histories in the colonies and across the British Empire. By locating medical and welfare histories together in this framework, this study draws on the significant overlapping pasts of these scholarly fields, also showing the common interests of historians in both. Historians examining welfare, like those interested in the histories of insanity, have argued for the productive power of 'cases' in the nineteenth-century lexicon of social description.[5] The practices of making individual subjects into 'cases' through the iterative processes of the case record and reporting statistics, and the way that the 'interpretative gestures' and conventions of case note records of individual people – and the fact that the information inside cases was then codified – reflect the analytical trend towards discursive analysis in social histories of both medicine and welfare.[6] However, this study draws more especially on a database of patients from hospitals for the insane since, for the most part, similar records of welfare 'cases' in the nineteenth century no longer exist.

Instead, the chapters in this book draw together regular concerns from welfare institutions as they reported their activities, and examine the many asylum inmates whose institutional careers included stays in other social institutions.

This book also features the histories of migrants who became vulnerable to confinement in colonial social institutions. While we know some facts about immigrant histories from letters, diaries, stories of long ship journeys and similar contemporary sources, this study shows that historians can find out additional information through looking at the institutional records of hospitals for the insane, and the reports of welfare institutions, which together provide another lens on the mobile peoples we are talking about.[7] If instances of insanity disrupted notions of settler success and also generated anxiety about whether settlements were healthy, the records of those immigrants and settlers who ended up inside these social (medical and welfare) institutions can possibly reveal more about the world of settlers and its use of social markers and distinctions, thereby shedding light on the core concerns of this colonial world. In part, then, this book also foregrounds migrants' experiences of the colonies through the prism of social welfare and medical care.

Historians have engaged with the structural imperatives of 'empire' and with the many and varied imperial meanings of gender, sexuality and medicine.[8] They have considered the movements of travellers, migrants, military bodies and medical personnel. They have also examined a variety of 'transnational lives', but they are yet to fully examine an empire-wide discourse of 'madness' as part of this inquiry.[9] Institutions for the insane were part of an imperial network of solutions to the problem of madness which followed Europeans to new places of settlement, and which continued to present colonisers with serious challenges in the form of ill populations among both settlers and their subjects. The bodies of both colonisers and the colonised have also attracted attention from historians interested in the meanings generated by gender and racial differences in imperial settings. Such histories include studies of prostitution and empire, and of gender and medicine in imperial contexts.[10] Yet this vein of scholarship has so far tended to neglect bodies inside psychiatric institutional settings. Similarly, while scholars have examined a range of different aspects of psychiatry and 'empire', an overarching history of knowledge about insanity across the many locations and institutions of the European empire is yet to be attempted, in part because the site and discursive field of 'empire' proves difficult and unwieldy.[11] In other words, scholars engaged with the 'imperial turn' have only scratched at the surface meanings of psychiatric institutions which operated across the British Empire, and as

INTRODUCTION

yet, few projects have attempted to investigate these institutions' own particular articulations of colonialism.

Specifically, in analysing processes of colonial social formation in the wider context of the British Empire, this study focuses on the patient populations of the Yarra Bend Asylum (Hospital for the Insane after 1905) and Auckland Asylum (Auckland Mental Hospital after 1905). Drawing upon the extensive records of these two institutions, it seeks to understand and situate the creation of institutional patient identities, and the relationships between different social welfare institutions in these two sites over time.[12] These were social institutions and must be understood as such: their accounts and representations of people are the records and stories of women and men who passed through the social worlds of their time and place, and who inhabited the assemblages of institutional worlds and practices described in this history.[13] Although these sites were separate imperial jurisdictions, and have different histories, they also had many characteristics in common, and they shared distinct approaches, not least their solutions to the problem of colonial insanity and its management, solutions well practiced across the British Empire from at least the 1860s, and part of an imperial form of governmentality.[14]

For some time, scholars have urged for both large-scale 'comparison' but also, 'close-up' analysis of places and populations to achieve a sense of how world processes had a bearing on our understanding of specific histories.[15] Historians have asserted the value of transcolonial studies of the past, and have argued for studies of different sites to be mobile, with an analysis that can move across places.[16] Penelope Edmonds situates two cities of empire in one analytical frame: Melbourne, and the city of Victoria in British Columbia, in *Urbanzing Frontiers*. Edmonds argues that these sites are ripe for a cross-examination of global imperial processes and local manifestations of imperial cultures, as well as local expressions of colonialism.[17] James Belich, too, starts his work about the Anglo-settler revolution with 'tales of two cities', including Melbourne as a precocious story of growth in the latter part of the nineteenth century in a world context.[18] Other scholars show the importance of linking 'urban modernity' and 'empire' to better illustrate the intertwined histories of imperial cities of the world.[19] If '[s]ettler cities were ... vitally important nodes in an imperial network through which capital and peoples moved', they were also places where colonial identities were formed and asserted.[20] Indeed, the very 'culture' of 'empire' was formed through the marking of bodily and social 'difference'.[21]

In particular, this book examines the themes of migration, relocation, ease of adjustment and transition by linking research about migration patterns to patient data from the colonial hospitals for the insane.

Although it focuses on two urban centres – Melbourne and Auckland – it also considers them within the wider politico-geographical and administrative spaces of the colony (later state) of Victoria, Australia, and the province of Auckland in the North Island of New Zealand. Many of the inmates of colonial social institutions came from the surrounding areas, and the mobility of colonial populations was a feature of colonial life, as I show in this book. This is especially significant, since contemporaries, including institutional medical superintendents, commented frequently on the problems of colonial societies and their dispersed populations, identifying immigration and geographical and social isolation as causes of mental breakdown.[22] Immigration 'produced new categories of need', categories based on the emergent identities of colonial subjects.[23] This research is therefore couched within broad historical and contemporary understandings of the knowledge about colonial society, migration patterns and experiences, and medical ideas about the vulnerability and susceptibility of new migrants to mental breakdown, illness and institutionalisation.

The process of 'transplanting communities' and creating new societies through immigration brought the fashioning of specific social groups into sharp focus for contemporaries.[24] 'Europeans everywhere', argues Alan Atkinson, 'struggled to know what they themselves were like, and what they were unlike.'[25] Colonial names for different kinds of people developed: 'grass widow', 'remittance man', 'new chum', to note a few. One contemporary account mentions 'old identities', meaning distinctions between immigrants as newcomers, and those who had been in the colonies for lengthy periods of time.[26] The 'old identity' who had fallen on hard times was seen as a deserving recipient of state welfare assistance.[27] It follows, then, that social groups inside institutions received specific forms of codification from asylum inspectors and doctors in the narrating of their cases of mental illness.[28] By examining specific groups through the analysis of patient casebooks and case studies, and by identifying patterns from a large amount of data, I aim to provide insight into the lives of the many patients confined inside institutions. Coupled with this, I highlight the body as a trope of colonial medical discourse.[29] These were the 'hidden colonists', those 'deviants' who formed a kind of social 'residuum' including prisoners, lunatics, the diseased Chinese, or morally ambiguous, as well as Aboriginal peoples.[30] Looking at the way some social groups were discursively constructed through class, gender and 'race' or ethnicity, as well as the other markers of bodily difference referred to in the past is important, not least because these constructs informed contemporaries' practices and treatments inside institutional spaces.[31] Social institutions produced commentaries on the people they confined, much of which stigmatised the institutionalised.

INTRODUCTION

The individual chapters in this book belong inside a wider intellectual project: establishing how colonial social identities were produced through medicine and its institutions, specifically through the hospitals for the insane. The term 'social identity' is taken here to mean the way that certain groups were formed inside specific social, cultural and political settings, and given meaning through social categories.[32] I distinguish this term from 'national identity', which is constructed and formed over time in relation to the nation state, and could be said to be invented and imagined.[33] Historians tend to agree that forms of 'colonial', 'imperial' and 'national' identities coexisted and overlapped in Australia and New Zealand for a long time, finding expression in the making of public histories through buildings, monuments, celebrations and commemorations, as well as in the rhetoric of daily civic life.[34] Australian historian Miriam Dixson visited the theme of 'identity' in *The Imaginary Australian*, a work which privileges 'national identity' as a form of subjectivity by using psychoanalytic concepts, and in it, she argues that late twentieth-century anxieties about immigration to Australia became a fertile ground for producing new and older forms of ethnic identity based in Australia's colonial Anglo-Celtic origins, as well as in the origins of Indigenous and 'new ethnic' Australians.[35]

Yet, as this book also demonstrates, the records of the hospitals for the insane are a problematic route to finding out about past 'subjectivities'. The focus is therefore on the creation of social identities as 'labels' which were then ascribed to people confined inside institutions. Although 'identity' can be explored as the manifestation of subjective feelings about ethnicity in this period, as suggested by Angela McCarthy in her work on Scottishness and Irishness in New Zealand, for the purposes of this study, I suggest that it is very likely that specific social groupings were formed inside institutions through medical knowledge and ideas about them.[36] The notion that 'society' and 'medicine' are interrelated is now well established.[37] To this we might add that colonial social institutions took their place among a system of assemblages for identity formation, with the intertwining roles for these institutions explicable in their similar reporting techniques, and in their modes of spatial and cultural ordering of people.[38]

While it does not focus on subjective identities so much as upon constructed social groups with projected 'identities', this book to some extent highlights the way that 'different spaces [are] historically formulated as conducive to some subjectivities and not others'.[39] In colonial settings, scholars suggest, specific forms of identity were performed, allowed or disallowed.[40] If settlers 'made' colonial space, they were also engaged in both violent and passive acts of distinction, separating out some bodies from others.[41] In such settings, gender was shot through with the categories of class and ethnicity as colonial identities were created, and new colonial subject positions occupied.[42] Spaces were differently occupied by women and men; the urban environments of new societies were imbued with the variegated meanings of gender, 'race' and ethnicity and class.[43]

One of the critical contributions of this book is its reading of two colonial sites and their institutions for the insane as central to this formation of settler identities. The copious institutional record-keeping of the colonial era ensured that traces of these social identities shaped by gender, class and 'race' or ethnicity, all of which reflected, reinforced and transformed relations of power in the colonies, remained (and continue to remain) in view. The institutional records of the mental hospitals discussed here provide us with new ways of understanding these identities because the institutions housed those who fell foul of the established social order, having buckled under the strain and pressures of colonial life.[44] The process of 'settling' engendered a world of intolerance towards 'disorder'.[45] It follows that institutional sites such as those examined in this study aimed to keep complete records of their populations; from these materials we can draw conclusions about colonial society at large.[46]

Perhaps surprisingly, there are no specific book-length studies of colonial social identities which explore the use of psychiatric patient records to discover more about the production of gender, 'race' or ethnicity and class in the colonial context. *Medicine and Colonial Identity*, a collection edited by Mary P. Sutphen and Bridie Andrews, considers the question of medicine and colonial identity in broad terms – without consideration of psychiatry – and several separate book-length studies of insanity in different colonial settings, including different African countries and India, raise issues around 'identity' but without framing a coherent and sustained argument around this problem.[47] In fact, Sutphen and Andrews point to the instability of the term 'identity', and to its wide intellectual deployment. Their collection signals that in colonial settings, 'colonial subjects' had to come to terms with the 'identity labels that colonizers applied to them'.[48] However, most of the essays in their book foreground non-white identities being produced through colonialist interventions into health in the nineteenth and twentieth centuries, whereas this study investigates 'white' identities more closely.

Likewise, 'colonial' itself was, and is, a term loaded with meanings, and conveyed a major social distinction within the imperial world; that is, 'colonial' could mean 'not British', somehow more difficult to place, lacking subservience, if viewed from the imperial centre.[49] 'Colonial' identities also arguably erased subtle but important differ-

INTRODUCTION

ences between the ethnicities of white Europeans; 'encompassed within the white colonial other were ... ambiguous and contradictory subaltern identities' such as the Irish and the Scots in the dominance of the white 'British' ideals of empire.[50] This idea of the erasure of differences among white Europeans is a contested one inside institutional spaces; at times the differences are made plain, and at other times they are less visible; separate parts of this book examine the ways that ethnicities are brought into view by the form of the patient casebooks. Warwick Anderson advocates looking at the culture of the coloniser to find out what kinds of 'anxieties and uncertainties' also shaped whiteness.[51] In the work of 'migrancy', white women's performances of gender identity reinforced notions of their superiority – in both racial and class terms – over the spaces and peoples they encountered and with whom they interacted.[52] In situating colonial identity, we can locate tensions in the so-called 'hegemonic' colonial project. Overall, this book suggests that by taking up these ideas – the need to think about 'race' and situate whiteness in this way, and the exploration of the construction of colonial identity through what threatened it – we can find out more about the operations of colonialism through its perceived weaknesses. In other words, the flaws of white men and women might provide us with a way of knowing more about colonial society's concerns around race and ethnicity.

Insanity, Identity and Empire also situates these questions about colonial identity inside a discussion of 'colonial psychiatry'. Historians propose that colonial psychiatry must consider the function and operation of 'race' as it explores the relationship between knowledge and power in colonial settings, including white settler colonies.[53] 'Colonial idioms' of madness are significant in our interpretation of forms of insanity. Colonial identities derived from meanings of gender and 'race' and aspects of colonial society, including immigration, could produce 'mad' identities among British men and women, some of whom succumbed to what Waltraud Ernst has called the threat of a 'debilitating and maddening life in an alien land'.[54]

Although much scholarship on the topic of colonial psychiatry has focused on non-white populations of the insane in India and parts of Africa, concerns around ethnicity and 'race' in asylum populations in settler colonies, where non-whites and whites occupied the same institutional spaces, were specifically directed towards the construction of a 'white' identity for institutional populations.[55] In settler colonies, the identities of white colonists, as well as non-whites, were also being inscribed and produced by medicine and its institutions.[56] Ethnicity, in particular, is a relatively under-developed theme in the history of psychiatry literature.[57] By interpreting ethnicity in relation to several significant categories of historical analysis, this book sheds light on the way that colonial identities were created through institutional confinement in white settler colonies.[58]

Hospitals for the insane in the colonies of Australia and New Zealand offer historians pertinent and specific examples of the institutions of the white settler colony, and provide a much needed focus on the development of ideas about whiteness in relation to insanity. Asylums in these places have attracted much historical attention. Institutions, patients, gender and the culture of institutions have all been well researched and examined in a range of the colonial spaces of Australasia. Although few studies have attempted comparisons between Australian and New Zealand institutions, there is broad evidence of a trans-Tasman engagement with the histories of insanity and its management across places, particularly in edited collections and research projects. Several studies of single institutions have privileged the two individual asylums featured here: the Yarra Bend and Auckland asylums, though ample scholarship about other colonial Australasian institutions exists, with studies of Queensland, New South Wales, South Australian and Western Australian institutions.[59] In the New Zealand context, scholarship has particularly focused on South Island institutions and places.[60]

The current book is in many ways a companion piece to both of my own previous studies of institutional confinement, but extends those works by deepening my engagement with the wider social worlds of which these institutions were part. It invokes aspects of my own earlier explorations of gender and the asylum in Victoria in *Reading 'Madness'*, but uses a broader canvas and sharper critical tools, including reading across gender, sexuality, ethnicity and class in a reading which might be described as a form of 'intersectional' analysis.[61] This study shows that colonial power operated across the axes of gender, class and 'race'/ethnicity, and included formations of sexuality.[62] While *Madness in the Family* demonstrates that families played important roles in colonial asylum processes, it does not include a sustained analysis of different social categories, instead articulating some of the under-represented features of familial roles.[63] By contrast, this book will elucidate identity construction in the institution with reference to aspects of the family, including, for instance, concerns over heredity, but without privileging its role.

Elsewhere, I have written about the ways historians might use patient records to understand and interpret the making of colonial social identities.[64] We require a new historical methodology, or at least, new ways of viewing and seeing existing archival sources, to recognise

INTRODUCTION

these categories of social identity in the second half of the nineteenth century.[65] *Insanity, Identity and Empire* is based on a large sample of nearly 4,000 patient case records kept by two major public institutions, the Yarra Bend Hospital for the Insane, and Auckland Mental Hospital between 1873 and 1910, with the majority of these taken from the records of the Yarra Bend, simply due to the greater population at that institution. The sample has been constructed by taking every patient in the casebooks for every third year in that period. The study deploys both quantitative and qualitative analysis of these records, an approach which stimulates new arguments about the relevant methodologies in the field by balancing the need to know about who was confined inside institutions – the asylum demographic – with an analysis of the spaces and tools of confinement, and the ways that these both produced and reproduced social identities.

There are productive methodological tensions in this book: grappling with large amounts of patient case data represents a departure from my earlier work described above, which deployed evidence to tell more detailed stories about patients. Yet this book also aims to reflect on the stories of the insane within this larger framework, and argues that the numbers themselves tell us little about 'colonial identity', and need to be read against and inside a much more finely grained analysis of sources. In fact, the numerical data, while useful, is unstable, given the many gaps in the official record, and the likely errors in transcription, as well as later researcher interpretations based on these absences. Moreover, institutions only reflect periods of time in peoples' lives. These periods were 'abnormal' for the people being described. Yet this study shows that if the work of the institutions being examined here did, for a time, eclipse the individual freedoms of the peoples they confined, by retrieving and reading the extant evidence, historians might find out more about colonial worlds and those who populated them.

The chapters

The book is arranged into six main chapters. A specific focus in this book is the importance of imperial and colonial mobility, and this is articulated in Chapter 1. Concentrated attention on the concept of 'mobility' through recent historical studies of social mobility, movement and intimacy across frontiers and between peoples foregrounds these new interpretations of both imperial and colonial worlds.[66] The 'moving subjects' of these scholarly accounts range from whalers and seafarers in the early phases of colonial encounters, to Europeans in close contact with Indigenous peoples during periods of colonisation, with research suggesting that 'mobility and intimacy operated at the forefront of colonial processes'.[67] Mobility has been the subject of a range of studies in geography and demography, and more recently has been used as an analytical tool by historians. Historical mobility has come to mean more than the movement of people, and includes the flow of ideas between different imperial sites, and the connections and cultural dissonances created through mobility.[68] This study examines the way that different populations of people were caught in social institutions, and also the impacts of mobile medical practices as these moved between sites – both in an imperial network of medical knowledge and practitioners, and across colonial spaces. Importantly, mobility is an elastic concept which allows the historian, too, to look across sites.

Chapter 1 situates Melbourne and Auckland as colonial cities inside the imperial world of medicine and institutional confinement, also outlining the significance of population movement and the mobility of ideas and practices. Within the 'age of mobility', insanity travelled: in the minds and bodies of emigrants from Britain and other parts of the world, in the knowledge about insanity and treatment for it, and in the circulating meanings of colonial health and models of welfare and social institutions. Insanity was also produced in the colonies, as later discussed in Chapter 6, but was known through this mobility of peoples and ideas. Chapter 1 seeks to incorporate a discussion of immigration and insanity by foregrounding this book's major analytical frameworks and concepts, such as mobility, instability, population health, empire's reach, and institutional records as a way of finding out about the problems of immigration and dislocation in the years leading up to and including the 1870s.

Primarily, it was the movement of people across the empire, and around the colonies, as feminist historians suggest, which also gave rise to specific forms of discussion around identity formation.[69] Histories of immigrants to the colonies, their fortunes and failings, are central to Chapters 2 and 3, as I uncover the histories and stories of white women and men: we might call these the 'internal "others"', among them, Irish and other white arrivals.[70] In Chapter 2, the worlds of migrants and their experiences of insanity, poverty, social institutions and the amelioration of their many difficulties in 'settling' provide the focus for an argument about the imperial networks of welfare institutions and medical care in the 1850s to the 1890s. Mobility is again featured as a way of explaining the movement of peoples between social institutions, concerns about newcomers or 'strangers', as well as contemporary representations of immigrants in cities and the way that they symbolised the inherent tensions of white European settlement.

Not all of the inmates in the two colonial institutions in Melbourne and Auckland were foreign-born or immigrants. Chapter 3 carefully analyses the many social identity categories produced through official records of the insane in the colonies, using the database of almost 4,000 patients sampled from the two sites for every third year between 1873 and 1910. The social characteristics of this sample population are outlined here to provide a foundation for later chapters, and to throw light on the book's theme of social identity. The data presented in this chapter simplifies the vast amount of detail gathered, showing how asking different questions can complicate its interpretation and thus our analysis. Chapter 3 asks to what extent ascribed social distinctions meant anything to their reporters and recorders, and why or why not. Is it possible, perhaps, that these institutions produced social identities unwittingly, and that modern scholars have unduly emphasised the significance of institutional labels? There were, for instance, contemporary slippages between ethnicity and sexuality, or class and disease. One answer is that their production also had power; social identities were mobilised by contemporaries in legislation and inside institutions, and were also expressed often through the outcomes of institutional confinement. The formation of what Joel Braslow terms 'the psychiatric body', writing about a later period of psychiatry and therapeutics, begins in these ways inside institutions of the nineteenth century.[71]

Chapters 4 and 5 of this book investigate the construction of gendered identities for the insane. Scholars of the colonial world assert the importance of gender and other categories of analysis to understanding the production of regimes of power that operate in place.[72] Insanity among white men in settler colonies 'threatened white supremacy and raised the spectre of degeneration and hereditary insanity'.[73] In addition, as historians of the complexities of race in empire assert, white women may indeed have been 'boundary markers' of the imperial project.[74] White women exhibiting forms of mental weakness, or presenting as socially disordered, arguably gave contemporaries opportunities to form specific attitudes about what might be appropriate versions of gendered identity for the colonial world. These versions reached deep into the store of imperial ideas and beliefs about femininity and womanhood in the period. Chapters 4 and 5 examine masculinity and femininity in turn, unpacking the way that sex difference gave rise to gendered categories of disease, theories of colonial insanity, and in particular, how notions of whiteness also cut across these gendered patient identities.

A focus on whiteness, by the end of this book, therefore, helps to make explicit the histories of non-whites who were perceived as marginal to the colonial project, as Chapter 6 asserts. In this way this work also highlights the deep and sustained connections between colonial sites within the British Empire and the ways that, in white settler colonies, 'whiteness itself accrued legislative, regulatory and cultural substance'.[75] The focus of Chapter 6 is on the marginalising effects of institutional practices of ascribing social difference in patient case records, and it takes non-white patients as its main subject. In addition, it revisits the focus on mobility by looking closely at the ways that some members of the colonial institutional population were confined through their own vulnerability to policing and regulation, their social identities signalling disorder in the colonial world. Indigenous, Chinese, the so-called 'half-caste' inmates, and other fine calibrations of ethnic identities inside the institutions are all discussed here. This chapter also returns to the contemporary medical preoccupation with the health of white subjects by examining the colonial-born, or 'hybrid' populations of the insane. In both Australia and New Zealand, the emergence of national discourses of mental hygiene by the early twentieth century shifted the focus from the immigrants of the nineteenth century to the colonial stock of the future national health. The chapter asks how these problems were played out in separate 'colonial' spaces, and whether the approaches to psychiatric institutional care and treatments changed as a result. Local practices of psychiatry took their place among the plethora of imperial ones, and insanity was now viewed as an inherent feature of all new societies.

This book establishes a new area of inquiry by investigating insanity, welfare and colonial identity-making, especially through the analytical categories of gender and 'race' or ethnicity. It draws upon a large body of empirical data, and deploys new ideas to test historical methods and theories in its evaluation of this data. In drawing together separate but interconnected fields of scholarly inquiry, including feminist and gender studies, ideas about 'race' and ethnicity and social and cultural histories of welfare and medical institutions, the book asks different and relevant questions about the ways that colonial mental health institutions and colonial society intersected and reinforced notions of colonial social identities. Overall, then, this book makes a fresh contribution to studies of the history of colonial medicine, histories of psychiatry and its institutions, and to gender studies, by drawing together arguments about the shaping of the colonial institutional populations through categories of 'social identity'.

Notes

1 Public Record Office of Victoria, Melbourne (PROV), Yarra Bend Hospital for the Insane Patient Casebooks (VPRS) 7399/P1, unit 4, folio 31, 20 November 1879.
2 PROV, VPRS 7399/P1, unit 10, folio 102, 6 August 1894.
3 James Belich, *Replenishing the Earth: The Settler Revolution and the Rise of the Anglo-World, 1783–1939* (Oxford and New York: Oxford University Press, 2009), p. 21; pp. 1–3.

INTRODUCTION

4 Ann Laura Stoler, *Along the Archival Grain: Epistemic Anxieties and Colonial Common Sense* (Princeton and Woodstock UK: Princeton University Press, 2009), p. 35.
5 On welfare history and 'the case', see Franca Iacovetta and Wendy Mitchinson (eds), *On the Case: Explorations in Social History* (Toronto, Buffalo and London: University of Toronto Press, 1998).
6 Jann Matlock, *Scenes of Seduction: Prostitution, Hysteria, and Reading Difference in Nineteenth-Century France* (New York: Columbia University Press, 1994), p. 140.
7 See also Angela McCarthy, 'A difficult voyage', *History Scotland*, 10:4 (2010), pp. 26–31.
8 Ann Laura Stoler (ed.), *Haunted by Empire: Geographies of Intimacy in North American History* (Durham: Duke University Press, 2006); Elizabeth A. Povinelli, *The Empire of Love: Toward a Theory of Intimacy, Genealogy, and Carnality* (Durham: Duke University Press, 2006).
9 See for example: Tony Ballantyne and Antoinette Burton (eds), *Moving Subjects: Gender, Mobility, and Intimacy in an Age of Global Empire* (Chicago: University of Illinois Press, 2009); Desley Deacon, Penny Russell and Angela Woollacott (eds), *Transnational Lives: Biographies of Global Modernity, 1700–Present*, Palgrave Macmillan Transnational History Series (Basingstoke and New York: Palgrave Macmillan, 2010).
10 See for instance, Philippa Levine, *Prostitution, Race and Politics: Policing Venereal Disease in the British Empire* (New York and London: Routledge, 2003); Alison Bashford, 'Medicine, gender, and empire', in Philippa Levine (ed.), *Gender and Empire*, Oxford History of the British Empire (Oxford: Oxford University Press, 2004), pp. 113–33.
11 See for example Sloan Mahone and Megan Vaughan (eds), *Psychiatry and Empire*, Cambridge Imperial and Post-Colonial Studies (Basingstoke and New York: Palgrave Macmillan, 2007). See also Waltraud Ernst and Thomas Mueller (eds), *Transnational Psychiatries: Social and Cultural Histories of Psychiatry in Comparative Perspective c. 1800–2000* (Newcastle upon Tyne: Cambridge Scholars Press, 2010).
12 The Hospitals for the Insane Branch was established in 1867 with the Lunacy Statute of 1867 in Victoria, and separate 'lunatic asylums' were established under the legislation. In other work, I have used the term 'Yarra Bend Hospital for the Insane' to distinguish the institution from other forms of institutionalised welfare in the colony of Victoria, including Benevolent Asylums. See for example, Catharine Coleborne, *Madness in the Family: Insanity and Institutions in the Australasian Colonial World, 1860–1914* (Basingstoke and New York: Palgrave Macmillan, 2010). This study of four institutions in four colonies to 1914 used the last official name for each institution in the latter part of the period under examination throughout the book. In addition, the use of the term 'lunatic' is too static for the developing ideas about insanity across the period, and proved offensive to some reading and listening audiences who have been interested in my scholarship. Here, I have tried to use the name of the institution specific to the time period of the case mentioned, or 'Yarra Bend' as a shorthand to avoid repetition. Sometimes in official reports the name 'Hospital for the Insane' was used prior to 1905.
13 Sally Swartz, 'Colonial lunatic asylum archives: Challenges to historiography', *Kronos*, 34:1 (2008), p. 297.
14 See Sally Swartz, 'The regulation of British colonial lunatic asylums and the origins of colonial psychiatry, 1860–1864', *History of Psychology*, 13:2 (2010), p. 172.
15 David Goodman, *Gold Seeking: Victoria and California in the 1850s* (Sydney: Allen & Unwin, 1994), p. xiii.
16 Tony Ballantyne, *Orientalism and Race: Aryanism in the British Empire* (Basingstoke and New York: Palgrave, 2002), p. 3; Durba Ghosh and Dane Kennedy (eds), *Decentring Empire: Britain, India and the Transcolonial World*, New Perspectives in South Asian History (Hyderabad: Orient Longman, 2006); Warwick Anderson, 'Postcolonial histories of medicine', in Frank Huisman and John Harley Warner

(eds), *Locating Medical History: The Stories and Their Meanings* (Baltimore and London: Johns Hopkins University Press, 2004), pp. 299–300.
17 Penelope Edmonds, *Urbanizing Frontiers: Indigenous Peoples and Settlers in Nineteenth-Century Pacific Rim Cities* (Vancouver and Toronto: University of British Columbia Press, 2010), p. 20.
18 Belich, *Replenishing the Earth*, p. 2.
19 Felix Driver and David Gilbert (eds), *Imperial Cities: Landscape, Display and Identity*, Studies in Imperialism (Manchester: Manchester University Press, 2003), p. 4.
20 Edmonds, *Urbanizing Frontiers*, p. 68.
21 On the empire as a 'cultural project', see Gavin Lucas, *An Archaeology of Colonial Identity: Power and Material Culture in the Dwars Valley, South Africa*, Contributions to Global Historical Archaeology (New York: Springer, 2006), p. 180; Catherine Hall, *Civilising Subjects: Metropole and Colony in the English Imagination 1830–1867* (Chicago: University of Chicago Press; Cambridge: Polity, 2002), p. 16.
22 See Catharine Coleborne, '"His brain was wrong, his mind astray": Families and the language of insanity in New South Wales, Queensland and New Zealand, 1880s–1910', *Journal of Family History*, 31:1 (2006), pp. 45–65. Many inmates of colonial institutions were, as Mark Finnane points out, 'socially isolated people'; Mark Finnane, 'The ruly and the unruly: Isolation and inclusion in the management of the insane', in Carolyn Strange and Alison Bashford (eds), *Isolation: Places and Practices of Exclusion*, Routledge Studies in Modern History (London and New York: Routledge, 2003), p. 98.
23 Beverley Kingston, *The Oxford History of Australia, Volume 3: 1860–1900, Glad Confident Morning* (Melbourne, Oxford and Auckland: Oxford University Press, 1988), p. 154.
24 A. James Hammerton, 'Gender and migration', in Levine (ed.), *Gender and Empire*, p. 156.
25 Alan Atkinson, *The Europeans in Australia, Volume 2: Democracy* (Melbourne and New York: Oxford University Press, 2004), p. 325.
26 John Murray Moore, *New Zealand for the Emigrant, Invalid, and Tourist* (London: Sampson Law, Marston, Searle and Rivington, 1890), p. 201.
27 Margaret Tennant, 'Elderly indigents and old men's homes 1880–1920', *New Zealand Journal of History*, 17:1 (1983), p. 13.
28 On the codification of mental illness narratives, see Coleborne, *Reading 'Madness': Gender and Difference in the Colonial Asylum in Victoria, Australia, 1848–1888* (Perth: Network Books, Australian Public Intellectual Network, 2007), pp. 57–79. See also Sally Swartz, 'Lost lives: Gender, history and mental illness in the Cape, 1891–1910', *Feminism and Psychology*, 9:2 (1999), pp. 152–8.
29 Stephen Garton, 'On the defensive: Poststructuralism and Australian cultural history', in Hsu-Ming Teo and Richard White (eds), *Cultural History in Australia* (Sydney: University of New South Wales Press, 2003), p. 63.
30 Raymond Evans, 'The hidden colonists: Deviance and social control in colonial Queensland', in Jill Roe (ed.), *Social Policy in Australia: Some Perspectives 1901–1975* (Melbourne: Cassell, 1976), pp. 74–100.
31 Deborah A. Stone examines the way that categories of person developed over a long period of time and contributed to much later twentieth-century meanings of disability in the law, also informing a hierarchy of classifications for the State; see Deborah A. Stone, *The Disabled State* (Philadelphia: Temple University Press, 1984), pp. 29–55; p. 55.
32 For a useful and pithy description of the way the term identity can be used, and disturbed, see Emma Robinson-Tomsett, *Women, Travel and Identity: Journeys by Rail and Sea, 1870–1940*, Gender in History (Manchester and New York: Manchester University Press, 2013), p. 11.
33 Richard White, *Inventing Australia*, The Australian Experience 3 (St Leonard's: Allen & Unwin, 1981); Benedict Anderson, *Imagined Communities* (London and New York: Verso, 1983).

INTRODUCTION

34 Peter Gibbons, 'The climate of opinion', in Geoffrey W. Rice (ed.), *The Oxford History of New Zealand*, 2nd edn. (Oxford: Oxford University Press, 1992); Jeanine Graham, 'Settler society', in Rice (ed.), *Oxford History of New Zealand*.

35 Miriam Dixson, *The Imaginary Australian: Anglo-Celts and Identity, 1788 to the Present* (Sydney: University of New South Wales Press, 1999), pp. 18–19.

36 Angela McCarthy, *Scottishness and Irishness in New Zealand since 1840*, Studies in Imperialism (Manchester: Manchester University Press, 2011), pp. 3–6; McCarthy, 'Ethnicity, migration and the lunatic asylum in early twentieth-century Auckland, New Zealand', *Social History of Medicine*, 21:1 (2008), pp. 47–65; McCarthy, 'Migration and ethnic identities in the nineteenth century', in Giselle Byrnes (ed.), *The New Oxford History of New Zealand* (Auckland and Melbourne: Oxford University Press, 2009).

37 Andrew Wear (ed.), *Medicine in Society: Historical Essays* (Cambridge, New York and Melbourne: Cambridge University Press, 1992).

38 For a discussion about Gilles Deleuze's theory of assemblages, see Daniel Smith and John Protevi, 'Gilles Deleuze', *The Stanford Encyclopedia of Philosophy* (Spring 2013 edition), Edward N. Zalta (ed.), http://plato.stanford.edu/archives/spr2013/entries/deleuze/, accessed 17 June 2014.

39 See Elspeth Probyn, 'The spatial imperative of subjectivity', in Kay Anderson, Mona Domosh, Steve Pile and Nigel Thrift (eds), *Handbook of Cultural Geography* (London: Sage, 2003), p. 290.

40 Dianne Lawrence, *Genteel Women: Empire and Domestic Material Culture, 1840–1910*, Studies in Imperialism (Manchester: Manchester University Press, 2012).

41 Penelope Edmonds, 'The intimate, urbanising frontier: Native camps and settler colonialism's violent array of spaces around early Melbourne', in Tracey Banivanua Mar and Penelope Edmonds (eds), *Making Settler Colonial Space: Perspectives on Race, Place and Identity* (Basingstoke and New York: Palgrave Macmillan, 2010), pp. 129–54.

42 Bridget Byrne, *White Lives: The Interplay of 'Race', Class and Gender in Everyday Life* (Abingdon and New York: Routledge, 2006), p. 12.

43 Bettina Bradbury and Tamara Myers (eds), *Negotiating Identities in 19th and 20th Century Montreal* (Vancouver and Toronto: University of British Columbia Press, 2005), pp. 1–2.

44 Phrase belongs to Penny Russell (ed.), *For Richer, For Poorer: Early Colonial Marriages* (Melbourne; Melbourne University Press, 1994), p. 6. See also Coleborne, *Reading 'Madness'*.

45 Bronwyn Labrum, 'The boundaries of femininity: Madness and gender in New Zealand, 1870–1910', in Wendy Chan, Dorothy E. Chunn, and Robert Menzies (eds), *Women, Madness and the Law: A Feminist Reader* (London, Portland, OR, and Coogee: GlassHouse Press, 2005), p. 68.

46 Institutions might also be sites for the exploration of colonial mobility; see also Angela Hawk, 'Going "mad" in gold country: Migrant populations and the problem of containment in Pacific mining boom regions', *Pacific Historical Review*, 80:1 (2011), pp. 64–96.

47 Mary P. Sutphen and Bridie Andrews (eds), *Medicine and Colonial Identity*, Routledge Studies in the Social History of Medicine (London and New York: Routledge, 2003); Lynette A. Jackson, *Surfacing Up: Psychiatry and Social Order in Colonial Zimbabwe, 1908–1968*, Cornell Studies in the History of Psychiatry (New York: Cornell University Press, 2005); Julie Parle, *States of Mind: Searching for Mental Health in Natal and Zululand, 1868–1918* (Scottsville: University of KwaZuku-Natal Press, 2007).

48 Sutphen and Andrews (eds), *Medicine and Colonial Identity*, p. 2.

49 Graham, 'Settler society', in Rice (ed.), *The Oxford History of New Zealand*, pp. 134–5.

50 Lindsay J. Proudfoot and Dianne P. Hall, *Imperial Spaces: Placing the Irish and Scots in Colonial Australia*, Studies in Imperialism (Manchester: Manchester University Press, 2011), p. 37.

51 Warwick Anderson, 'Postcolonial histories of medicine', in Huisman and Warner (eds), *Locating Medical History*, p. 298. See also Anderson, 'The trespass speaks: White masculinity and colonial breakdown', *American Historical Review*, 102:5 (1997), pp. 1343–70.
52 Lawrence, *Genteel Women*, pp. 236–7.
53 Richard Keller, 'Madness and colonization: Psychiatry in the British and French Empires, 1800–1962', *Journal of Social History*, 35:2 (2001), pp. 295–326.
54 Waltraud Ernst, 'Idioms of madness and colonial boundaries: The case of the European and "Native" mentally ill in early nineteenth-century British India', *Comparative Studies in Society and History*, 39:1 (1997), p. 168.
55 On colonial psychiatry, see Mahone and Vaughan, *Psychiatry and Empire*. For a discussion of the 'poor white' insane in late colonial Kenya, see Will Jackson, *Madness and Marginality: The Lives of Kenya's White Insane*, Studies in Imperialism (Manchester and New York: Manchester University Press, 2013).
56 Catharine Coleborne, *Madness in the Family: Insanity and Institutions in the Australasian Colonial World 1860–1914* (Basingstoke and New York: Palgrave Macmillan, 2010).
57 For extended commentary about the relevant historical work and those historians who have examined this theme, see Angela McCarthy and Catharine Coleborne, 'Introduction: Mental health, migration and ethnicity', in McCarthy and Coleborne (eds), *Migration, Ethnicity, and Mental Health: International Perspectives, 1840–2010* (New York and Abingdon: Routledge, 2012), pp. 1–14. See also McCarthy, 'Ethnicity, migration and the lunatic asylum in early twentieth-century Auckland, New Zealand', *Social History of Medicine*, 21:1 (2008), pp. 47–65.
58 On categories of historical analysis, the best summary of how a 'category of analysis' functions is Joan W. Scott's 'Gender: A useful category of historical analysis', *American Historical Review*, 91:5 (1986), pp. 1053–75.
59 See for example Catharine Coleborne and Dolly MacKinnon (eds), *'Madness' in Australia: Histories, Heritage and the Asylum*, UQP Australian Studies (St Lucia: University of Queensland Press, 2003).
60 See for example Barbara Brookes and Jane Thomson (eds), *'Unfortunate Folk': Essays on Mental Health Treatment 1863–1992* (Dunedin: Otago University Press, 2001).
61 Coleborne, Reading 'Madness'.
62 Mrinalini Sinha, *Colonial Masculinity: The 'Manly Englishman' and the 'Effeminate Bengali' in the Late Nineteenth Century*, Studies in Imperialism (Manchester: Manchester University Press, 1995).
63 Coleborne, *Madness in the Family*.
64 Catharine Coleborne, 'Locating ethnicity in the hospitals for the insane: Revisiting casebooks as sites of knowledge production about colonial identities in Victoria, Australia, 1873–1910', in Angela McCarthy and Catharine Coleborne (eds), *Migration, Ethnicity, and Mental Health: International Perspectives, 1840–2010*, Routledge Studies in Cultural History (Abingdon and New York: Routledge, 2012), pp. 73–90.
65 'Social identity' is a term used by social psychologists, including Henri Tajfel, to describe the way that group consciousness determines self-identification into categories. As the journal *Social Identities*, first published in the late 1990s, proclaims, scholarly concerns around identity including ethnicity and 'race' have arisen in tandem with social change and new forms of nationalism and racism. I use the concept to show how identity 'labels' are applied to individuals who occupy specific social groupings, and are used in often disabling ways, rather than assuming self-identification, although this process may also have been occurring in the past.
66 Tony Ballantyne, 'On place, space and mobility in nineteenth-century New Zealand', *New Zealand Journal of History*, 45:1 (2011), p. 58.
67 Ballantyne and Burton (eds), *Moving Subjects*, p. 11.
68 Ballantyne and Burton (eds), *Moving Subjects*; Tony Ballantyne and Antoinette Burton (eds), *Bodies in Contact: Rethinking Colonial Encounters in World History* (Durham, NC: Duke University Press, 2005); Marilyn Lake and Henry Reynolds,

INTRODUCTION

Drawing the Global Colour Line: White Men's Countries and the International Challenge of Racial Equality, Critical Perspectives on Empire (Cambridge and New York: Cambridge University Press, 2008); Radhika Viyas Mongia, 'Race, nationality, mobility: A history of the passport', in Antoinette Burton (ed.), *After the Imperial Turn: Thinking With and Through the Nation* (Durham, NC, and London: Duke University Press, 2003), pp. 196–214; and James Belich, *Replenishing the Earth*.

69 Antoinette Burton, 'Introduction: The unfinished business of colonial modernities', in Antoinette Burton (ed.), *Gender, Sexuality and Colonial Modernities*, Routledge Research in Gender and History (London and New York: Routledge 1999), p. 2.
70 Laura Tabili, 'A homogeneous society?' Britain's internal "others", 1800–present', in Catherine Hall and Sonya O. Rose (eds), *At Home with the Empire: Metropolitan Culture and the Imperial World* (Cambridge: Cambridge University Press, 2006), pp. 53–76.
71 Joel Braslow, *Mental Ills and Bodily Cures: Psychiatric Treatment in the First Half of the Twentieth Century* (Berkeley, Los Angeles, and London: University of California Press, 1997), pp. 1–13.
72 See for example Antoinette Burton, 'Introduction: The unfinished business of colonial modernities', in Burton (ed.), *Gender, Sexuality and Colonial Modernities*, pp. 1–16.
73 Harriet Deacon, 'Insanity, institutions and society: The case of the Robben Island Lunatic Asylum, 1846–1910', in Roy Porter and David Wright (eds), *The Confinement of the Insane: International Perspectives, 1800–1965* (Cambridge and New York: Cambridge University Press, 2003), p. 27.
74 Anne McClintock, *Imperial Leather: Race, Gender and Sexuality in the Colonial Contest* (New York and London: Routledge, 1995), p. 24.
75 Angela Woollacott, 'Whiteness and "the imperial turn"', in Leigh Boucher, Jane Carey, and Katherine Ellinghaus (eds), *Historicising Whiteness: Transnational Perspectives on the Construction of an Identity* (Melbourne: RMIT Publishing, in association with the School of Historical Studies, University of Melbourne, 2007), p. 10.

CHAPTER ONE

Insanity in the 'age of mobility': Melbourne and Auckland, 1850s–1880s

Picture the city of Melbourne in the late 1860s and early 1870s. Its European character and population had begun to take shape in the 1850s with the Victorian goldrushes, and in subsequent decades there had been further waves of free immigrant settlers. The act of 'settling' had been brutal, rapid and charged with the imperial prerogatives for land and the preeminence of white settlement. Aboriginal peoples had to a large extent been forcibly removed from what was the centre of the city, and dispersed to the fringes of the colony of Victoria, but they were still visible in the city and surrounds.[1] The city was in many respects wealthy, promising opportunity, a centre of business, commerce, and a major port, a destination. The wide streets were imposing and gave the city a feeling of grandeur and space, although laneways and dark alleys provided spaces for lurkers and those people with nefarious purposes who were hiding from view. The European population, estimated at more than 200,000 in the 1870s, had swollen quickly from the 1850s, when it was around 20,000, as a result of the goldrushes.[2] And, as a corollary, it had a population of the needy, as social commentators always noted: there was, in fact, a pronounced and obvious poverty in Melbourne, if you knew where to look beyond the 'magnificent' streets described by contemporaries, such as the visiting writer Anthony Trollope, who was impressed by the urban grid and its symmetry.[3] While Trollope noticed the Chinese and Irish city quarters, he did not dwell on these in great detail, and the overwhelming impression left by his account of colonial Victoria is his excitement about the energy of colonial mobility, in part because of his own status as a traveller.[4]

Now imagine the New Zealand city of Auckland in the same period. Auckland's urban population was much smaller: in 1871, while it was not the largest New Zealand city in terms of its population, the province of Auckland boasted more than 62,000 people and in terms of its land mass, took up around one half of the entire North Island, with its boundaries drawn from the Waikato region to the far north.[5] This population figure, though, excluded Māori.[6] After the turn of the century the city grew fast, and the total North Island population overtook that of the South Island, with Auckland's population 103,000 by 1911. The surge in population growth for New Zealand came in the mid-1870s, and specifically to the province of Auckland, with the Pākehā population of the colony increasing from 256,393 to 489,933 between 1871 and 1881.[7] As the administrative centre of the region, and the seat of provincial government before 1876, Auckland was an important city. As Trollope wrote, Auckland was 'the leading province' of New Zealand, and, being an older city than the cities in the South Island, and the place where Europeans had first established significant relationships with local Māori from the 1840s, he regarded it as 'the representative city of New Zealand'.[8] It had two harbours and ports, making it accessible to inter-colonial trade and travel. It had its own versions of gold fever in the Thames and Coromandel areas, south east of Auckland, after the mid-1860s, as well as circulating populations of men working as kauri gum diggers in Northland.[9] As for the city, Trollope wrote, 'Auckland is redolent of New Zealand. Her streets are still traversed by Maoris and half-castes, and the Pakeha Maori still wanders into town from his distant settlement in quest of tea, sugar, and brandy.'[10] For surgeon John Murray Moore, grateful to New Zealand for the 'renovation' of his health, this was a 'Neapolitan-like city', a 'balmy Eden of the South Pacific'.[11]

In order to understand insanity as one aspect of the imperial age, this chapter takes urban Melbourne and urban Auckland as two sites of imperial and colonial connection. Represented through images of new arrivals, as depicted in Figure 1.1, and busy colonial city streets, as in Figure 1.2, these places signalled adventure, excitement and success. For Trollope, and other writers, these places were imperial possessions, with writers often declaring their lack of doubt that England had a 'moral right' over these places, although some writers did doubt the rights of Europeans to assert violent power and take the lands of Indigenous peoples.[12] Their writings were part of the larger discursive process of rendering the colonies as a 'coherent site' for imperial readers, despite the apparent 'instability' of new colonies for those same audiences.[13] These were colonial cities, where ships docked, and to which new immigrants flocked, as this chapter explains, but the cities are also situated in this discussion within their wider geographical and cultural locations to show how mobility was experienced across space and beyond urban centres. The colonies had significant rural populations, evidenced by the growth of towns and centres and the spread of the pastoral economy following the goldrush era. There were differences, too, between the colony of Victoria and the province of Auckland, which also highlight the role of geography and place, and the attitudes to place, in colonial invasion and settlement. However, this chapter places particular emphasis on the urban populations of these cities and their hospitals for the insane as institutions, given the metropolitan status of the specific institutions for the insane discussed here, while also suggesting that many people moved in and around the colonies and also spent time in different institutions, highlighting their vulnerability as mobile people as well as the role mobility played in social and institutional formation.

Colonial Victoria and the province of Auckland are brought here into the scholarly framework of the mobile imperial world. Local expressions of mobility shaped reactions to the movement of people, and therefore also formed colonial practices of the regulation of this movement.[14] While Melbourne has been the subject of a vast amount of urban history, and is also more readily compared with other colonial cities in the British Empire, Auckland is not often drawn into this framework, though it can and ought to be. The 'empire' is not a single site, but a plurality of spaces and places for investigation, and therefore this chapter moves between cities and rural locations.[15] This chapter also describes the populations of the mobile in these places: immigrants, sojourners, travellers and nomads and finally the immigrant insane.[16]

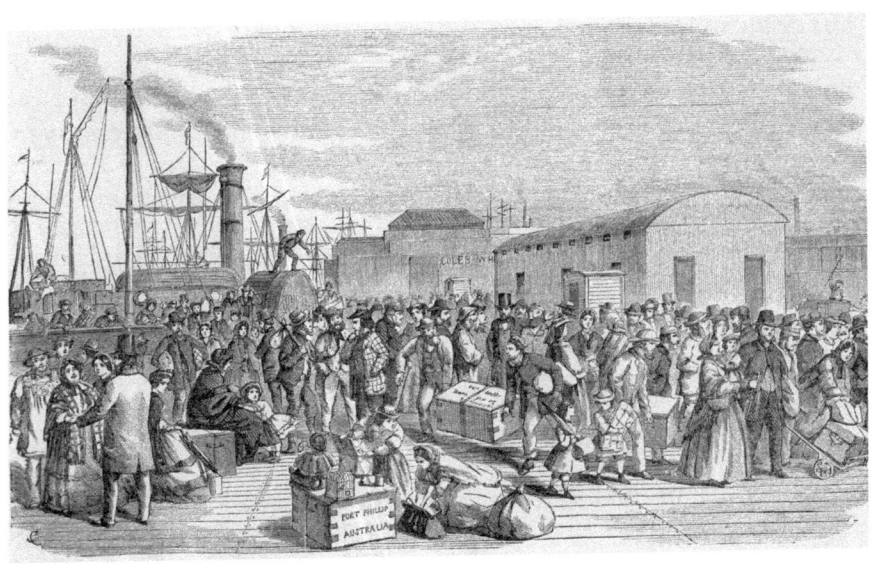

1.1 'Emigrants landing at the Queen's Wharf, Melbourne'

INSANITY IN THE 'AGE OF MOBILITY'

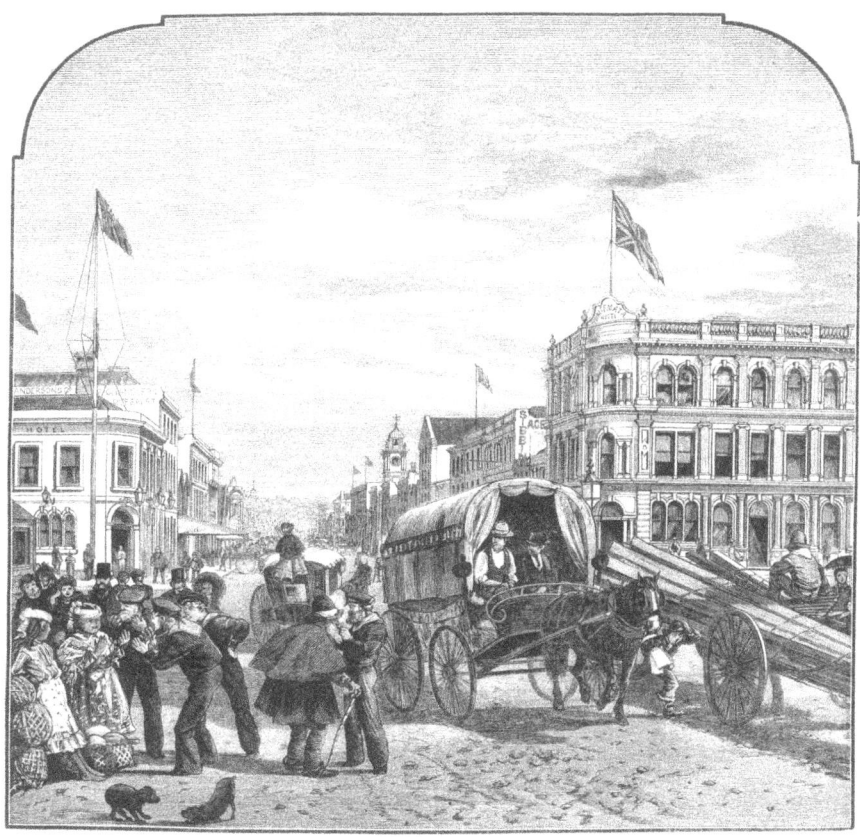

1.2 'Queen Street, Auckland', 3 October 1883

Migrants to colonial Victoria in Australia, and to the province of Auckland in New Zealand, traversed imperial and colonial spaces, including institutional spaces, as they ventured to the growing cities of Melbourne and Auckland from the 1850s (see Map 1.1). Their histories, many evoked in institutional records by the 1870s and the 1880s, provide a clear example of the way notions of 'mobility' were formed in the colonial context. While insights into the worlds of immigrants emphasise patterns of familial networks, or the lack thereof, with some exceptions, their very mobility, and the effects of this on their mental health, have not often been examined as a feature of their identities inside the imperial and colonial worlds they occupied during this period.[17] The 'chaos of humanity' in early Melbourne matches the chaotic, lonely frontiers of New Zealand.[18] This chaos

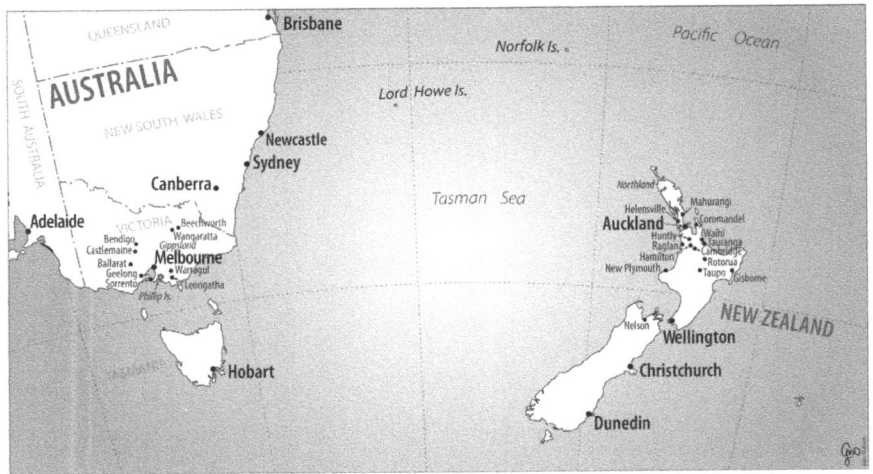

Map 1.1 Map of south-eastern Australia and New Zealand, showing major places mentioned in the text

would be the 'enemy' of the 'ideal society' imagined for colonial places. Migrants could become dissatisfied and broken by their poor luck.[19]

The region of colonial Victoria is most productively explored alongside other colonies in settler jurisdictions which found their populations swollen after the goldrushes. Victoria, known as Port Phillip before 1851, when several districts were 'settled' by squatters and pastoralists, and coastlines exploited by sealers and others, experienced a flow of immigrant populations in the 1850s, which also severely affected the movement and livelihoods of Aboriginal peoples.[20]

Auckland, meanwhile, was built from 1840 following the Crown purchase of Māori lands. In 1842 the plan of Auckland showed the military, colonial government and its institutions all situated south of Point Britomart around Commercial Bay.[21] This act of 'purchase' came some five years after a failed purchase in colonial Port Phillip, where John Batman attempted to negotiate with local Aboriginal peoples in 1835 and came to an agreement about a land sale which was later disallowed by the Crown, as Batman did not represent Crown government. Nonetheless, in either place, the 'sale' of Māori and Aboriginal land was problematic: European entrepreneurs eyed parcels of land keenly and with a view to the later uneven distribution of its resources.

Mobility in the colonies

Forms of imperial mobility, with thousands of hopeful emigrants searching for new worlds beyond their experiences of early nineteenth-century Britain, took shape in the colonies of Australia and New Zealand soon after they became destinations for migration.[22] Not only did these factors of a long sea journey and the prospect of a new life drive conceptions of population movement, but also internally colonies were imagining 'movement' across space, with migration and its attendant dimensions of seeking rightful places for this new 'imperial' existence driving many individuals. By the middle of the nineteenth century in the Australian colonies, 'imagined webs and networks of movement, as in a factory, were overwhelmingly common'.[23] 'Webs' of interaction and communication were also formed in, across, and beyond New Zealand, placing settlers inside empire.[24] Such networks – of communication, transport, cultural forms and organisations – were also real, and colonial populations, many of them becoming 'settlers', lived in a highly mobile world of interactions and movement. Settler society was a 'random and motley collection' formed through and by people and their 'possessions, attitudes and ideas'.[25] Not only was there a vast movement of peoples from the imperial centre to the colonial ports, but there was also much internal movement of immigrants in the colonies themselves, both between Australian colonies and across the Tasman sea to New Zealand and back. Rollo Arnold terms these 'two way trans-Tasman population movements' the 'Perennial Interchange'.[26] This 'interchange' comprised both formal and informal connections and movement of people, commodities and finance.

There were also trans-Tasman exchanges of ideas about social policy in the late nineteenth century, including the discussions around Old Age Pensions in the colonies.[27] Labour migration was an important aspect of the flow; in the mid- to late 1880s, New Zealand's population experienced a large exodus to the Australian colonies, with over 20,000 people going across the seas in search of work or a new life.[28] And yet many also came in the opposite direction, as Arnold notes, especially during the period of the Thames and Otago goldrushes and including those who stayed into the early twentieth century.[29] These patterns of movement ebbed and flowed as opportunities came and went; as Jeanine Graham writes of settler society in New Zealand, '[u]nderlying this mobility was a sense of opportunity, if not in one part of the colony, then in another'.[30] Internal population movement in the Australian colonies in the final two decades of the nineteenth century can be summarised as a flow of people to the north and to the east of the main population centres in the south-eastern part of the continent, with the largest centre of population in Melbourne in 1888.[31]

'Mobility' and 'settlement' operated in a dynamic and dialectical relationship in the past, and both were forces for social change. Social institutions in the past, such as families, the Law and the Church, were not immutable in the wake of new populations. Travellers, sojourners, internal migrants and strangers moved through 'settled' spaces and featured in everyday life.[32] Mobility could be said to have characterised the colonial period, and was especially, as Graham notes about early colonial New Zealand, a feature of the 'adjustment and establishment years', with 'establishment' considered normative and underpinned by the concept of stability.[33] Most of New Zealand society was transient, yet by the early 1870s, as census figures reveal, most people were connected in some way to a family unit.[34] However, the spectre of movement or transience was often evoked. It was watched, written about, regulated, and policed by-law makers and institutional authorities, and it shaped places and peoples. It was 'the unspoken assumption behind many everyday customs and beliefs', also characterising the economic relationships between peoples and places.[35] It was through the management of mobility that colonial settlement defined itself, with power residing in the social institutions and practices of the colonial state, which were shaped through class, gender and ethnicity.

In colonial patterns of movement, we can identify forms of mobility which pushed against colonialism's imperative to settle.[36] The ways in which new settlers, themselves immigrants to the colonies, created institutional solutions for the social problems posed by these increasingly mobile peoples during a period of intense colonisation warrants further investigation. Contemporaries, too, noted this as 'a travelling age', in the words of John Murray Moore, who published his *New Zealand for the Emigrant, Invalid, and Tourist* in London in 1890.[37] Moore was a doctor trained in both Edinburgh and at the New Zealand University, and he was a member of various imperial and colonial societies and institutes including medical and botanical societies. Moore's account of travelling to New Zealand suggests that the figure of the 'globe-trotter' was a creation of this age of travel.[38] Frances Steel provides an engaging account of Pacific Island shipping trade routes by the 1870s, including trans-Pacific travel.[39] By the late nineteenth century, travel by the leisured classes became increasingly prized as the idea of sea travel transformed, partly through new boats which included recreational activities and spaces.[40] However, emigrants often travelled on more basic ships. Conditions could be cramped for passengers in steerage class, just below deck, where people slept in bunks.[41]

Expressions of mobility can be found in accounts of voyages and in travellers' writings more generally, which were embedded within an imperial relationship.[42] Colonial narratives of travellers depicted colonial Melbourne as both an inversion of the metropolis, but also as a new site for the development of ideas about manhood and class mobility. It is in this narrative that we see the colonial subject depicted 'as both more manly and more unruly than the metropolitan'.[43] This ambiguous narrative positioned gender as central to settler discourses. Furthermore, deeper anxieties were caused by the apparent failures of the mobile. Although travellers were not always themselves intending to settle, and nor were they strictly emigrating, their insights do offer something in the way of commentary about life in the colonies. They often observed immigrants, writing about the throngs of people waiting for mail or looking for work at the docks. Some other 'travellers', as contemporaries also commented, attracted attention for their transience and 'wandering life', as noted by John Hunter Kerr's writing about colonial Victoria, first published in the 1870s.[44] There were, among emigrants, many 'unsuitables' who were unskilled and unlucky with prospects for work.[45]

Forms and practices of mobility were gendered. By the middle of the nineteenth century, deserted wives were at the centre of debates about a raft of colonial social problems, including the stability of marriage and the family.[46] Undoubtedly, these women did feature in representations of the destitute and discussions of the 'houseless' immigrant in the period before 1870.[47] Yet by the later period – and emanating from the goldrush era of the 1850s onwards – mobile, white immigrant men were the real locus of anxiety about settler stability. In particular, fears surrounding the future of white masculinity in the period under examination highlight the gendered meanings of mobility in the white settler context. Many poor, white male immigrants were perceived as members of both the welfare and health institutional network, and treated as depleted specimens of the male colonial citizenry. Like their non-white counterparts, these men disappointed expectations of settler success and a more confident form of mobility in the context of the colonial narrative of the quest for both settler control and white masculine prowess.

Male settlers who came to the Australian colonies as hopeful immigrants sometimes disturbed notions of settlement through their eventual lack of success, either in the rush for land or gold, or as male heads of families and providers. Some of these men – fugitives, restless wanderers, men without women, remittance men, alcoholics, the desperately lonely and dislocated – ended up in social institutions.[48] White men in institutions had arguably failed to meet expectations of strong, white masculinity in a variety of respects; as robust fathers, marriage partners, providers and economically productive citizens. As later chapters of this book also show, these men were, perhaps, 'unsettlers'[49] and exhibited aspects of both the 'settler' identity but also occupied the space of the 'exogenous other' through their instability.[50] Of course, 'success' itself could involve deeply unsettling practices, especially on frontiers, as historians have illustrated.[51] The behaviour of men on colonial frontiers – their efforts to 'show a bold front' to Māori, in the words of Samuel Butler, writing about the Canterbury settlement in 1863 – was becoming a style of interaction among Europeans 'settling' and farming in lands owned and occupied by Indigenous peoples.[52] Similarly, women immigrants sometimes became the deserted, the unmarried mothers, the poor, and fell victim to lives of destitution, prostitution and vagrancy, all themes which are further articulated in later chapters of this study.

Mobility and opportunity were also shaped by class and ethnic differences. Poor and non-white or non-English speaking migrants, too, were part of these stories of migration networks.[53] Melbourne became a highly diverse city in terms of the faces on the streets, as contemporary writers often commented. In the mid-1850s, William Howitt described it as being 'mottled with the people and costumes of nearly all nations, amongst them Americans, Persians, and Chinese'.[54] Trollope had pointed out that the lives of the Chinese were filled by '[g]ambling, opium-smoking, and horrid dissipation seemed to prevail among them constantly'.[55] It is well known that anxieties about the Chinese, in particular, and about Chinese immigration, in both the Australian colonies and in New Zealand between the 1850s and the 1870s were pronounced, and shared many of the same characteristics. Howitt's view was not unusual when he suggested that the Chinese 'were a very worthless class of immigrants' in his opinion.[56] Public and official commentaries alike conflated Chinese male behaviour with vice and sometimes disease. The fact that single men came unaccompanied by women meant that they were perceived as 'unsettlers', and were also vulnerable to police surveillance and sometimes, institutionalisation. The goldrush era brought threats from other places, too. Howitt went on to mention 'Turks, lascars, Negroes and black natives ... Englishmen, Frenchmen, Germans, Poles, Swedes, Danes, Spaniards, Californians, Yankees, and men of other nations'.[57] Later, by the 1880s, it was perceived by contemporaries that social problems stemmed from the presence of non-whites on the streets of Melbourne, and also in New Zealand: male Afghan hawkers, Chinese grocers, dark-skinned 'foreigners' ... the fears of heterogeneity were ever-present in the popular press.[58]

That mobility was gendered, and was also patterned by racial and ethnic differences, is relevant because, as feminist scholars of the many colonial worlds assert, colonial regimes are, historically, always 'in process', with the production of 'gendered and sexualized orders' consequently precarious; far from being all-powerful, the supervision of the state is uneven and has limitations.[59] These scholars emphasise the 'persistent mobility of bodies' across the imagined communities of the empire.[60] It was this movement of people, and bodies, which occasioned anxiety about identity. In 'making identity' through institutional confinement and the official records of this, colonists, working within an imperial framework, strained against inappropriate forms of mobility and against certain forms of social fluidity. This was particularly so if such inappropriate mobility upset the dominant prescriptions for settler life. As examples, mixed-race marriages or forms of so-called aberrant sexual practices, as well as those people who disappointed expectations around gender, could find their mobility curtailed. For their part, many individuals who came to be confined in social institutions were also perceived to have transgressed the borders of place, and it became impossible to situate them except as outcasts.

Melbourne and colonial Victoria

One-tenth of all of those leaving Britain as emigrants worldwide between 1860 and 1900 were lured to the colony of Victoria.[61] Victoria was attractive to emigrants because of the constant portrayal of the colony as a place of plenty, a destination for workers, which also promised good futures for families. Melbourne was its own 'empire', and was at the centre of the Tasman world's economic growth and pre-eminence in the region by the 1890s.[62] A million emigrants arrived in Australia between 1860 and 1900. Over 60 per cent of these were from England, 20 per cent were from Ireland, and just 13 per cent were from Scotland. Victoria took roughly 40 per cent of all of these immigrants in much the same ethnic proportions, though it is difficult to be precise about their origins.[63] Ethnicity looms large in the account of peoples 'mixing in' during these years of 'settling', with sectors of the Irish population dispersed around the colony but also forming strong urban enclaves in inner Melbourne.[64] The English, too, constituting one-third of Victoria's population in 1861, were widely scattered around the colony but also lived in the urban city areas with their pronounced working-class dimension.[65] Around three-quarters of all immigrants who arrived in Victoria from 1860 were unassisted, meaning they paid their own way to come to the colony.[66] Among those arriving in Victoria on ships were people from other Australian colonies, as well as travellers and visitors.[67]

By the 1870s, where this study begins, around half of Victoria's population had been born in the colonies, while 23 per cent were from England and Wales, almost 14 per cent from Ireland, only 7 per cent from Scotland, 2.5 per cent from China, and a tiny group came from elsewhere in Europe or the wider world, with the German-born constituting just over 2 per cent of the population.[68] By 1871, on average, the male population of Victoria was both larger, with men outnumbering women between the ages of twenty and forty, but also slightly older.[69]

'Mobility' among these new arrivals took many forms and carried different meanings. Together with the colonial-born, immigrants possessed a 'certain restless mobility'.[70] Priding themselves on the egalitarian nature of their new society, nineteenth-century colonists in Victoria made much of the possibilities of class mobility. As one contemporary writer put it, in such a place, servants could be 'the real masters and mistresses',[71] contrasting this class fluidity with that of Britain. However, the local expressions and social meanings of 'mobility' were highly layered. Both desirable and undesirable forms of mobility, according to contemporary European observers, can be discerned in patterns of colonial settlement and its regulation. By the 1860s, for example, it is now well-documented, Aboriginal peoples had already been confined to mission stations in eastern and western Victoria at Corranderk and Lake Condah, among other mission sites, their movement restricted by laws surrounding Aboriginal 'protection'.[72] Settler colonial histories provide another angle on the 'unsettling' process of colonial population movement and expansion across frontiers. Aboriginal-European relations are inscribed here in scholarship which relates the conditions of the settler world as confining, restraining and preventing Aboriginal mobility.[73]

Victoria's capital of Melbourne developed around Port Phillip Bay. Europeans already in New South Wales had earlier moved in every direction to settle the land, especially after an influx of free settlers and assisted immigrants from Britain in the 1830s and subsequent decades. The rapidity of European settlement was dramatic. In the goldrush years to 1861 the European population was significantly higher, with more than 500,000 immigrants arriving in that decade.[74] Gold miners were more mobile than most, and were followed by storekeepers, bankers, pub-keepers, prostitutes and many others who followed the goldrushes, and it is in histories and accounts of gold mining that historians have found much of the social anxiety surrounding forms of mobility.

Mobility was also regulated and controlled, and even prohibited, because it was regarded as an implicit threat to colonial order. The very 'containment' of the mobile insane was a primary aim of law makers and police across the colonial world.[75] Police were explicitly involved in the maintenance of meanings around 'mobility' and engaged in restricting urban movement and the occupation of public and private spaces in the period under examination.[76] Between the 1850s and the 1890s, Melbourne became a thriving urban centre which was known for its sharp contrast between poverty and wealth. Melbourne was also notable for its different spaces and areas which were marked by social class and differentiated social groupings.[77] But some individuals and groups transgressed the invisible borders between these spaces. Vagrants, among others, appeared in the many different city spaces, thereby becoming vulnerable to the attention of police.[78] Indeed, police in Melbourne were particularly visible and noted for their roles in managing the different people who could be said to be examples of the 'undesirably mobile': street urchins, lunatics, paupers, those who indulged in the 'popular vices', soldiers, spies and prostitutes.[79] Male homosexuality, which involved crossing the boundaries of proper masculinity received surveillance; the 'immoral conduct' of men in the city was policed more discreetly, perhaps, but was, nonetheless, another aspect of police work.[80]

Police performed a wide range of roles in the period. These included removal and escort functions; lunatics were taken to institutions, and trouble-makers on goldfields were removed.[81] Aboriginal people were sometimes removed for their own 'protection' from specific communities, as in the case of the request from the Central Board for Aborigines, in Melbourne, made on 22 August 1860 to Captain Standish, the Chief Commissioner for Police, for the removal of an Aboriginal girl from the care of Mr Banfield, a hotel keeper at Benalla in northern Victoria, in the escort cart.[82] Police were asked to look for 'missing friends', many of whom were immigrants. In 1868, for example, Melbourne police were contacted by an Immigration Agent seeking John King, who had left his wife and child after arrival in the colony on a ship the *White Star*.[83]

Police were often asked to carry out operations to 'clean up' city spaces. Police were responding to a newspaper article on 28 November 1868, when they examined the complaints about the 'infestation' of the Botanical Gardens walk, particularly the 'wattle-grove and a portion of the bank', by 'dirty frowsy vagabonds of both sexes, who, at all hours of the day and night, are to be found there indulging in a sort of unsavoury pic-nic, and engaging in conversation unfit for decent ears to listen to'.[84] The police responded often to similar requests about the 'incorrigible class', even when the area was outside the police beat; directives in the notes talk about police including the area in their beat walk after being asked to do so by the Council of the City of Melbourne. Distinctions were drawn between the 'deserving poor' and the 'incorrigible', with frequent arrests made in the Domain gardens area in the late 1870s, while in other poor communities, the police offered assistance rather than punitive measures.[85] These policing practices suggest a close, and even intimate, level of urban policing of mobility in urban areas.

Auckland and the wider province

New Zealand experienced different phases of migration. For at least forty years the migrant population outnumbered the European colonial-born population, making it a society of newcomers.[86] Like Melbourne, Auckland 'centred around the port'.[87] The growth of the small settlement situated on Officials Bay in 1840 meant that by 1842, it had become a township of 2,895 people.[88] Although there was some population decrease in the late 1840s with the rush for gold across the Pacific to California, Auckland continued to grow.[89] By 1874, it was a city with a population of 21,590.[90] And the wider province, too, grew as different people came, attracted by the commercial centre. By 1891, the population of the province of Auckland was 133,159 and by 1896, it had grown further to 153,564.[91]

Like other colonial settlements including Melbourne, men outnumbered women.[92] Most Christian worshippers were Anglican, with some Catholic, and smaller populations of Presbyterian, Church of Scotland and Wesleyan. There was also a very small population of Jewish people.[93] The Jewish community was respected, and as in Melbourne, many from its ranks came to hold senior positions in local government.[94] Yet some trans-Tasman travel narratives, just as they singled out the Irish for comment, or the Māori, also signalled the presence of 'the Jew', drawing attention to social, religious and ethnic differences in colonial society.[95]

One-third of the population of the province lived in the city of Auckland or its hinterland. Smaller centres of population clustered in the villages of Auckland city: Howick, Panmure, Remuera, Epsom, Mt Eden and Avondale, the final site of the Auckland Asylum by 1867.[96] In the 1880s and 1890s the rate of the population growth of Auckland was faster than the rate of growth in Otago.[97] This is important because Otago had always been a centre of population growth, but by 1891, Auckland and its surrounds had overtaken Dunedin as the centre of population.[98] The increasing Auckland population was due to immigration, but also to expanding families.

Auckland was full of workers' cottages. Contemporaries pointed to the poor origins of many immigrants in early Auckland, and viewed Auckland's inhabitants as constituting a 'London slum'.[99] Locals saw Auckland as 'shapeless', full of 'tortuous alleys, and huddled-up lanes'.[100] Yet immigrants came to New Zealand to escape worse conditions in the industrialising cities of Britain. Auckland had stronger minorities of Irish and Scottish than other New Zealand settlements, too, making for a diverse society, although the southern city of Dunedin was the most Scottish of New Zealand's places.[101] In 1864, over 70 per cent of the population of New Zealand was immigrant, but by 1901, the native-born constituted 65 per cent of the population.[102]

Class structures accommodated the elite and the poor, with less opportunity for social mobility. The differences between social groups were more noticeable as suburbs emerged in the township, with the wealthier members of society living around the elevated areas of the city, and places like Parnell and Epsom.[103] As well as the cottages and 'slums', more substantial buildings were erected, showing Auckland as the respectable cousin city of Melbourne across the Tasman. Both had impressive institutions, such as public libraries, and main streets, and both boasted a network of suburbs. Auckland's Queen Street, bustling and alive with commerce and transport, was the 'commercial heart' of the city.[104]

Photographic depictions of Auckland in the late nineteenth century show the development of land once rough, dirty and from a contemporary European perspective, 'empty' of landmarks.[105] Despite its 'picturesqueness' for some observers, apparent 'in the sky, in the air, in the turrets and spires … [and] in the suburban villas peeping coquettishly from bowers of evergreens', like Melbourne, Auckland was 'dismal' after dark, with few gas lamps and dark streets.[106] Auckland city's Domain, a place for the public to wander through gardens, take picnics and celebrate, was also the site of unsavoury characters, and a refuge for vagrants.[107] In his novel *Spur of Morning*, New Zealand writer Alan Mulgan depicted Auckland at the turn of the century as a 'a straggling, quickly growing city'.[108] It was a city peopled by 'a queer mixture of types'.[109]

Colonial cities in an imperial world

Both of these colonial cities could be said to have rationalised 'settlement'.[110] In both places, their dominant British immigrant populations and political influences embodied specific discourses which characterised their identities as places and as populations.[111] For instance, as noted earlier in this chapter, laws controlling immigration were shared across the imperial world, with both Victoria and New Zealand involved in immigration restriction of non-whites by the 1880s.[112] Melbourne, in particular, offers an example of a city ripe for examination of global imperial processes and local manifestations of imperial cultures, as well as the local expressions of colonialism. Tensions over space, population and society were ever-present in the push to settlement. If cities were part of the 'consummation of empire' through their commercial and cultural roles as centres of population, they were also places of 'anxiety and bewilderment' and ultimately 'places of dislocation' for many of their inhabitants.[113] Those wandering, 'half-caste' Māori noticed by Trollope in his account of Auckland remind us of this dislocation from the point of view of the Indigenous subjects rendered to a large extent as outsiders in the colonial city of the Europeans in New Zealand.

The dislocation experienced by immigrants was another aspect of this process, and another result of the tensions inherent in colonialism. That people found themselves mixing with so many 'strangers' in the colonial worlds they now inhabited was often remarked upon and became a feature of reportage and commentary about colonial places. In his *Hints Upon Health*, a pamphlet published by the Immigrants' Aid Society (IAS) in Melbourne in 1853, Dr H. Earley, who was medical officer to the IAS, warned new immigrants that the already overcrowded city of Melbourne had 'unhealthy' tendencies. He advised immigrants to seek work in the country towns, or on stations, in advice probably directed at single men.[114] Likewise, in his pamphlet *Hints to Immigrants Upon Colonial Life and Its Requirements*, published in the same year, the Reverend William Jarritt counselled immigrants to seek different forms of work, beyond the goldfields, and to avoid work for which they were 'unsuited'. It was 'rough labour', said Jarritt, which could turn honest men into discouraged men, and cause them to abandon patience and hope.[115] In these early years of the colony of Victoria the call to 'settle' was juxtaposed with these exhortations to newcomers to seek work in a variety of places, to become peripatetic in search of both stability and personal fulfilment, and to avoid placing a strain on the new city of Melbourne and its rapidly expanding population. In New Zealand, a similar trend to short-term labour, seasonal work, geographical distance and population mobility gave rise to fears that transience could become the main feature of colonial life, rather than settling down. Contemporaries wondered if transience might result in 'a mentality of ceaseless striving', and could mean that men, in particular, became 'derelict', a theme later examined further in Chapter 4.[116]

In the 1850s, local observers scorned the notion that great wealth could be found in the colonies. Destitution, and tales of utter desperation, were both common. William Howitt's haunting 1855 account of the cold Melbourne winter with '2000 souls' set to arrive at the ports and descend upon 'Canvass Town', or seek lodgings in the already crowded urban spaces, hints at the lunacy of the speed of population growth in that period.[117] 'Distressing scenes', noted traveller John Askew, were often witnessed 'upon the wharfs among the new arrivals from home, who had been accustomed to live in comfortable houses'.[118] These scenes included his memory of entering Canvas Town for the first time and encountering a group of women:

> They were fresh arrivals. Some of them were weeping, and their husbands were trying to console them. This place had the appearance of a regular encampment. Tents made of canvass and brown calico were planted over a considerable space of ground. This suburb was then called Canvass Town, but since then it has been named Emerald Hill.[119]

Figure 1.3, from a sketch by S. T. Gill, is an 1853 engraving later published in a supplement to the *Illustrated Australian News* which depicts the basic and makeshift world of tents and new arrivals. This world was 'Canvas Town'.

By the 1870s, Melbourne's inner city urban areas were visibly dirty and overcrowded. There were higher child mortality rates in the densely populated suburbs of North Melbourne, Fitzroy and Collingwood than in other areas of the city.[120] John Hunter Kerr suggested that emigrants intending for Melbourne were somewhat deluded in their expectations of instant wealth or comfort: they would instead encounter 'the same scene of struggling for a livelihood as goes on daily in the great towns of the old world'.[121]

Residents and observers of Auckland had for some time signalled some of the same problems for their city. In the 1850s Auckland was

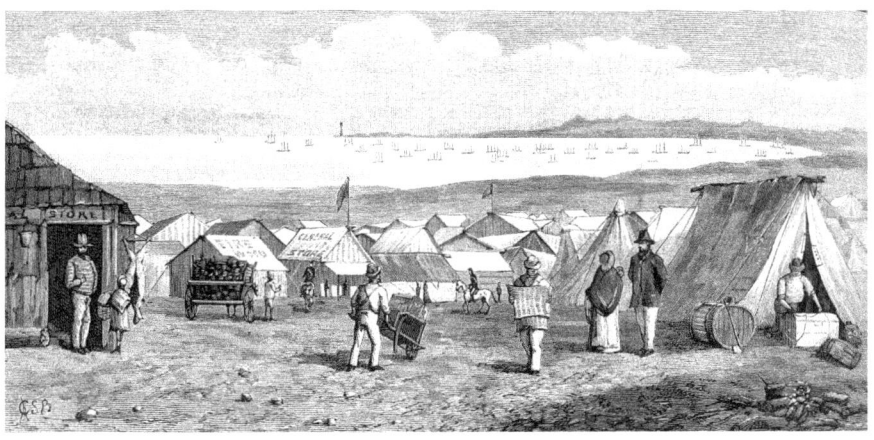

1.3 'Canvas Town in 1853'

known for its 'poorly constructed hovels, overflowing outhouses, and cramped yards' and, like Melbourne and Sydney in these decades, it possessed slums, poor sanitation and an inadequate water supply.[122] Auckland regulated its street hawkers and porters using city by-laws in 1871, and in the 1870s, debate about the city's young street 'arabs' attracted social research and journalistic commentary.[123] John Murray Moore pointed out the 'conspicuous blemishes' in New Zealand's social life, noting the 'prevalence of gambling, immoderate drinking, and excessive smoking'.[124] Drinking was particularly worrying, with Moore singling out the 'injurious colonial habit of treating friends and acquaintances to a drink at any hour of the day they may chance to meet'.[125] Moore ended his account of New Zealand with some sobering comparative statistics on the incidence of insanity in the colonial population, although his intention, as he sets it out, was to correct popular erroneous beliefs that colonial insanity was rife. Like other travel writers and social commentators, Murray was exercising his observational powers to foster better health practices. Coming as it did in 1890, Murray's text was both a useful corrective, and a companion to earlier enticements to emigrants who arrived in the Australasian colonies from the 1850s.

Urban environments, then, were places where the 'classing gaze' operated to good effect.[126] It was in the cities that authorities took interest in specific populations: of the poor, of the sick, of the able, and of those who were likely to be a burden on society. The ideas and practices of imperial professions, including medicine, were themselves highly mobile, and also shaped experiences of the insane and the institutions which they inhabited.[127] Regular assays of the population and institutional populations evident in colonial reporting to parliaments through its 'vital statistics', with all manner of inspectors visiting and noting aspects of the life of cities and towns, tell us that the health of the population was of utmost importance.[128] The emphasis here is on the forms taken by imperial and colonial mobility, rather than population control. However, the contemporary concerns over immigration and the health of immigrants highlight the growing discourse of population control and restriction, as this chapter and Chapter 6 both show.

Immigration provided social investigators everywhere with material. Patterns of urban surveillance of the immigrant had been fashioned in imperial cities before colonial places and authorities took up this habit of watching newcomers. In urban nineteenth-century London, for example, Jewish immigrants in the East End presented an interesting social, religious and 'racial' group for study. Medical writers were concerned to identify the effects of external influences, such as the urban city environment, on specific sectors of society, following theories about racial degeneracy and hereditary illnesses.[129] It was possible, argued Francis Galton in 1865, that urban life could exacerbate the predisposition of Jewish people to mental and nervous diseases, given their levels of poverty, a characteristic of most immigrants.[130] Likewise, as later chapters of this book also show, the Irish were often singled out as being at risk of mental disease, especially given their diasporic movement, with vast numbers of Irish immigrants seeking work in England, especially around Liverpool, and accessing the English poor relief system. In this way the Irish became very visible as a needy population. There were 'staggering percentages' of Irish in Lancashire asylums, where they were portrayed as weak bodies which signalled degenerative tendencies. Although Irish labour was sought after, once inside social institutions, the Irish were no longer seen as strong and capable working bodies, but were more likely to be represented as diseased and susceptible to mental breakdown. It was their mobility and movement which seemed to cast doubt on their suitability as migrants.[131]

Increasing numbers of Irish inmates in these asylums during the 1870s and 1880s were diagnosed with General Paralysis of the Insane (GPI) or the tertiary stage of syphilis. Writing about the specific diagnosis of GPI in the 1880s, William Julius Mickle posited that urban life played a role in exposure to the exciting cause of the disease, syphilis, and commented that Irish people had far lower rates of the disease 'at home'.[132] Later, Thomas Clouston, who was known for his *Clinical Lectures on Mental Diseases* (1883), suggested that the modern city itself was responsible for some mental degeneration.[133] Clouston's book *The Hygiene of the Mind* was reprinted several times after it first appeared in 1906, and in it he argued that cities encouraged numb, mindless activity: 'the street, the shop, the electric car, the factory bell and the policeman keep life going for many dwellers in the city without any thinking on their part'.[134] He advocated parks, gardens, camping trips for active thought and reflection.[135]

Trollope, too, did not confine his observations of the urban spaces of the colonies to the solely decorative, but also wrote about the socially ameliorative institutions of these places, and the swollen populations of cities which presented challenges to their elegance and sophistication. He noted that, in time, the colonial-born population would surpass that of the immigrant population, but was curious as to whether the 'race' would 'deteriorate or become stronger by the change'.[136] His remarks may have been stimulated by his abhorrence at the lives of the 'dissipated' Chinese, as well as the interest he took in the rates of insanity and destitution in the colonies.[137] Certainly, views about the possibility that the rush for gold had attracted a sickly population, including the diseased, 'idle', 'neuralgic' and those with 'worn-out constitutions', were already in circulation in Victoria.[138] The heavy reliance on alcohol, a tendency from which no class seemed immune, meant that the colonies were awash with drink; Dr John Singleton, who established the Melbourne City Mission in 1854, faced a 'torrent of drunkenness' in 1850s Melbourne, citing numerous cases of families ruined and torn apart by alcoholism and deaths due to drinking.[139]

The two large, public urban institutions for the insane at the centre of this study both reflected their urban populations but also provided shelter and refuge for the insane from their wider catchment areas. Established in the late 1840s, the Yarra Bend Asylum drew its substantive patient population from the suburban areas of Melbourne, with some patients from rural areas. After institutions were established in the rural towns of Ararat and Beechworth in the 1860s, and the Kew Asylum was built in the 1870s, inmates at the Yarra Bend were most likely to be poor and living in the inner city areas with many admitted from Fitzroy, Collingwood, Carlton, North Melbourne, St Kilda and the city itself.[140] The Provincial Auckland Lunatic Asylum was first established in the 1850s in the buildings of Auckland Hospital but was moved in 1867 to new brick buildings set inside vegetable gardens and pasture on sixteen acres outside the urban centre on Great North Road, Avondale.[141] Known informally and locally as Te Whau because it was located some three to five miles outside of Auckland City near Te Whau Creek, the institution took inmates from all over the North Island, especially the upper North Island. It was a wide catchment area.

In the Annual Report of the Inspector of Asylums in Victoria for 1870, produced by then Inspector of Asylums, Dr Edward Paley, the short history of the institutions for the insane in the colony no doubt made for startling reading. In only two decades, the asylums had become 'the refuge for all who can be declared lunatics, idiots, or of feeble or unsound mind in any shade or degree; without discrimination as to their suitability for asylum treatment', Paley declared.[142] The population of the Yarra Bend that year was 986.[143] Moreover, the asylum was usually easier to access than other social institutions for a variety of reasons Paley outlines; and it also became the final destination for many of the colony's most desperate people.[144] The impact of emigration, and the age structure of the colony, also played a role in the growing reliance on the asylum, as well as determining rates of mental illness which tended to strike people in their middle age. Paley's detailed account of immigration, the gendered makeup of the immigrant population, and the changing age structure of the colonial and institutional population, shows that much thought was given to the way that the institution was itself bound up with concerns about social structure and population.[145]

The situation at Auckland was different in that the asylum was at that time relatively small and catered to less than one hundred inmates, most of them male. Yet like Paley and his contemporaries in the Australian colonies, concerns about the immigrant insane struck notes of uncertainty among doctors. In 1870, John King, Inspector of Asylums, wondered at some length if some of those insane at the Auckland Provincial Asylum, as it was known, might be better served if removed and sent back to their 'native country'.[146] King even proposed that the cost of such voyages to return the insane home to their 'native' places might be defrayed by the government. To place these comments in a wider context, the point of returning the insane inmates to their countries of origin was part of a wider discussion about the value of patients being cared for by families in familiar contexts, as asylum authorities debated the various colonial and imperial models of boarding-out or extra-institutional care across the period.[147]

Immigrants and insanity

Some immigrants to colonial Victoria 'lived out dissatisfied lives, plagued by the loneliness that comes from old age, far from one's family and roots'.[148] This isolation dogged immigrants of all walks of life and was exacerbated by poverty and need, and was particularly obvious among those receiving charity and indoor and outdoor welfare in the new cities and towns of the colony.[149] Popular views of insanity existed and were commented on in newspapers and other colonial publications.[150] Yet the stories of the unsuccessful migrants to the colonies appear in only some historical accounts of colonial settlement and life. The '"other" pasts' of the mobile peoples traversing empire are often occluded.[151] Some migrants returned 'home' after a period of time, as private and official sources can tell us, and these stories of the returnees of the period might also provide insights into the mental health of migrants.[152]

Instances of mental breakdown in colonial family letters, private diaries and similar sources are fleeting; mental illness is often silent in the private record.[153] Accounts such as the one by Danish woman Ingeborg Stuckenberg who arrived in Auckland in 1903 and who found New Zealand 'still in embryo', and – judging by her views of the town and its people – was horribly alienated before her eventual suicide, are rare.[154] Similarly, studying migration stories through letters, shipping records and related sources with a view to uncovering mental illness presents challenges, with mental illness either muted in descriptions or too rarely noted to be of significance. Among the colonial working class in New Zealand, there are numerous examples of insanity, from evidence of mental breakdowns which occurred on the voyage out, to reports of lunacy among labouring men on the West Coast of New Zealand in the 1870s, as well as suicides among colonial men.[155] 'Maggie', a 'hopeful' immigrant writing letters to her brother in Canada from New Zealand which were published in 1887, commented on the rates of insanity in the colonies and suggested it was no surprise that the emigrants suffered grief, 'utter disappointment' and 'bitter regrets' about their new lives, which sometimes failed to measure up to expectations.[156] Her absolute certainty that the mind could become 'quite unhinged' in such environments led 'Maggie' to construct advice about 'classes' of people who should 'come out' to the colonies and those who should not, suggesting that contemporaries gave thought to the way that innate characteristics combined with environmental factors in the production of mental health and illness.[157]

Institutional records, then, provide more detail about insanity as it manifested among immigrants.[158] In May of the year 1900, James Waddell, an artist aged forty-six, was admitted to the Yarra Bend Hospital for the Insane. Waddell had been hospitalised at the Beechworth Asylum in the previous year. At the Yarra Bend he was diagnosed with delusional insanity, reporting he heard people calling him a 'who', and he exhibited other paranoid tendencies, among them, the belief that he suffered from syphilis, and that his pelvis was 'diseased'. Like a number of other insane admitted to institutions in Australia and New Zealand, Waddell had a longer history of mental illness; in his case, dating back fifteen years prior to his emigration to the colonies from Scotland.[159] In 1906 he was again admitted to the Yarra Bend, this time designated as having dementia, with his brother requesting he be transferred to Sunbury Asylum in Melbourne's outer western fringe that year.[160] Waddell's institutional mobility – he spent time in several institutions in the colony of Victoria, as well as the suggestion that he had done so earlier in Glasgow – is also instructive. Insanity was a kaleidoscope of mental diseases which defied national borders, despite earlier attempts by colonial authorities to safeguard the colonies from its presence, or the expectation from some medical writers that new places would somehow be immune from mental diseases.

Although a relatively small number of direct references to patients having spent time in individual institutions outside Australia can be found in the total number of patients at the Yarra Bend, and a similar number of references to patients having spent time in individual institutions outside New Zealand in the total number of patients at Auckland, there are many more hints that other inmates at both of these colonial institutions had longer histories of mental disturbance. This is important, as it indicates that the stresses of mobility and migration were not always the sole trigger for mental illness, even if these experiences exacerbated the existing tendency to mental illness, as contemporaries noted in their official observations and commentaries in asylum reports. In 1871, for instance, the report of the Joint Committee on Lunatic Asylums included comments by Dr M. Grace, who cited 'oppressive loneliness' among new arrivals as one cause of insanity. 'Many immigrants too', he added, 'form the most extravagant anticipations of their new home, and are proportionably depressed by the result of actual experience.'[161]

Most of the foreign-born inmates who had definitely spent time in asylums before migrating, according to their committal papers, had spent it in English institutions, with some in Irish or Scottish asylums and a handful in European hospitals, the European asylums in India, or in the American mental hospitals. Their stories tell us something of the travails of mental illness in time and space, the way it patterned individual experiences of mobility and movement across and within the imperial world, and the knowledge about institutions that was gained by families and friends in the process. At the Yarra Bend, for instance, Frances Phillips supplied information about her sister, Miss Rose Stanley, aged thirty, admitted to the institution in 1903. Rose had been in asylums 'at 25 years of age at Calcutta and Colombo'. She had never worked, had lived in India for the 'last 16 years', and her sister suggested that her state was 'a relapse of similar troubles in India', going on to describe her delusion that she 'believe[d] she has been bayonetted and that bits of iron are lodged in her body'.[162] Mrs Ellen Clark, admitted in the same year aged sixty-five, continued to 'express an exaggerated regret for all her past life', with her son-in-law explaining that she had been in a Scottish asylum thirty years before.[163] In an earlier period of the Yarra Bend's history, between the 1870s and 1880s, even less information was gathered in many cases. James Jones, admitted in his forties in 1882, had come to the colonies already exposed to the vicissitudes of poor mental health, if his record is indicative. A blow to the head in England had made him unpredictable, violent, and he had suffered a previous instance of 'insanity': his notes comment that he had delusions relating to land selection near Lake Boort in Victoria, the district where he was apprehended as insane.[164]

Prior institutionalisation, however, did not always mean that more detail could be amassed about individual inmates or cases by medical authorities. At Auckland, apart from sparse notes about a few institutions, such as Staffordshire Asylum or Kilkenny District Asylum, very little detail was known about the patients who had spent time in asylums in England, South Africa, Ireland, or America. Aged sixty-five in 1900, Mary Jackson had been admitted to Auckland Asylum on numerous occasions in the 1890s with mania, and her records note that she had previous attacks of insanity in England, but no institution is noted. Perhaps her daughter, Harriet Wills, had no knowledge of the specific prior committals, making it impossible for the asylum to trace any paperwork about Mary.[165]

Still others had been transferred between colonial institutions. In 1894, Margaret Page, who 'fell down a mine when 5 years old', had already spent eight years in a private asylum in New Zealand.[166] This institution, while unnamed in the patient notes and described only as 'P.A.', was probably Ashburn Hall. Another woman inmate at the Yarra Bend had been in Seacliff Asylum in Dunedin fifteen years before with a personal history of murder and suicide attempts.[167]

Immigrants of all kinds – assisted, poor, ordinary and otherwise – became recipients of a newly formed web of institutional measures, and were later inscribed in the institutional record. This chapter has described two colonial sites, placing urban locations within their wider geographical contexts, and has examined the way mobility shaped the lives of immigrants and settlers in these imperial and colonial spaces. Although institutional confinement curtailed the mobility of some immigrants and settlers, in the process of containing mobile peoples within the walls, spaces and textual apparatus of their confines, institutional records can tell us something about who these people were. These case records allow us, usefully, to partially locate immigrants in the 'age of mobility', and provide us with small glimpses of the experiences of people who might ordinarily be less visible in the colonial record.

At the same time these colonial records allow us to understand the implications of mobility for colonial society. The archival record of the institutions for the insane is also a record of imperial modes of governance; it is through this record that we can begin to locate some aspects of the contemporary imagining of the problem of mobility. The colonial world operated inside an imperial and global world of movement of which migration to the Australasian colonies was but one aspect. Peoples who were mobile across many other geographical sites met similar fates and were made subject to a range of legal and state controls, with specific patterns of jurisdiction in white settler colonies reflecting shared anxieties about mobility.

As the next chapter demonstrates, a range of welfare, medical and legal institutions was quickly established in the Australasian colonies, including New Zealand, by the mid- to late nineteenth century. Immigrants, the sick, the mentally ill, the impoverished, the

Indigenous and the wayward were segregated and housed in different institutional spaces. By looking at the movement of people *between* social institutions, as well as at the exchanges of ideas about mobility itself, the following chapter suggests that we might open up new ways of seeing and interpreting immigration as a form of mobility that was also regulated and circumscribed by the welfare and health institutions which were part of the fabric of the state.

Notes

1 It is important to note that by talking about Aboriginal peoples as being on the 'fringes' of white society and spaces, historians do not perpetuate perceptions of their absence from history, as Penelope Edmonds also points out. See Edmonds, 'The intimate, urbanising frontier: Native camps and settler colonialism's violent array of spaces around early Melbourne', in Tracey Banivanua Mar and Penelope Edmonds (eds), *Making Settler Colonial Space: Perspectives on Race, Place and Identity* (Basingstoke and New York: Palgrave Macmillan, 2010), pp. 130–1.
2 For population figures and estimates, see Peter McDonald, 'Demography', in Andrew Brown-May and Shurlee Swain (eds), *The Encyclopedia of Melbourne* (Cambridge, New York, and Melbourne: Cambridge University Press, 2005), p. 201.
3 Anthony Trollope, *Australia and New Zealand*, Vol. 1 (London: Dawsons of Pall Mall, 1873), pp. 384–5.
4 Trollope, *Australia and New Zealand*, Vol. 1, pp. 384–5; p. 386. For perceptive comments about Trollope as travel writer, see Lydia Wevers, *Country of Writing: Travel Writing and New Zealand 1809–1900* (Auckland: Auckland University Press, 2002), pp. 140–6.
5 Jeanine Graham, 'Settler society', in Geoffrey W. Rice (ed.), *The Oxford History of New Zealand*, 2nd edn (Oxford: Oxford University Press, 1992); Sir Julius Vogel (ed.), *The Official Handbook of New Zealand: A Collection of Papers by Experienced Colonists on the Colony as a Whole, and on the Several Provinces* (London: Wyman & Sons, 1875), p. 243.
6 Vogel (ed.), *The Official Handbook*, p. 250. David Hamer finds that the population of Auckland nearly doubled between 1846 and 1911; see Hamer 'Centralization and nationalism (1891–1912)', in Keith Sinclair (ed.), *The Oxford Illustrated History of New Zealand* (Oxford: Oxford University Press, 1990), p. 140.
7 Margaret Tennant, *Paupers and Providers: Charitable Aid in New Zealand* (Wellington: Allen & Unwin/Historical Branch, 1990), p. 22.
8 Trollope, *Australia and New Zealand*, Vol. 2, pp. 455, 456.
9 Trollope, *Australia and New Zealand*, Vol. 2, pp. 459, 461. See also J. H. M. Salmon, *A History of Gold-Mining in New Zealand* (Wellington: Government Printer, 1963).
10 Trollope, *Australia and New Zealand*, Vol. 2, p. 456.
11 John Murray Moore, *New Zealand for the Emigrant, Invalid, and Tourist* (London: Sampson Law, Marston, Searle and Rivington, 1890).
12 The phrase is used by W. J. Woods, *A Visit to Victoria* (London: Wyman & Sons, 1886), p. 41.
13 See Trollope, *Australia and New Zealand*, Vol. 1, pp. 1–3, on the imperial responsibility for the colonies and their white populations in particular. See also Helen Gilbert and Anna Johnston (eds), *In Transit: Travel, Text, Empire* (New York: Peter Lang Publishing, 2002), p. 5.
14 In particular, I am departing from earlier social history studies of 'persistence' and 'transience'; Tom Brooking, Dick Martin, David Thomson and Hamish James, 'The ties that bind: Persistence in a New World industrial suburb, 1902–22', *Social History*, 24:1 (1999), p. 60. I am also reinterpreting older histories of migration:

see Richard Broome, *The Victorians Arriving* (Sydney: Fairfax, Syme and Weldon, 1984).
15 Philippa Levine, *Prostitution, Race and Politics: Policing Venereal Disease in the British Empire* (New York and London: Routledge, 2003), p. 4.
16 Graeme Davison, J. W. McCarty and Ailsa McLeary (eds), *Australians 1888* (Broadway: Fairfax, Syme & Weldon, 1987), Chapter 12, pp. 230–49.
17 Brooking *et al.*, 'The ties that bind'; Miles Fairburn, *The Ideal Society and Its Enemies: The Foundations of Modern New Zealand Society, 1850–1900* (Auckland: Auckland University Press, 1989).
18 Alan Atkinson, *The Europeans in Australia*, Vol. 2: *Democracy* (Melbourne and New York: Oxford University Press, 2004), p. 269; see also the arguments in Fairburn, *The Ideal Society*.
19 Broome, *The Victorians Arriving*, p. 127.
20 This theme is taken up in the comparative study of the cities of Melbourne and Victoria in British Columbia, Canada, by Penelope Edmonds. Both of these places attempted forms of control over the mobility of Indigenous subjects and tried to contain their populations: Edmonds, *Urbanizing Frontiers: Indigenous Peoples and Settlers in Nineteenth-Century Pacific Rim Cities* (Vancouver and Toronto: University of British Columbia Press, 2010), p. 12.
21 See the Plan of Auckland at 1842 in G. W. A. Bush, *Decently and in Order: The Government of the City of Auckland 1840–1971* (Auckland and London: Collins, 1971), p. 23.
22 For histories of immigration to the Australian colonies, see Eric Richards, 'Migrations: The career of British white Australia', in Deryck M. Schreuder and Stuart Ward (eds), *Australia's Empire*, The Oxford History of the British Empire Companion Series (Oxford and New York: Oxford University Press, 2008), pp. 163–85; Broome, *The Victorians Arriving*. For New Zealand studies, see Angela McCarthy, 'Migration and ethnic identities in the nineteenth century', in Giselle Byrnes (ed.), *The New Oxford History of New Zealand* (Auckland and Melbourne: Oxford University Press, 2009), pp. 173–95; Lyndon Fraser and Katie Pickles (eds), *Shifting Centres: Women and Migration in New Zealand History* (Dunedin: University of Otago Press, 2002). See also the Special Issue of the *New Zealand Journal of History* focused on Migration and the Nation, 43:2 (2009).
23 Atkinson, *The Europeans in Australia*, p. xiv.
24 Tony Ballantyne, *Webs of Empire: Locating New Zealand's Colonial Past* (Wellington: Bridget Williams Books, 2012).
25 Graham, 'Settler society', p. 112.
26 Rollo Arnold, 'The Australasian peoples and their world, 1888–1915', in Keith Sinclair (ed.), *Tasman Relations* (Auckland: Auckland University Press, 1987), p. 53.
27 Philippa Mein Smith, 'The Tasman world', in Byrnes (ed.), *The New Oxford History of New Zealand*, p. 299. William Pember Reeves, *State Experiments in Australia and New Zealand*, Vol. 2 (South Melbourne: Macmillan of Australia, 1969 [1902]).
28 Arnold, 'The Australasian peoples', p. 60.
29 Arnold, 'The Australasian peoples', p. 64.
30 Graham, 'Settler society', p. 113.
31 For a representation of internal population movement, see the table/diagram in Davison, McCarty and McLeary (eds), *Australians 1888*, p. 232.
32 David Rollison, 'Exploding England: The dialectics of mobility and settlement in early modern England', *Social History*, 24:1 (1999), p. 10.
33 Graham, 'Settler society', p. 113.
34 Dean Wilson, 'Community Violence in Auckland, 1850–1875', unpublished Masters Thesis in History, University of Auckland, 1993, p. 39.
35 Davison, McCarty and McLeary (eds), *Australians 1888*, p. 230.
36 Damon Salesa, 'New Zealand's Pacific', in Byrnes (ed.), *New Oxford History of New Zealand*, p. 153; Tony Ballantyne and Antoinette Burton (eds), *Moving*

Subjects: Gender, Mobility, and Intimacy in an Age of Global Empire (Chicago: University of Illinois Press, 2009).
37 Moore, *New Zealand for the Emigrant*, p. 1.
38 Moore, *New Zealand for the Emigrant*, p. 2.
39 Frances Steel, *Oceania under Steam: Sea Transport and the Cultures of Colonialism, c. 1870–1914*, Studies in Imperialism (Manchester and New York: Manchester University Press, 2011), pp. 24–5.
40 Steel, *Oceania under Steam*, pp. 54–5.
41 Angela McCarthy, 'Migration and madness in New Zealand's asylums, 1863–1910', in Angela McCarthy and Catharine Coleborne (eds), *Migration, Ethnicity and Mental Health: International Perspectives, 1840–2010*, Routledge Studies in Cultural History (New York and Abingdon: Routledge, 2012), pp. 62–5. For an account of emigrants' voyages to Victoria, see also Broome, *The Victorians Arriving*, pp. 50–6.
42 David Goodman, 'Reading gold-rush travellers' narratives', *Australian Cultural History*, 10 (1991), p. 99.
43 Goodman, 'Reading gold-rush travellers' narratives', p. 102.
44 John Hunter Kerr, *Glimpses of Life in Victoria, by 'A Resident'* (Melbourne: Melbourne University Press, 1996 [1876]), p. 163.
45 Frederic Algar, *A Description of the Province of Victoria: Australia* (London: Algar and Street, 1858), p. 22.
46 Christina Twomey, '"Without Natural Protectors": Histories of Deserted and Destitute Colonial Women in Victoria 1850–1865', unpublished Ph.D. thesis History, University of Melbourne, 1995.
47 Twomey, '"Without Natural Protectors"', p. 81.
48 These social 'types' were observed by contemporaries and studied by historians, featuring in accounts of the mobile: see the account of different 'nomads' in Davison, McCarty, and McLeary (eds), *Australians 1888*, p. 249. Miles Fairburn's transient and itinerant men also form the basis of some of these ideas; see Fairburn, *The Ideal Society*, pp. 204–6; pp. 246–7. On remittance men in Auckland, see Jack Adam, Vivien Burgess and Dawn Ellis, *Rugged Determination: Historical Window on Swanson, 1854–2004* (Auckland: Swanson Residents and Ratepayers Association, 2004), pp. 51–2.
49 See Daiva Stasiulis and and Nira Yuval-Davis (eds), *Unsettling Settler Societies: Articulations of Gender, Race, Ethnicity and Class*, Sage Series on Race and Ethnic Relations (London and Thousand Oaks: Sage, 1995).
50 Lorenzo Veracini, *Settler Colonialism: A Theoretical Overview* (Basingstoke and New York: Palgrave Macmillan, 2010), pp. 26–7.
51 See for example the now extensive literature describing the Australian colonial frontier(s), including Bain Attwood and S. G. Foster (eds), *Frontier Conflict: The Australian Experience* (Canberra: National Museum of Australia, 2003). National histories including the following title have since the 1990s incorporated revisionist histories of the Australian frontiers: see for example, David Day, *Claiming a Continent: A New History of Australia* (Sydney: HarperCollins, 2001 [1996]).
52 Samuel Butler, *A First Year in Canterbury Settlement, With Other Early Essays*, edited by R. A. Streatfeild (London: A. C. Fifield, 1914), p. 127.
53 Eric Richards (ed.), *Poor Australian Immigrants in the Nineteenth Century*, Visible Immigrants: Two (Canberra: Australian National University, 1991), p. 3.
54 William Howitt, *Land, Labour, and Gold, or, Two Years in Victoria with Visits to Sydney and Van Diemen's Land* (Sydney: Sydney University Press, 1972 [1855]), p. 285.
55 Trollope, *Australia and New Zealand*, Vol. 1, p. 415.
56 Howitt, *Land, Labour, and Gold*, p. 285.
57 Howitt, *Land, Labour, and Gold*, p. 286.
58 Andrew Brown-May, *Melbourne Street Life: The Itinerary of Our Days* (Melbourne: Australian Scholarly Press/Arcadia and Museum Victoria, 1998), p. 163.

59 Antoinette Burton, 'Introduction: The unfinished business of colonial modernities', in Antoinette Burton (ed.), *Gender, Sexuality and Colonial Modernities*, Routledge Research in Gender and History (London and New York: Routledge, 1999), p. 2.
60 Burton, 'Introduction: The unfinished business', p. 2.
61 Broome, *The Victorians Arriving*, p. 95.
62 James Belich, *Replenishing the Earth: The Settler Revolution and the Rise of the Anglo-World, 1783–1939* (Oxford and New York: Oxford University Press, 2009), pp. 356–7.
63 Broome, *The Victorians Arriving*, p. 98.
64 Broome, *The Victorians Arriving*, p. 102.
65 Broome, *The Victorians Arriving*, p. 100.
66 Nicole McLennan, 'Glimpses of unassisted English women arriving in Victoria, 1860–1900', in Eric Richards (ed.), *Visible Women: Female Immigrants in Colonial Australia*, Visible Immigrants: Four (Canberra: Division of Historical Studies and Centre for Immigration and Multicultural Studies, Australian National University, 1995), p. 59.
67 Broome, *The Victorians Arriving*, p. 96.
68 Broome, *The Victorians Arriving*, p. 98.
69 For detailed representations of historical statistics in the colonies, see Wray Vamplew (ed.), *Australians: Historical Statistics* (Melbourne: Fairfax, Syme & Weldon, 1987), pp. 25–37.
70 Broome, *The Victorians Arriving*, p. 99.
71 Goodman, 'Reading gold-rush travellers' narratives', p. 105.
72 Broome, *The Victorians Arriving*, pp. 49–51. A sad example of the ways in which Aboriginal people were caught inside institutional and legal networks which challenged their movement is set out by Bain Attwood's search for the story of Brataualung man Tarra Bobby. See Bain Attwood, 'Tarra Bobby, a Brataualung man', *Aboriginal History*, 11:1–2 (1987), pp. 41–57.
73 Lynette Russell (ed.), *Colonial Frontiers: Indigenous-European Encounters in Settler Societies*, Studies in Imperialism (Manchester: Manchester University Press, 2001).
74 Broome, *The Victorians Arriving*, p. 72.
75 Hawk is interested in 'mad migrants', especially the miners who become caught in institutional settings across gold-mining regions of the Pacific. See Angela Hawk, 'Going "mad" in gold country: Migrant populations and the problem of containment in Pacific mining boom regions', *Pacific Historical Review*, 80:1 (2011), pp. 64–96.
76 Dean Wilson, '"Well-set-up men": Respectable masculinity and police organizational culture in Melbourne 1853–c.1920', in David G. Barrie and Susan Broomhall (eds), *A History of Police and Masculinities, 1700–2010* (Abingdon and New York: Routledge, 2012).
77 Frank Fowler's *Southern Lights and Shadows* remarks on the many cultural activities available to dwellers in Melbourne, leaving him at a loss to explain the way excessive drinking was a hallmark of Melbourne colonial life; see Frank Fowler, *Southern Lights and Shadows* (Sydney: Sydney University Press, 1975 [1859]), pp. 42–3.
78 Susanne Davies, '"Ragged, dirty ... infamous and obscene": The "vagrant" in late-nineteenth-century Melbourne', in David Philips and Susanne Davies (eds), *A Nation of Rogues? Crime, Law and Punishment in Colonial Australia* (Parkville: Melbourne University Press, 1994), pp. 141–65.
79 Dean Wilson, *The Beat: Policing a Victorian City* (Melbourne: Circa, 2006), p. 110; see also Catharine Coleborne, 'Passage to the asylum: The role of the police in committals of the insane in Victoria, Australia, 1848–1900', in Roy Porter and David Wright (eds), *The Confinement of the Insane: International Perspectives, 1800–1965* (Cambridge and New York: Cambridge University Press, 2003), pp. 129–48.
80 Wilson, *The Beat*, pp. 209–10.

81 Coleborne, 'Passage to the asylum'.
82 PROV, VPRS 937/P4, Inwards registered Correspondence 1853–1894.
83 PROV, VPRS 937/P4, Bundle 2.
84 PROV, VPRS 937/P4, Bundle 2. A cutting of the newspaper can be found in the records, but no date or newspaper title is included.
85 Wilson, *The Beat*, p. 129.
86 Angela McCarthy, 'Migration and ethnic identities in the nineteenth century', in Byrnes (ed.), *The New Oxford History of New Zealand*, pp. 177–80.
87 Bush, *Decently and in Order*, p. 32.
88 Wilson, 'Community Violence', p. 7.
89 Bush, *Decently and in Order*, p. 32.
90 Wilson, 'Community Violence', p. 7. Wilson also cites G. T. Bloomfield, *New Zealand: A Handbook of Historical Statistics*, Reference Publication in International Historical Statistics (Boston: G. K. Hall, 1984), p. 57.
91 Margaret Mutch, 'Aspects of the Social and Economic History of Auckland, 1890–1896', Unpublished Masters thesis, University of Auckland, 1968, p. 107.
92 Bush, *Decently and in Order*, p. 32.
93 Bush, *Decently and in Order*, p. 32.
94 Judith Elphick, 'Auckland 1870–74: A Social Portrait', unpublished Masters thesis, University of Auckland, 1974, p. 17.
95 See for example, John Askew, *A Voyage to Australia and New Zealand Including a Visit to Adelaide, Melbourne, Sydney, Hunter's River, Newcastle, Maitland, and Auckland; With a Summary of the Progress and Discoveries Made in Each Colony From its Founding to the Present Time. By a Steerage Passenger* (London: Simpkin, Marshall and Co., 1857), pp. 326–7.
96 Mutch, 'Aspects of the Social', p. 98.
97 Mutch, 'Aspects of the Social', p. 107.
98 Raewyn Dalziel, 'Railways and relief centres (1870–1890)', in Keith Sinclair (ed.), *The Oxford Illustrated History of New Zealand*, Oxford Illustrated Histories (Auckland and Oxford: Oxford University Press, 1990), p. 108.
99 Note that Wilson draws upon work by Jock Philips, Erik Olssen and others: see Wilson, 'Community Violence', p. 7.
100 Bush, citing the *Southern Cross* (26 February 1850), p. 2; see *Decently and in Order*, p. 33.
101 Wilson, 'Community Violence', p. 8.
102 See a table on birthplaces at 1874 in Elphick, 'Auckland 1870–74', p. 16.
103 Wilson, 'Community Violence', pp. 9–10.
104 Elphick, 'Auckland 1870–74', p. 3. Auckland's Public Library dates from 1887; see Dalziel, p. 108.
105 William Main, *Auckland Through a Victorian Lens* (Wellington: Millwood Press, 1977).
106 E. E. Morris (ed.), *Pictorial New Zealand* (London, Paris and Melbourne: Cassell & Company, 1895), pp. 11, 113.
107 Caroline Daley, 'A gendered domain: Leisure in Auckland, 1890–1940', in Caroline Daley and Deborah Montgomerie (eds), *The Gendered Kiwi* (Auckland: Auckland University Press, 1999), p. 89. See also 'Charge of vagrancy', *New Zealand Herald* (24 June 1911), p. 5.
108 Alan Mulgan, *Spur of Morning* (London: Whitcombe and Tombs, 1934), p. 8.
109 Mulgan, *Spur of Morning*, p. 43.
110 Edmonds, *Urbanizing Frontiers*, p. 69.
111 Edmonds argues that 'discourses of Britishness' produced and strengthened identities of 'settlers and cities'; Edmonds, *Urbanizing Frontiers*, p. 69.
112 New Zealand's immigration laws of the 1880s place it within this frame; see Edmonds, *Urbanizing Frontiers*, p. 231.
113 Edmonds, *Urbanizing Frontiers*, pp. 228, 246.
114 Dr H. Earley, *Hints Upon Health, Addressed to Newly Arrived Immigrants* (Melbourne: B. Lucas, Collins Street, 1853), p. 1.

115 Reverend William Jarrit, *Hints to Immigrants Upon Colonial Life and Its Requirements* (Melbourne: Argus, Collins Street, 1853), pp. 2–3; p. 4.
116 Fairburn, *The Ideal Society*, p. 134.
117 Howitt, *Land, Labour, and Gold*, p. 279. Howitt provides an account of population growth in the short period he examines, p. 283.
118 Askew, *A Voyage to Australia and New Zealand*, p. 37.
119 Askew, *A Voyage to Australia and New Zealand*, pp. 131–2.
120 Atkinson, *The Europeans in Australia*, p. 269.
121 Kerr, *Glimpses of Life in Victoria*, p. 247.
122 Wilson, 'Community Violence', p. 11.
123 Elphick notes that a journalist interviewed boys in their teen age years about living on the streets and published the work in 1872, 'Auckland 1870–74', pp. 91–2. See also *Weekly News* (16 March 1872), cited in Elphick.
124 Moore, *New Zealand for the Emigrant*, p. 215.
125 Moore, *New Zealand for the Emigrant*, p. 216.
126 Lynette Finch, *The Classing Gaze: Sexuality, Class and Surveillance* (Sydney: Allen & Unwin, 1993).
127 On travelling knowledge cultures, including medical and legal cultures, see David Lambert and Alan Lester (eds), *Colonial Lives across the British Empire: Imperial Careering in the Long Nineteenth Century* (Cambridge and New York: Cambridge University Press, 2006); Lauren Benton, *A Search for Sovereignty: Law and Geography in European Empires, 1400–1900* (Cambridge and New York: Cambridge University Press, 2010), pp. 3, 23; and M. Anne Crowther and Marguerite W. Dupree, *Medical Lives in the Age of Surgical Revolution*, Cambridge Studies in Population, Economy and Society in Past Time 43 (Cambridge and New York: Cambridge University Press, 2007).
128 Both the colonies under examination here, Victoria and New Zealand, produced Yearbooks published by the government which contained vital statistics of the colony's population, health, institutions, economy and other details. From 1893 until 1914, the New Zealand Official Year Book was published by the Registrar-General's office, and was popularly known as the *New Zealand Year-book*. In Victoria, the *Victorian Year Book* was published from 1873 by the Government Statistician.
129 Carol Anne Reeves, 'Insanity and Nervous Diseases Amongst Jewish Immigrants to the East End of London, 1880–1920', unpublished Ph.D. thesis, University of London, 2001, pp. 18–20.
130 Carol Anne Reeves, pp. 23–4. Reeves cites Francis Galton, 'Hereditary talent and character', *Macmillan's Magazine* 12 (1865).
131 The wider context circulating about poverty, the workhouse and the movement of people in and out of the social and medical institutions helped to reinforce negative views of the Irish. See Hilary Marland and Catherine Cox, 'Emaciated and exhausted: Irish minds and bodies in nineteenth-century Lancashire asylums', unpublished conference paper, European Association for the History of Medicine and Health (EAHMH) Body and Mind Conference, Utrecht, September 2011; see also Catherine Cox, Hilary Marland and Sarah York, 'Itineraries and experiences of insanity: Irish migration and the management of mental illness in nineteenth-century Lancashire', in Catherine Cox and Hilary Marland (eds), *Migration, Health and Ethnicity in the Modern World*, Science, Technology and Medicine in Modern History (Basingstoke and New York: Palgrave Macmillan, 2013).
132 Marland and Cox, 'Emaciated and exhausted'; William Julius Mickle, *General Paralysis of the Insane* (London: H. K. Lewis, 1886 [1880]), pp. 259–60.
133 T. S. Clouston, *Clinical Lectures on Mental Diseases* (London: J. & A. Churchill, 1883).
134 T. S. Clouston, *The Hygiene of Mind*, 7th edn (London: Methuen & Co., 1918 [1906]), pp. 262–3.
135 Clouston, *The Hygiene of Mind*, p. 263.
136 Trollope, *Australia and New Zealand*, Vol. 1, p. 479.
137 Trollope, *Australia and New Zealand*, Vol. 1, p. 415; pp. 393–4.

138 Michael Cannon, *Melbourne After the Gold Rush* (Main Ridge: Loch Haven Books, 1993), p. 44. Cannon quotes from Dr Mingay Syder's tract published as *The Voice of Truth in Defence of Nature: And Opinions Antagonistic to Those of Dr Kilgour, Upon the Effect of the Climate of Australia Upon the European Constitution in Health and Disease* (Geelong: Heath and Cordell, 1853), in which Syder suggests that the colonial world was a magnet for the weak and degenerate; see p. 5. Colonial women were particularly diseased, according to Syder, as discussed in Chapter 5.
139 John Singleton, *A Narrative of Incidents in the Eventful Life of a Physician* (Melbourne: M. L. Hutchinson, 1891), p. 121.
140 Stephen Garton presents a similar finding about the patterns of admission for the inmates of the hospitals for the insane in Sydney; see Garton, *Medicine and Madness: A Social History of Insanity in New South Wales, 1880–1940* (Sydney: New South Wales University Press, 1988), p. 121.
141 Elphick, 'Auckland 1870–74', p. 176.
142 *Report of the Inspector of Asylums on the Hospitals for the Insane for the Year 1870*, in *Victoria Parliamentary Papers (VPP)*, 1871, p. 9.
143 *Report of the Inspector of Asylums on the Hospitals for the Insane for 1870* (Melbourne: John Ferres, Government Printer, 1871), Appendix B, Table 1, p. 38.
144 *Report of the Inspector of Asylums*, p. 10.
145 *Report of the Inspector of Asylums*, see pp. 25–7.
146 *Reports on Lunatic Asylums in New Zealand*, D-29, *Appendices to the Jourals of the House of Representatives (AJHR)*, 1870, pp. 2, 4.
147 See Catharine Coleborne, *Madness in the Family: Insanity and Institutions in the Australasian Colonial World, 1860–1914* (Basingstoke and New York: Palgrave Macmillan, 2010), pp. 137–9. At the same time, the New Zealand government, like that of Victoria, deliberated about the efficiencies of the asylum system across the colony and debated whether New Zealand might be better served by a central asylum, with the report of the Joint Committee on the subject published as a government document in 1871; see *Report of the Joint Committee on Lunatic Asylums*, AJHR, H-10 (Wellington, 1871).
148 Broome, *The Victorians Arriving*, p. 127.
149 Broome, *The Victorians Arriving*, p. 127.
150 Coleborne, *Madness in the Family*, pp. 69–72.
151 Desley Deacon, Penny Russell, and Angela Woollacott (eds), *Transnational Lives: Biographies of Global Modernity, 1700–the Present* (Basingstoke and New York: Palgrave Macmillan, 2010), p. 2.
152 An extended discussion of this theme is beyond the scope of the present study. Angela McCarthy has examined this question; see McCarthy, 'A difficult voyage', *History Scotland*, 10:4 (2010), pp. 29–30.
153 See for example the archival research illustrating the theme in Coleborne, *Madness in the Family*, pp. 43–51.
154 John Kousgård Sørensen, 'Ingeborg Stuckenberg in New Zealand', in Henning Bender and Birgit Larsen (eds), *Danish Emigration to New Zealand*, translated by Karen Veien (Aalborg: Danes Worldwide Archives, 1990), p. 50.
155 Julia Millen, *Colonial Tears and Sweat: The Working Class in Nineteenth-Century New Zealand* (Wellington: Reed, 1984), p. 18; pp. 48–9.
156 'Hopeful', *'Taken in'; Being, a Sketch of New Zealand Life*, 2nd edn (London: W. H. Allen & Co., 1877; reprint 1974), pp. 167–9.
157 'Hopeful', pp. 170–84.
158 Angela McCarthy, 'Ethnicity, migration and the lunatic asylum in early twentieth-century Auckland, New Zealand', *Social History of Medicine*, 21:1 (2008), pp. 47–65; Angela McCarthy, 'Migration and madness in New Zealand's asylums, 1863–1910', in McCarthy and Coleborne (eds), *Migration, Ethnicity and Mental Health*, pp. 55–72.
159 PROV, VPRS 7399/P1, unit 12, folio 281, 12 May 1900.
160 PROV, VPRS 7399/P0, unit 15, folio 520, 8 October 1906.

161 Dr Grace, Appendix, *Report of Joint Committee on Lunatic Asylums*, *AJHR*, H-10 (Wellington, 1871), p. 10.
162 PROV, VPRS 7400/P1, unit 13, folio 346, 3 May 1903.
163 PROV, VPRS 7400/P1, unit 13, folio 329, 9 June 1903.
164 PROV, VPRS 7399/P1, unit 5, folio 72, 29 March 1882.
165 National Archives New Zealand, Auckland, Auckland Mental Hospital, (YCAA) 1048/9, 351, patient 2846, 1 June 1900.
166 PROV, VPRS 7400/P1, unit 11, folio 43, 15 November 1894.
167 PROV, VPRS 7400/P1, unit 10, folio 128, 24 December 1891.

CHAPTER TWO

Immigrants, mental health and social institutions: Melbourne and Auckland, 1850s–1890s

In May of 1882, William McDonald was removed from the Immigrants' Home in Melbourne by a warder of the Home and brought to the Yarra Bend Asylum. Aged forty-five, William was a gardener, originally from Glasgow. At the new institution he was described as 'feeble and paralysed', and was diagnosed as 'delusional', though he was mostly quiet. The admission details noted that he had no friends or relatives in the colony.[1] Miss Margaret Mears was admitted to the Auckland Mental Hospital in 1903 aged sixty-three. She had been living at the Costley Home for the Aged Poor in Epsom, Auckland, and by the time of her committal to the mental hospital she had been suffering from 'senile decay' for at least two years. Margaret arrived in New Zealand from Ireland in the early 1860s aged twenty-three.[2]

These two institutional inmates were both, like large numbers of men and women, colonial dwellers who had traversed the world of the huge migrations of the nineteenth century, and had arrived in the cities of colonial Australia and New Zealand. Their short, limited life stories, available for historical scrutiny only through extant institutional records, tell us different things about imperial mobility, the mental diseases of the colonies, the relationships between institutions and the inscription of detail about the immigration process itself, among other themes. The questions outlined in this chapter are couched within broader understandings of the knowledge about colonial society, gendered migration patterns and experiences, as well as medical ideas about the vulnerability and the susceptibility of new migrants to mental breakdown, illness and institutionalisation.

While many of the patient notes are as brief as those described above, these can also reveal something of the patterns of life of mobile immigrants in the colonies. Their stories also gesture to an imperial and colonial web of social institutions. This system of colonial institutions in an imperial context has been partially described and explored by Australian and New Zealand social and legal historians, who draw links between charity and health institutions, policies and practices, also referring to the impact of poverty and sickness on immigrants.[3] Arguably, as this chapter shows, there was a web *within the web* of welfare provision signalled by the relationship between institutions of health and welfare, or, to use New Zealand historian Margaret Tennant's phrase, a 'fabric' of welfare organisations and modes in the colonial state.[4] Tennant provides an overview of the role and power of the voluntary sector and the tireless work of agencies and groups in nineteenth-century New Zealand, also arguing that welfare provision was 'patchy' and less elaborate than the charitable assistance offered in parts of Australia and Britain.[5] Responding to the very poor was not just a matter of policy and practice; it also spoke volumes about the meanings of new settlements and their populations in the colonial world. The civilising mission or purpose of welfare was apparent in both colonies – Victoria and New Zealand – as evidenced by the emphasis on the 'deserving poor' as recipients of welfare assistance in both places, and the interaction between the State and the voluntary sector, with pressure on the State to provide and support public charitable institutions a continual refrain during the period under examination.[6] The use of the term 'fabric' also highlights the way that the interaction of the State and voluntary sector functioned in the colonial context.[7] On the other hand, though, contemporaries lamented the way that the colonial asylum as an institution became the most obvious solution to poverty, illness and need; large numbers of asylum admissions in New Zealand, Dr Frederick Skae noted in 1881, were due to the lack of other forms of charitable and official provision for the poor.[8]

Although hospitals for the insane had a relationship to other colonial welfare provisions and, like other authorities, provided a form of outdoor relief (meaning forms of institutional relief for the needy), these institutions have not often or readily been understood or historicised in this manner. However, there 'was a link ... between the high hopes of immigrants and the crowded asylums'.[9] Links between health and welfare organisations figure in the social landscape of early colonial Melbourne. In his description of the state of 'public health' in post-goldrush Victoria, Michael Cannon notes the array of social groups who found help and solace in the various medical and welfare institutions operating from as early as the 1850s. Among the institutions in his survey, Cannon includes the lying-in hospital, the asylum at the Yarra Bend, the treatment of paupers in the benevolent asylums, as well as charities like the Melbourne City Mission.[10] From the 1850s, doctors at the Yarra Bend had to contend with very hopeless medical cases who were literally left at the doorstep of the asylum when all other avenues of care had failed, with frequent transfers from the Melbourne Hospital and later the Melbourne Gaol, leaving Cannon to wonder if the aim was to ensure that 'the obloquy of their deaths would fall upon the Yarra Bend'.[11]

This chapter examines some of the forms of institutional care and relief relevant to immigrant populations in Melbourne and Auckland. The fact that social and medical relief was offered to immigrants in these new societies in a variety of forms is significant. In particular, the chapter describes the specific concerns over the mental health of immigrants, or the foreign-born, inside medical and welfare institutions. It explores the histories of the Victorian Immigrants' Homes established by the Immigrants' Aid Society in the 1850s, and touches on the roles of other welfare institutions in Victoria, and homes for the aged poor, including the Costley Home in Auckland, New Zealand. It shows how, in the absence of a Poor Law in the colonies, certain institutions for indoor and outdoor relief functioned to ameliorate social conditions for immigrants. These homes for the aged poor and immigrants became *de facto* colonial poorhouses.[12] Furthermore, the asylums and later mental hospitals were themselves often seen as 'workhouses' by contemporaries, hinting that these institutions simply captured the overflow population of the socially needy.[13] When the various mechanisms of charitable aid in the colonies failed, 'there was always the gaol or the lunatic asylum'.[14]

Immigrants and welfare in the colonies

Established in the early 1850s to cope with the influx of recent arrivals to the colony of Victoria, the Immigrants' Aid Society in Melbourne published advice booklets, administered the records of the persons seeking relief and shelter in the Immigrants' Homes, and maintained reports over the second half of the nineteenth century.[15] Together with contemporary travel writing and memoirs, these advice books, guides and reports, including those produced specifically for immigrants, form the basis of arguments in this chapter about a culture of assistance provided to immigrants in colonial Victoria. Similarly, the province of Auckland was a place where charitable institutions also took their place as social institutions for immigrants, though no specific immigrants' homes existed. New Zealand's field of welfare was nowhere near as well developed in the 1850s as the 'highly organised philanthropic activities already apparent in Australia'.[16] This was despite the fact that similar socio-economic conditions prevailed in both colonial Victoria and the province of Auckland, with growing pauperism evident in Auckland in the 1860s. The phenomenon of deserted wives, whose men left for work opportunities in other parts of the colony of New Zealand, as well as a drift of men across the Tasman to Victoria's goldfields, and an influx of immigrants looking for work, food and shelter, also contributed to the increasing visibility of poverty.[17] In fact, the presence of new migrants made these two societies very similar, with the only major difference being the large disparity between the numbers emigrating to and arriving in the two centres of Melbourne and Auckland.

Like the women and men inside asylums, those who entered the Immigrants' Home in the city of Melbourne, or institutions in urban Auckland such as the Costley Home, were ethnically diverse, but with the common distinction of poverty. Yet differences between the populations of such welfare institutions in Melbourne and Auckland are notable: separate systems of colonial welfare and charitable aid determined the contours of these institutions, a fact also noted by contemporaries, and worthy of more discussion.[18] That so many people foundered so terribly in the early years of Melbourne's settlement, for instance, was remarked upon by contemporary writers in descriptions of the many charitable institutions established there, as discussed further below.[19] Mental health authorities were puzzled by the growing incidence of insanity in the colonial populations over time, and found it challenging to accommodate them, in both a literal and a metaphorical sense.[20] In 1871, the official report presented to the Victorian Parliament from the Inspector of the Insane, Dr Edward Paley, commented that the rate of insanity among the immigrants was, thus far, not alarming, but that an 'accumulation' of insanity among Victorians was anticipated as the population both increased and hereditary insanity became more identifiable among the colonial-born.[21]

Migrants were also among those whose lives over time in the colonies had not yet fully taken hold; the full process of 'settling' was not immediate and, as the evidence deployed here suggests, sometimes included long stays inside social institutions. In Victoria, by 1901, just over 78 per cent of the population had been born in the colonies, but in the 1870s and 1880s, still only half of the general population was colonial-born.[22] Contemporaries, too, pondered this question of the long-term migrant status of some inside its social welfare homes, including the Immigrant's Home in Melbourne, as the chapter describes further below. Therefore this chapter's use of the term 'immigrant' is broadly inclusive of foreign-born asylum inmates. The changing character of the Immigrants' Aid Society's dependent population in Victoria, as reported by contemporaries, also tells us something about the shifting uses of colonial welfare over time. In 1870, Dr James Saunders Greig, then Secretary to the Immigrants' Aid Society (IAS), was interviewed by the commissioners of the Report into the Royal Commission into Charitable Institutions, published in 1871. Greig commented that originally, in the 1850s, the 'class' of persons primarily relieved by the IAS were the 'new arrivals', but that by 1870 the group of applicants had been largely composed of the 'destitute of all society', including internal migrants from other 'sister' colonies: these people thus continued to be 'migrants'.[23] Although many had been in the colony for twelve months, this could still be considered a very short time during the years of colonial development.[24]

Immigrants were, of course, still entering the Australian colonies after the initial wave of 1850s and 1860s immigrants. Dr Greig continued to defend his position in 1890 at a later Royal Commission on Charitable Institutions in Victoria, suggesting that there was a place for such an institution in a city like Melbourne, as the chapter later expands.[25] More impatiently, by 1890, Dr Walter Balls-Headley dismissed the notion that the Immigrants' Home was really for immigrants any longer, remarking, '[i]t is just for the poor'.[26] Historian Jean Uhl asserts that the IAS became known as a 'national relieving association for the poor' as early as the 1860s.[27] In New Zealand, Duncan MacGregor produced articles on the problem of poverty in New Zealand. MacGregor produced a three-part extended discussion of 'the problem of poverty' in the *New Zealand Magazine* in 1876.[28] In these essays and in his later official reports as Inspector-General he tended to link the immigrants of the 1870s with poverty and social decay, calling them a 'social residuum'.[29] Paupers were, historians remind us, regarded as an 'undesirable burden on the community'.[30]

Large numbers of the inmates inside the colonial asylums referred to here were foreign-born or immigrants, and not colonial-born. As Table 2.1 shows, at least one-third of the Yarra Bend population sampled for this study was born outside Australia, and over a third of the Auckland Asylum population was born outside New Zealand. Of the 402 women in the total sample from the records of the Yarra Bend Lunatic Asylum where 'birthplace' was recorded, 176 were from Ireland, 122 from England, 56 from Scotland, and 6 from Wales, with 17 from Germany.[31] At Auckland, 33 women were from Ireland, 66 from England, 13 from Scotland and only 2 were from Germany. Women in both institutions also hailed from European countries in very small numbers. The overseas-born populations of men inside these institutions mirrored those of the women.[32] Official commentaries about the birthplaces of the insane, found in both medical writings and statistical profiles of institutional populations, formed a specific aspect of the institutional reporting on the state of asylums in the colonies.[33]

In general, new arrivals to the colonies brought concerns about transmissible disease, if not mental instability. In New Zealand, the Immigration Officer J. Edwin March reported in 1872 on the passengers

Table 2.1 Overview of patient sample

Institution	Women	Recorded birthplace outside Australian/NZ colonies	Men	Recorded birthplace outside Australian/NZ colonies	Total sampled (with foreign-born as total and as % of total)
YBA	1321	402	1747	792	3068 (1194) (38.9%)
AA	310	125	558	270	868 (395) (45%)

Note:
No place was recorded for 1834 at the Yarra Bend, and for 282 at Auckland; at the Yarra Bend, 74 were said to have been born in Australia. At Auckland, 191 were said to have been born in New Zealand.
Source:
Database of all patients sampled for every three years from patient casebooks from the Yarra Bend Asylum and the Auckland Asylum, 1873–1910, showing number of foreign-born where a birthplace was recorded. Yarra Bend figures include entries of New Zealand-born; Auckland figures include entries of Australian-born. Large numbers of patient cases include no information on place of birth.

who became ill on the ship *Charlotte Gladstone*, which arrived from London, noting that 21-year-old Rosa Mills, who had been subject to 'hysterical fits' since the age of seventeen, was one of three young women who had obviously embarked the ship already ill. Rosa had severe convulsions and paralysis, and although she gradually improved, it was determined that she would leave 'the tropics', given her propensity to 'sentimental dreaming'.[34] The hint here of an unstable nature was enough to suggest her return to Britain.[35] The policing of women and gender boundaries on board ships during voyages to the colonies also signals a concern about the sexual health of women and the risks to their well-being, but also, as discussed below, the question of morality and the female immigrant.

Immigrants and colonial institutions in Melbourne, Victoria

Although all Europeans had been, at one time or other, themselves newcomers to the colonies, the rapid phases of settlement in Port Phillip, known as Victoria after 1851, meant that existing older populations of 'Victorians' watched with interest the many new arrivals to the growing city. 'Strangers' and 'foreigners', especially those who wandered out of place, attracted the attention of commentators in the press, perhaps more so because they were potential settlers.[36] Marked by accent and sometimes language itself, as well as clothing, customs and names, these strangers were visibly mobile. The colonial press made daily comments about 'strangers', highlighting the 'discomfort old colonists felt about the congregation of large numbers of people unknown to them on the wharves and in the backlanes'.[37] Immigrants – now new 'strangers' – were known, by virtue of their seeking temporary lodgings in the shanty town of tents known as Canvas Town, as 'The Houseless'.

Melbourne was patterned by a 'map of social inequality', with boarding houses, lodging houses and charitable agencies such as the Immigrants' Home, in close proximity.[38] Located at Princes Bridge, St Kilda Road, the Immigrants' Home was established in 1852 by the Immigrants' Aid Society, and by the middle of 1853, this home and other shelters had already provided temporary lodging for more than 10,000 immigrants.[39] These were relatively expensive to run, and were supported through voluntary contributions and a government grant, and in the tradition of welfare institutions, they had rules: no alcohol or fraternisation was allowed, and fires and lights had to be out by nine at night. Inmates needed to practise obedience and had duties to clean the place.[40]

The 'strange place' of 'Canvass Town', as it was known in the 1850s, was, in the words of Frederick Mackie, 'exposed to the full blaze of the sun, the power of the wind and the clouds of dust'.[41] Mackie was right to suggest that behind benevolence lay a desire for immigrants to come to view the colonial port of Melbourne as one that would welcome and comfort them given its need for immigrants, especially women immigrants. So much depended upon it, said Mackie, that these immigrants were 'looked for anxiously as each vessel arrives'.[42] Continuing his visits to immigrant families, Mackie spoke to people who had been reduced from affluence to poverty by emigrating.[43] More than this, over time, Canvas Town became a 'resort for vicious characters', making the lives of those decent immigrant families more stressful and highlighting the dangers of such transient communities, including, as Mackie observed in 1854, a large group of newly arrived young Chinese men, presumably bound for the goldfields.[44]

Missionaries and Christian ladies found the inner city suburbs of Melbourne fertile ground for rescue work, religious charity and presumably a source for attracting followers. Interestingly there were distinct roles for religious charitable groups and institutions such as the Melbourne City Mission. Where the IAS performed the express role of supporting new arrivals and those colonials born overseas who never succeeded, the Melbourne City Mission, which began in the same decade as the IAS as the Ladies' City Mission, visited the poor and neglected, ran meetings to evangelise, established mothers' meetings and distributed food, clothing and blankets. Many of the poor were, of course, also immigrants in the 1850s. In the 1870s and 1880s, city missionaries made it part of their regular work to visit the Immigrants' Home, Benevolent Asylum and Sailors' Homes, offering separate religious services to male and female immigrants in the Homes.[45]

The apparent poverty of inner-urban Melbourne was the subject of much commentary by missionaries. Mission sisters were appointed in the early 1860s, and tended to visit 'fallen' women and opium dens in specific parts of the city. By 1887, the Mission to the Streets and Lanes, founded by women to help relieve the stress of poverty in inner-city Melbourne, also worked in the city's streets.[46] Among the histories produced from female missionary accounts is Colonel Percival Dale's history of the Melbourne City Mission, which recounts the impact of poverty and drunkenness following the goldrush era.[47] The increase in crime was noticeable, writes Dale, and changes in population led to new forms of social disturbance:

> The permanent residents of the town were harassed by the influx, and the elderly men, widows with families and spinsters, huddled in the small houses in narrow thoroughfares with the buildings in many cases right on the street line, lived in terror of rough fellows demanding accommodation.[48]

By the 1860s and 1870s, the immigrants waiting to be 'housed' included aged and infirm men waiting for admission to Benevolent Asylums, men suffering from chronic diseases, convalescents, single and pregnant women, and deserted wives and children. Immigrant men, many of whom came to the colonies from Britain in pursuit of social improvement, were among the 'outcasts of Melbourne'. Often bachelors, they mixed among the poor and criminal, and who formed part of the 'itinerant street economy'.[49] Poor, infirm and older men were vulnerable to institutionalisation.[50] Many men arrested under vagrancy laws were also immigrants, with the policing of vagrancy in Victoria peaking in the 1880s.[51] The *Illustrated Australian News* ran a story on the Home in 1868 with two images of male inmates: an image of the night refuge where the men sit picking oakum (reproduced here as Figure 2.1), and another featuring men waiting in the 'casual room'.[52] The text pronounced that all classes of men and women sought help here – from the 'street-arab' who was a familiar sight in the main streets of the city, to the labouring man. Others included the women and children who had become the 'unhappy objects' of institutional life because of their poor luck in life. Poverty could also strike the educated and the highly trained among professional men. As the author commented, 'it would be difficult to enumerate the various classes of persons' seeking shelter here.[53]

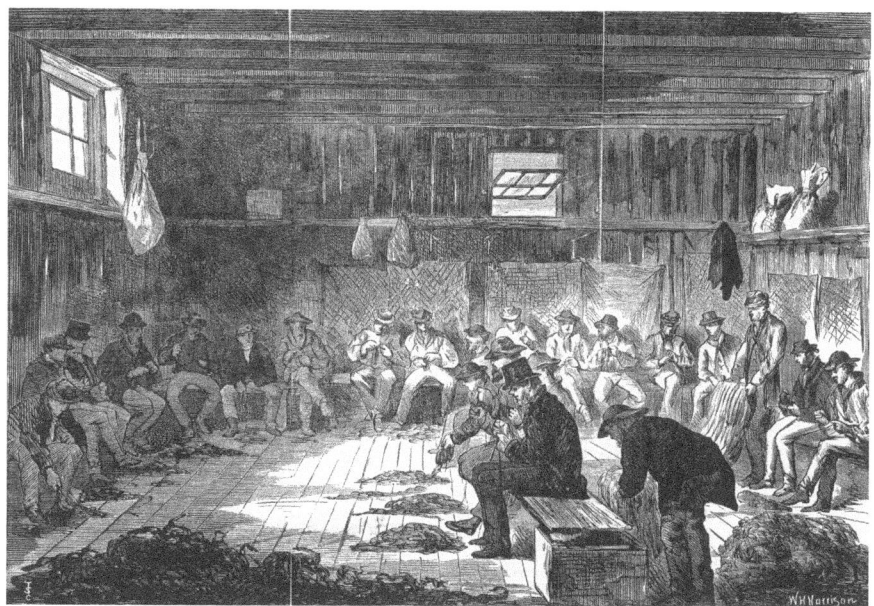

2.1 'Night refuge at the Immigrants Home'

The Immigrants' Home, then, was a place where need was ever-present. It catered to the freshly arrived immigrants who were yet to venture far beyond the city, and it served as a shelter for men and women whose ambitions to settle respectably in Victoria had not been realised. The roving journalist John Stanley James spent a night in the Home in the 1860s and wrote of the 'sickening smell' of 'unwashed humanity', with everything 'foul': 'rugs, mattress, floor, and walls'.[54] The inmates were mostly old men, and many of them had been in the Home for many years, as the Annual Reports of the Immigrants' Aid Society and its Home show. For 1874 the society reported that:

> The male adult inmates were of the most helpless class, the majority suffering from disease, and requiring medical treatment and hospital care. The really able-bodied who sought as 'casuals' temporary relief were comparatively few, and these only applied in any number during the severe period of our winter season.[55]

In fact, throughout the 1870s, the annual reports of the society, including the reports of the medical officer and the special committees, began to complain about the problem of men in particular. Sick, disabled, living unstable lives, they were often 'utterly helpless' and were a burden on the community. Increasingly, the reports also remarked upon a class of 'imbecile' women.

From the 1850s, despite circulating knowledge about the instability of colonial life, new arrivals to the colony of Victoria continued to be attracted by the promise of wealth and prosperity, especially following the news of the discoveries of gold, but also because migration from parts of Britain and Europe had become one response to poverty and overcrowding. Contemporaries had already produced discussions about the effects of immigration on mental health. Medical superintendents of institutions drew attention to immigration as a source of social breakdown, commenting frequently on the problems of dispersed populations in colonial society. They also pointed to immigration and geographical isolation as causes of mental breakdown.[56] The 'Hints upon Health' for the new arrivals by Dr Earley, discussed briefly in the previous chapter, stressed the importance of 'judicious conduct' among immigrants. Earley's pamphlet specifically noted the mental risks of immigration, gesturing towards single men in particular:

> Mental influences ... of no ordinary character, present difficulties in the case of immigrants: from the period they decide upon quitting the mother country until arrival, their minds are subjected to the extremes of hope and doubt, and who shall define the extent of these upon the health? They are advised most strenuously to exert themselves to resist the depression of spirits, which is the natural consequence of so much previous excitement, and to strive for that calmness, self-possession, and reliance, so essential to success ... in a new country.[57]

Similarly, the advice offered in a separate pamphlet by the Reverend William Jarritt, *Hints to Immigrants Upon Colonial Life and its Requirements*, also appeared to be levelled at male immigrants; Jarritt emphasised the value of good 'character'. Character was important given the presence of 'persons of plausible manners but of worthless principles, as well as ... desperate and abandoned ruffians'.[58] Jarritt reminded new immigrants to be wary of strangers, advice tinged with irony given that they too would be strangers in their new environments.

However true it was for some migrants, the popular myth of the Australian colonies as a 'working man's paradise' was being questioned at the very time of its construction.[59] Contemporary colonial statisticians 'neglected the extent of poor living and working conditions and their relation to illness and mortality'.[60] There were very poor health conditions of the inner city in Melbourne and Sydney for the working classes and those out of work. As the Immigrants' Aid Society noted in the 1870s, the 'loose kind of life' being led by women added to the burdens of the colonial welfare network, with local charities in smaller, rural communities in Victoria sending these women back to Melbourne, usually single women who found themselves pregnant in these communities. Immigrant men were possibly more vulnerable to isolation in the colonies, as Frederic Norton Manning, Inspector General of Asylums in New South Wales, noted in 1880: they operated a 'peculiar mode of life' as bushmen and miners, they were often unmarried, they were peripatetic and lured by seasonal work, and they were inherently restless.[61] In addition, according to Manning, there was a marked tendency towards introspection, suspicion, distrust and selfishness among colonists who could not fall back on support from associates and family.[62] In the comparable economic and social setting of New Zealand, men who had disappointments and failures in work experienced severe alienation, leading them to commit suicide.[63]

Following its establishment in the 1850s, the number of immigrants who needed to use the available welfare services such as the Immigrants' Home continued to swell in Victoria. William Howitt's account of 1850s Melbourne describes how 'thousands [were] suffering in the tents of Canvass Town, and in the most miserable lodgings'.[64] Even families who arrived with money deemed sufficient for them could be reduced to destitution, according to contemporary observers like Howitt.[65] The author of *Glimpses of Life in Victoria*, published in 1876, noted that Victoria and its institutions harboured 'much misery' for such a young colony.[66] Over time, the IAS reports produce a prevailing sense that all the 'unwanted' cases from hospitals were being turned over to the Immigrants' Home. Of the women discussed in a special report of 1873, '[a] good many who had no family ties were incapable from mental defect of caring for themselves'.[67] This is important: if housed in the Immigrants' Homes, some individuals remained among the unwanted; the asylum then became a final and last resort for these individuals.

The asylum or mental hospital became part of this 'web' of colonial health and welfare provision, characterised by the intersecting agencies of the fledgling state, as well as religious charitable institutions, in the absence of a Poor Law in the colonies.[68] In 1861, new emigrants to the Australian colonies could read or consult N. W. Pollard's *Homes in Victoria, Or, The British Emigrant's Guide to Victoria*, and find out more about the social and political world of their destination, as well as about its attitudes to charity and benevolence.[69] Pollard's advice provided to emigrants to Victoria in the 1860s noted the presence of a range of charitable institutions, where these 'flourished' in the metropolis and in rural areas, because despite Victoria's 'brilliant colours', 'sickness and calamity' could affect men and women everywhere.[70] His text established the idea that institutions were in place to support immigrants who did not immediately succeed:

> A 'new chum' may be laughed at, but he is sure to find those who will soothe his anxiety, and put him in the way of taking his stand among the industrious classes of the country, if he be willing and able to work; and if he be not; if incapacitated by sickness, if not fortunate in at once finding employment, he will still find either the public hospital or the philanthropist in any part of Victoria he may select as his abiding place.[71]

By the late 1870s, this web included industrial or reformatory schools, benevolent homes, institutions for the blind, deaf and dumb, orphanages, the Immigrants' Home, and the 'Old Colonists' Association' home which by 1876 took in infirm 'new arrivals' whose landing in the colony dated back as far as 1851.[72] Indeed, in 1878, the Immigrants' Aid Society discussed the length of time immigrants under their care had been in the colonies, also showing that immigrants could retain their status for some time for the purposes of charitable aid or indoor and outdoor relief. The majority of cases seen by the IAS had been in the colonies for between twenty and thirty years, with the vast majority of these cases male immigrants, as Table 2.2 indicates.

Already by 1870, the Medical Officer's report for the Immigrants' Home mentioned that its accommodation space was poor. On the male side, the accommodation was 'utterly inadequate', and on the women's side, even worse, and at risk of creating epidemic disease conditions.[73] These views contrast with an earlier newspaper report in 1868 from the *Illustrated Australian News* which made much of the fact that women at the Home looked 'healthy' but had taken a 'wrong step' in life.[74] Popular representations of the Immigrants' Home included women and children, as Figure 2.2 shows. The William Ralston wood engraving of 1872 published in London depicts some women with

Table 2.2 Length of time in the Australian colonies from IAS report

Length of time in the Australian colonies	Men	Women
Over 50 years	7	12
Between 30 and 50 years	60	38
Between 20 and 30 years	128	30
Between 10 and 20 years	69	32
Under 10 years	83	25
Total	347	137

Source:
Twenty-fifth Annual Report of the IAS (Flinders Lane West: Mason, Firth & McCutcheon, General Printers, 1874), 8.

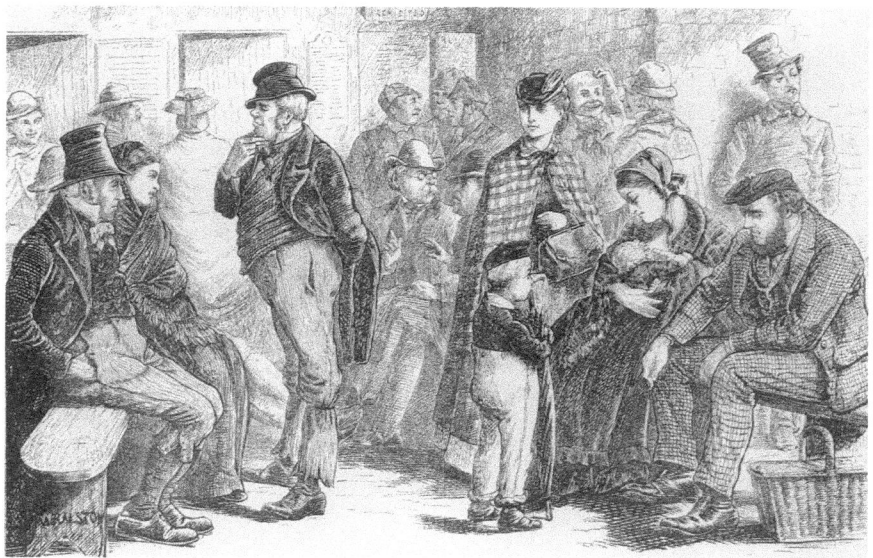

2.2 'Australian Sketches: The Melbourne Immigrants' Home', London, 1872

infants, a particular area of concern to the IAS. In 1869, these women were described as a class of immigrant in an extended discourse about the Immigrants' Home published in the *Argus* newspaper, and collated in a report for the IAS in the early 1870s. 'Of the female inmates', the *Argus* pronounced, there were, like male immigrants, poor, sick and injured, in smaller numbers than the men, but 'there are other classes in addition – namely, deserted wives and poverty-stricken widows, with young children to provide for, and women who have children without ever having been wives'.[75] This 'class' of women presented a pernicious problem, reported the *Argus*, since they could not easily be moved on when children were also involved in the care situation.

The Annual Reports of the Immigrants' Aid Society made regular comments about the profile of women inside its institutions in Victoria.[76] In 1870, both the desperate condition and 'problem' of 'delinquent' women attracted the attention of the committee of its board.[77] Among the female inmates were deserted wives, young women with infants, the aged and infirm, and incurable sick 'imbeciles'.[78] Those women who, as the report noted, had been living a 'loose kind of life' had often been removed by local charities from smaller rural communities and ended up in the urban environment, where they also sometimes found their way into the Yarra Bend Lunatic Asylum.

Among these women, a 36-year-old Irish Catholic woman from Belfast, Ellen B., left an eight-year-old daughter at the Home when she was taken to the asylum in 1873.[79] She died at the Yarra Bend after an epileptic fit four years later, leaving no further information about the welfare of her child. Three of the women who came from the Salvation Army or Benevolent Homes in Victoria were recorded as having infants or children. Annie O., a 19-year-old prostitute, gave birth in the asylum in 1894.[80] Another woman, Augusta H., was brought by police from the Salvation Army Maternity Home, in Fitzroy, Melbourne to the Yarra Bend in 1903, with the police commenting that she had two children 'though unmarried'.[81]

Those women who had come to the asylum from similar institutional settings, such as Salvation Army Homes, were also perceived as 'unwanted' in those spaces, though so far this research has not uncovered institutional reports for those sites. They, too, suffered from imbecility, feeble-mindedness, or similar diagnostic designations, and presumably presented real challenges for the welfare settings from whence they came. The IAS supported a Medical Officer whose work entailed the assessment of individual inmates. Over time, among the concerns of the Medical Officer for the IAS was the fact that some women came to the home utterly beyond rehabilitation.[82] One example of this type of female immigrant is found in the case of 30-year-old Sarah M., who came from the Immigrants' Home to the Yarra Bend Lunatic Asylum in July of 1879 in a very 'weak' bodily state. A widowed and Catholic Irish woman from Donegal, Sarah was described in the case notes at the Yarra Bend as having been 'daily troublesome' at the Immigrants' Home, partly because of her 'incessant' talking.[83] Her diagnosis was GPI, and she died of brain disease at the institution only a few months later.

There was, then, a strong relationship between immigration and women's perceived vulnerability, and the threats posed to the social order by their possible 'disorder'. The unhealthy physical state of a number of these women stands out in the detail collected by the institution at the time of committal. Their bodies were in 'delicate' health, or bore 'extensive scars' from burns. Other women were 'feeble' and suffering from pain or 'declining'.[84] Some had distinct disabilities which caused them to worry about their physical safety, such as Ann S. who was blind in both eyes and worried that people from the Immigrants' Home came into her room at night.[85] She was not the only woman who came to the Yarra Bend Lunatic Asylum concerned about the safety of the Home: 42-year-old Kate H. claimed the asylum was a much more secure place for her in 1885.[86] Women came as possible victims of abuse and violence: Jane W. had old wounds on her breast and chest area when examined at the asylum in 1897.[87] These immigrant women – some with infants, pregnant, battered, homeless and sick – were colonial welfare dependants. Their diseases were both organic and the result of harsh life conditions in the wake of their migrations. This aspect or 'melancholy result' of immigration drew comment from the IAS more generally over time.[88]

Their stories illustrate the gendered nature of the migration experience, but also the way that social institutions rendered migrants both visible and invisible at different times.[89] Jean Uhl notes that double the number of women, in comparison with men, were also called before the official committee of the IAS to explain disorderly conduct, most likely due to more narrow conceptions of orderly conduct for women in the period.[90] Other institutions formed in the mid-1850s saw a specific group of women as particularly needy: as M. J. Kernot's *Reminiscences of the Carlton Refuge* noted in the early twentieth century, these were the 'weak, the wasters and the undesirables' who needed the protection of a home.[91] Although a relatively small number of women were explicitly designated as 'prostitutes' or 'dissolute' or even as 'vagrant' in these records, in general, many women attracted institutional attention for their perceived 'hopelessness', based on notions of middle-class respectability and growing sensibilities about colonial health, especially women who became an increasing burden on the fledgling system of welfare established in the colonies. This was a problem which had surfaced at least two decades earlier in the 1850s as new waves of (free) immigrants arrived. Poor, white women, especially immigrant women who had been labelled as promiscuous, helpless or diseased, could also become, like non-whites, the 'casualties of colonialism'.[92] This theme is further elaborated in Chapters 5 and 6 of this book.

Particular sectors of the settler immigrant population were, then, seen to be more susceptible to problems of ill health, including mental breakdown. The evidence for this growing need can be found in the reports of social institutions. These reports convey a sense that all the unwanted cases from hospitals were being turned over to the Immigrants' Home, an important point, since the asylum then became the final and last resort, making it, too, part of this 'web' of welfare provision. The reports noted not only the aged and infirm men whose lives were damaged by age and disease, but also a group of younger men, disabled and diseased and utterly dependent upon welfare.

The men who had recourse to these institutions, simply by virtue of their need for forms of charity in hard times, were working-men and poor men who lived hard and drank heavily. Men were more affected by 'drink, drugs and violent accidents'.[93] Like the older men eking out their existence in boarding houses and homes, young men, too, were likely to fall on hard times, especially in the 'excitement' of the 1850s, as Dr John Singleton suggested; he saw a number who, because of the 'heat' and drink, ended up in the Yarra Bend Asylum.[94] Vagrancy also loomed as a social category which highlighted fears about the failures of settler masculinity, as Chapter 4 examines in more detail.[95] Many men had perhaps lived between institutions and the outdoors, both visible and invisible as the rough, houseless strangers in the developing urban world of colonial Melbourne, as the case of John R. suggests: he was covered in 'bruises and abrasions' when he arrived from the Immigrants' Home.[96]

The evidence suggests that in the Australian colonies, as in other white settler colonies, it was institutions that were increasingly seen as the appropriate places for the treatment of the mentally ill, although families also played important roles.[97] Medical superintendents and inspectors guessed that the relative 'popularity' – or perhaps, acceptability – of institutions was due to several factors, among them, the lack of a poorhouse system, as existed in Britain, and the large number of itinerant persons pursuing work in the colonies.[98] Figures 2.3 and 2.4 illustrate the great variety of people who both sought refuge in the Immigrants' Home, and who presented colonial society with concerning behaviours.

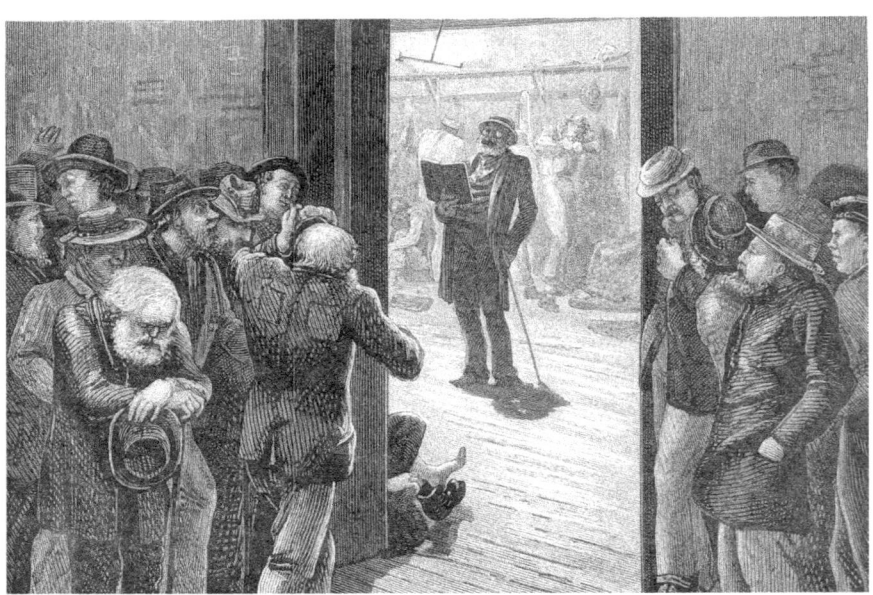

2.3 'Casuals at the Immigrants' Home', 19 June 1880

IMMIGRANTS, MENTAL HEALTH, SOCIAL INSTITUTIONS

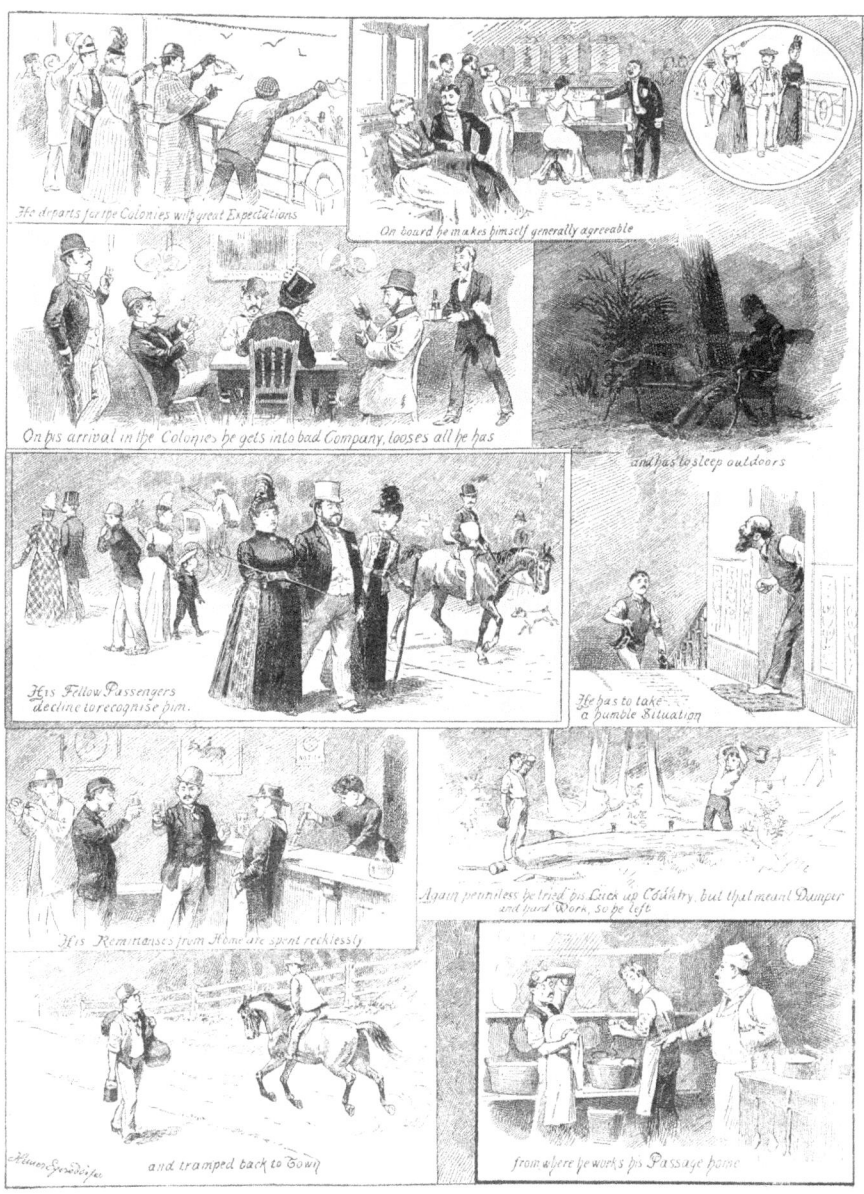

2.4 'The Ne'er-Do-Well in the Colonies', 1 October 1890

In addition, and suggesting more reasons for transfers to the asylum, there were some challenging users of the Home and its services. Many people seeking shelter, both women and men, presented with aggression, drunkenness and general 'insubordination'.[99] A continual refrain of concern over the ability of the Home to provide for cases of 'chronic disease, debility, and old age – cases turned out of the Melbourne and provincial hospitals, and sent from the country generally', as noted in the report for 1872, shadowed the Immigrants' Aid Society.[100] This may account for some of these transfers of men from the Home to the Yarra Bend who were perhaps not cases of mental breakdown, but rather cases of men malnourished and feeling the physical effects of poverty. However, in addition, by 1880, the Medical Officer's report for the Society noted 'revolting' cases among the ranks of the male immigrants, perhaps hinting at cases of paresis or GPI, the tertiary stage of syphilis, as Chapter 4 describes. Mental defects among women were also causing great anxiety. The Society's own medical work was being privileged and a system of diagnosis and classification had generally improved over the decades, but this was still not the aim of the Society, nor was it ever intended to be. Migrants' transitions from the Immigrants' Home, the Salvation Army homes, or the street, to the hospital for the insane were triggered by this sense of hopelessness, including advanced age or incurable illness.

By 1890, suggesting that colonists had begun to reflect on the social problems that began with the large population growth of the 1850s and 1860s, Victoria's Inspector of Asylums, Thomas Dick, reported that a 'large proportion of ... admissions were of a chronic and incurable type, received principally from gaols, hospitals, benevolent asylums and the Immigrants' Home'.[101] Other organisations and social institutions, including the Melbourne City Mission (1854) linked the experiences of poverty and destitution among colonial population to mental health problems. In her report of visiting houses in the South Richmond area in the early 1900s, Sister Thompson wrote of the 'nearly starving' young family with a baby, and the man 'much depressed'.[102] In his various encounters with the sick, poor and destitute of Melbourne, Dr John Singleton averted suicides, met with drunkards, and witnessed cases of neglected children. Among those he met was 'the constant influx of immigrants *en route* for the goldfields, most of them young men not long arrived in the colonies; and of these, great numbers, between the heat of the climate and strong drink, were deprived of reason and sent to the lunatic asylum'.[103]

Immigrants and the fabric of welfare in the province of Auckland, New Zealand

Similar concerns about the health of immigrants were raised in Auckland in the 1870s. In 1874, the Provincial Surgeon, Thomas Philson, commented:

> It may be remarked that not a few of our hospital patients are derived from the recently arrived immigrants, in the shape of consumptives, imbeciles, and cripples, evincing the necessity of more stringent selection by home agents.[104]

New immigrants, it was alleged, arrived in 'destitute' circumstances, also placing a burden upon the local health and welfare services.[105] By 1875, Auckland boasted a range of social and charitable institutions, some of which were financed by the provincial government, such as the public hospital and the lunatic asylum, and the Old Men's Refuge (established in 1867).[106] There were denominational homes, such as Anglican and Catholic orphanages, as well as homes for neglected and criminal children, and a female refuge, which, as in Melbourne, was created for the welfare of women working in prostitution and was relatively short-lived. The Ladies' Benevolent Society, founded in 1857, managed an old women's home and contributed much in the way of ongoing welfare provision, mostly in the fields of child welfare and deserted women.[107] This society most likely catered to new arrivals and to poor immigrants, just as its sister organisation did in Melbourne. The Auckland City Mission was founded in 1863 and had a broad remit, taking in the poor and needy as well as visiting the institutionalised.[108]

Immigrants, who arrived in smaller numbers than the notable influx to Victoria, but who still posed considerable challenges to new settlements and their physical and social infrastructure in the colonial era, dispersed from the major arrival ports of Lyttleton in the South Island, and later Auckland in the North Island, and came to urban Auckland and the areas north and south of the city.[109] John Murray Moore's account of migration, discussed briefly in Chapter 1, also made several arguments about the medical and welfare support available to immigrants to New Zealand. Hospitals and public lunatic asylums rate a mention, as did the body overseeing their work, the Hospitals and Charitable Aid Board.[110] But despite his cheerful account of the positive aspects of New Zealand society, including its various limitations, in his 1890 publication Moore was also still promulgating the belief, which circulated about the colonies and the imperial world, that people with incipient mental illness – 'lunatics' – were regularly 'shipped off from England to the colony by their relatives, in order to get rid of them, and so throw the burden of their support upon the colony'.[111] Immigrants thus came to the colonies under suspicion. There was so much potential for many of them to succeed – and yet so many preordained failures for a few.

Though not the same kind of institution as the Immigrants' Home, the Costley Home in Auckland provides a useful comparable site to investigate welfare assistance. The Costley Home for the Aged Poor was established in Auckland with a bequest from Edward Costley as a wing of the Auckland Hospital in the 1880s, and run by the Auckland Hospital and Charitable Aid Board, a publicly funded entity.[112] It became the largest of the homes established for the aged poor in New Zealand.[113] Edward Costley had been a generous benefactor to Auckland, and his bequest supported a range of institutions, including the Free Library, the Museum, the Sailors' Home and the Parnell Auckland Home.[114] The Costley Home featured, along with many imposing buildings and scenes of Auckland, in a series of photographic illustrations of Auckland published in 1910, indicating its role in public life.[115] While seven and a quarter acres of land was left in Costley's original endowment of £8,000 for the purposes of a home for the elderly and destitute, by 1919 it occupied more than twice this space and was self-sufficient with a piggery and farm.[116] In the late 1880s, the Home provided for around 190 inmates of both sexes.[117] In the absence of homes specifically designed for poor immigrants, institutions such as the Costley Home were one landing place for elderly migrants who, like those living in colonial Victoria, sometimes later found themselves sent to the hospitals for the insane. The Costley Home transferred inmates to the Auckland Asylum, as the institutional records illustrate. Dogged by controversy in the late 1890s, inmates were also, at least once, transferred from the Costley Home to the asylum during an 'authoritarian' period of administration of charitable institutions under the leadership of Duncan MacGregor, who highlighted the suitability of the asylum for 'pauper lunatics'.[118] MacGregor was the Inspector-General of Hospitals and Charitable Institutions from 1886, and was formerly Professor of Mental and Moral Science at the University of Otago.[119] His contributions to debates about poverty among new immigrants sheds light on contemporary attitudes towards 'the immigrant', a social category of person under scrutiny in the colonies.

The presence of immigrants in larger numbers by the 1870s certainly influenced ideas about welfare provision in the colonies, and specifically in Auckland. There was a 'reframing' of benevolence in the early 1870s in Auckland, the result of new debates about the social landscape and tensions over the responsibility for 'a range of social outcasts'.[120] And yet there was also a noticeable lack of social compassion exhibited by colonial welfare authorities in some cases. The Charitable Aid Board, to which the Costley Home reported, enforced Costley Home regulations and stipulated funding strictures, with 'meanness' and adherence to obedience, a signal that the Home was run like a prison.[121] The scandal at the Home in the late 1890s, which highlighted the poor treatment of inmates and bad management practices at the Home, resembled similar debacles in earlier periods at lunatic asylums in the colonies.[122] In fact, the slur on a member of the attendant staff at the Costley Home – that she 'had been in the asylum in attendance on lunatics and was only fit to be in attendance on lunatics' – echoes the conflict over the reputation of attendants in hospitals for the insane over the second half of the nineteenth century, as Lee-Ann Monk has so effectively demonstrated.[123]

Some of these events took place against the backdrop of welfare reform in the mid-1880s. The Hospitals and Charitable Institutions Act (1885) set out a system of dual responsibility for charitable aid between the State and voluntary contributions, putting pressure on some institutions to define themselves as charitable and others as State-run entities.[124] By the 1890s, the colonies faced severe economic depression, which perhaps explained the attitude of the Charitable Aid Board to some seeking welfare assistance. The economic depression of the 1890s was a time of 'mental anguish' for many. It affected working men, families and the wealthier set, many of whom also lost investments and were forced to declare bankruptcy.[125] There was, then, a perception that men and women needed to make themselves useful, even when they were facing economic disaster. Some were forced out of the institutions that had offered them temporary respite. Gum diggers, known to be 'an assorted lot', were often 'vagrants ordered out of the cities by the police; [and] "useless men" from the Costley Home for the Aged, sent out by the Charitable Aid Board in an endeavour to make them earn their living'.[126] Before the introduction of the Old Age Pension in both Victoria and New Zealand, the elderly indigent were forced to rely on institutions, homes and charity when family networks failed or were absent.[127] Tennant shows that growing numbers of persons aged sixty-five and over were housed in institutions across New Zealand between 1885 and 1920, even though she suggests this evidence needs to be put in perspective, and that many elderly people were cared for in the community.[128] Some others received the 'imperial pension' which was paid by colonial treasury departments to individuals who had previously been employed by the Imperial Government, including men employed in the constabulary and other professions.[129]

The men and women who were transferred from the Costley Home and other homes in Auckland to the Auckland Asylum in this period

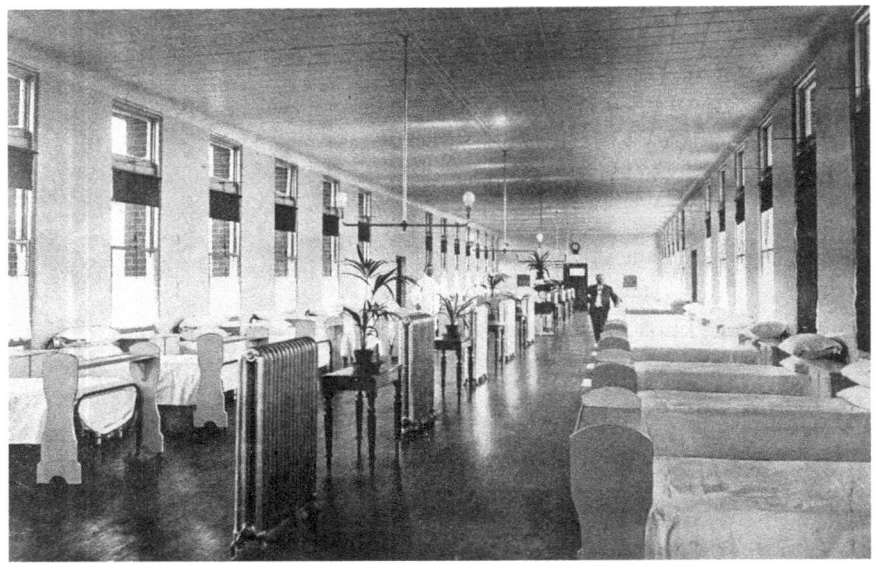

2.5 An interior view of the Costley Home New Infirmary Ward, Auckland, 9 December 1906

left bare traces of their lives in either institution. Very few images of the Costley Home in the nineteenth century exist to depict and remind us of the place itself; a sketch in the *Auckland Star* published in December 1898 showed an unremarkable and pleasant, well-kept house and garden, and an elderly gentleman sitting outside the front fence.[130] By 1907, images of the new infirmary and interior of the home (see Figure 2.5) belied the turmoil that had earlier beset its management, as described below in this chapter. Although this study's sample of asylum records includes only a small number of inmates from these homes, including Costley, the Salvation Army Homes, nursing homes in Auckland and Hamilton, and Old Men's Homes, many more were transferred, according to the official reports of the period. Their stories are full of contrasts about the lives of immigrants over time. Taken to the Auckland Mental Hospital from the Costley Home in 1903, 70-year-old Herman Henricksen, who came to New Zealand from Denmark in 1858 aged twenty-five, was suffering from pneumonia. Henricksen was a farmer, but he had been sick with dementia and worry over his wife's death when admitted to the Yarra Bend. Born in 1833, Henricksen had been in New Zealand for forty-five years and yet the institutional record identified him as foreign-born.[131] In fact several of the Costley Home inmates transferred to Auckland Asylum had been in the colony for lengthy periods of time at committal: one had arrived in 1846, and others arrived in the 1860s and 1870s. Most arrived at the asylum in the 1890s. Luke MacDonald, a 45-year-old pauper, was sent from the Costley Home to the asylum in 1891 where he was recorded as suffering from GPI and died two years later.[132] Although his birthplace was not recorded, he was born in 1847. Mrs Martha Jane Nicol went from the Costley Home to the asylum in 1903 with senile decay. Aged sixty-two, Martha's 'family troubles' were highlighted as one reason for her mental state, and these might also explain her dependence upon these two colonial welfare and medical institutions.[133]

By the early 1900s an atmosphere of fear and distrust pervaded the Costley Home and its administration. Although the previous Manager of the Home, Mr Moss and his wife, who was the Matron, had been removed in the 1890s, problems remained. The *Report of the Commission on the Costley Home* (1904) revealed that in 1903, investigators found squalid conditions, with the mostly elderly, sick and bedridden inmates 'requiring constant attention', and yet a Medical Officer came only three times per week. More troubling was the presence of at least five 'mentally deranged' inmates who were at once examined and taken to the asylum.[134] Moss and his wife gave evidence and presented witnesses at the 1903 hearing in an attempt to exonerate themselves. The very fact of homes for elderly, unwell and impoverished people seemed to make for impossible institutional conditions, especially without adequate support and funds. In 1909, the report of the Inspector-General of Hospitals and Charitable Aid in the Dominion reported separately on a range of charitable institutions, among them, the Costley Home. The brief summary, when read alongside summaries of other social welfare institutions, shows that Costley was not alone in experiencing difficulty in managing social outcasts.[135] Certainly the visibility on the streets of Auckland of the needy and destitute, as seen through the eyes of new immigrants, paint a stark picture of the worlds of colonists in New Zealand. Danish immigrant Ingeborg Stuckenberg, mentioned in the first chapter, commented that the people of Auckland were 'the most broken-down, tired, wrinkled workers' or 'dressed up, dirty, shabby women', and she wrote of contemporary reports about madness, suicide and homelessness.[136]

At the end of the nineteenth century in Auckland, in 1894, the Mission to the Streets and Lanes was established to provide for the poor, ill and wayward in inner-city Auckland.[137] The women Missioners worked from a cottage in Grey Street, central Auckland, and went from place to place in urban areas of Auckland to offer assistance. As Margaret McClure writes, these women 'spent a life of constant movement'; wearing the Anglican nun's dark habits, they were visible to city dwellers who needed their ministrations. Like the Melbourne female missionaries, these women set out to tackle urban problems of poverty, slums, ill-health and family breakdown. Influenced by the Melbourne Mission to the Streets and Lanes founded in 1887, the Auckland missionary women worked alongside the Anglican church of St Matthews on the corner of Hobson and Albert Streets. Their 'Church Mission to the Lanes' consisted of work among the poor and destitute, rescue work and visiting institutions, specifically the Costley Home.[138] This pattern of city missions to the poor – with Melbourne and Auckland sharing distinctive urban environments and approaches to the amelioration of slum poverty – provides evidence that the larger institutions for the confinement of the insane also took in a population of people who were likely to have been exposed to this fabric of welfare in the colonies, albeit on a modest scale.

Dispossession

A focus on immigrants should not obscure the fact that in colonial societies, Indigenous peoples and their spaces were severely disrupted by newcomers over time. This was a gendered disruption as well; new social formations also generated questions about women as vulnerable agents more widely. Among the women at the Immigrants' Home in Melbourne were internally displaced women, including 'Aboriginal native' Margaret Shaw, who also attracted the attention of the committee of the Immigrants' Aid Society in 1870. Shaw was admitted in 1870 following an application made on her behalf.[139] There were few Aboriginal women, or men, in the Yarra Bend Lunatic Asylum, with official reports rarely mentioning their presence, although commentaries on the presence of the Chinese were more regular.[140] In the total sample for this research, only one male inmate is designated 'Aboriginal', though other inmates were possibly also Aboriginal, as the following chapter suggests. The histories of Indigenous peoples in colonial Australia, and specifically Victoria, can shed light on this. Aboriginal peoples had been dispersed and segregated from the European populations in the colony by the 1860s, and were already living in other forms of institutions including missions under the management of the Aboriginal Protectorate.[141]

At Auckland, a different story about the dispossession of Māori peoples is visible in the records of the institution.[142] In the total sample for Auckland, there are forty-nine Māori or 'Aboriginal' inmates, and of this number, fourteen are female inmates. Like immigrants, these women, too, attracted attention for their poverty, poor health and transience, and were arguably also drawn into imperial discourses around the gendering of insanity. Racial designations increasingly defined notions of 'difference' inside institutions.[143] Mrs Ellen Lynch, an alcoholic aged forty-eight who had an episode of insanity at the Costley Home, was transferred to the Auckland Asylum where her delusions were described: although the record suggests she was born in New Zealand, she thought 'she [wa]s on board a ship when in a cell'. Interestingly, she also said that 'all of Auckland should belong to her and her people (the Maoris)', although she was not Māori herself.[144]

Conclusions

Discussions about the quality and plight of immigrants, the numbers seeking assistance and the problems which arrived with immigrants as they came to the colonies in successive waves, form a distinct pattern across the extent of the nineteenth-century public and private discussion of mental health and welfare. The different parliamentary inquiries, including royal commissions, and their ensuing public reports into charitable aid in both colonies in the period, serve to illustrate the way this web was imagined from the 1870s onwards. These reports also indicate how absences in the contemporary debate about welfare institutions might be highlighted to show that there were some aspects of institutional care which deserve more detailed scholarly attention, including the relationships between hospitals for the insane and other forms of 'asylum' for the poor in the colonies. Annual Asylum Inspectors' Reports for both Victoria and New Zealand also tell us about how many institutional transfers took place.

Official and archival sources, then, tell us much about formal attitudes to welfare and institutions, as well as providing glimpses of the immigrants who were caught in this 'web' of institutional relationships, however loose these were at the time. The records of the institutions discussed here contain absences and gaps, and silences about immigrants' experiences, but also disclose much about their vulnerability in relation to welfare and charity in the period. Travel writing about the health and welfare institutions of empire might be viewed as another 'domain' of imperial practice.[145] Glimpses of institutional life for the insane can also be found in the many travellers' accounts of visits to the colonies. Trollope was impressed, in general, with the care of the sick insane and the needy in Victoria.[146]

This chapter has sought to make clear the connections between debates about colonial systems of welfare and the specific identities of colonial dependants – such as women who moved between forms of institutional care in the colonies, or whose welfare needs were first identified in the institutions for the insane – as well as the developing language of institutional confinement for inmates of the asylum system. By describing the worlds of migrants to colonial Victoria and New Zealand, and the social welfare institutions available to them when their ambitions to settle in the colonies were dashed by bad fortune and illness, it has also suggested that social institutions worked together, providing a semblance of welfare for the needy, but also showing that institutions were interrelated and presented 'alternatives' for some individuals or their societies, given their unwanted status. Inside the institutions, immigrants' lives were captured and their movement stopped. Understanding and interpreting who they were was pretty basic in many respects, as authorities sought to grasp who the needy were and how to best handle them as social dependants.

Institutionalised people, including many immigrants – already at the margins of colonial society in a number of respects – were further marginalised inside institutional populations. Gender differences helped to categorise immigrants as recipients of colonial welfare and institutional care. For instance, contemporaries highlighted fears about weak men: or made the links between immigrants and an unhealthy white male population. Unemployed men were regarded as the 'unpopular objects' of charity.[147] Colonial masculinities were also shaped through ideas about the weakness of men who also found their way into welfare institutions.[148]

Women represented specific forms of social disorder and were positioned in different ways from men in the discourses around need, illness and dependency. Writing about the histories of women and welfare, Shurlee Swain notes that 'despite the demographic imbalance that marked most of the Australian colonies, women predominated amongst the poor' and that women came to 'signify a threat to the social order well beyond their individual plight'.[149] This 'threat' was embodied by the sometimes violent or disruptive female asylum inmate, but also by the physically weak and demoralised figure of the insane woman whose responsibilities to home, husband and family could not be met. Women who sought welfare support in the nineteenth century, having been deserted by male breadwinners, became the focus of social unease, and were ascribed their own 'class' in the discussions around the female immigrants occupying institutional spaces.[150]

Gender, ethnicity and social class all played significant roles in the construction of the range of 'colonial identities' inside social institutions. The following chapter examines patient identities in these two sites through a more careful analysis of the patient population data. The discussion centres on how these women and men were characterised in patient case notes through specific categories including gender, ethnicity, class and occupation, religion, marital status and disease, and on how these facts about them become part of the historical narratives of mental illness produced by contemporaries and by later historians. By using patient records in the Australian and New Zealand colonial contexts, and by teasing out the ways in which these records worked, it aims to highlight the way that migration and colonising experiences, evinced through the mobility of institutional inmates, are 'inseparable from class, gender, labour, politics, property and empire building'.[151]

Notes

1. PROV, VPRS 7399/P1, unit 5, folio 82, 23 May 1882.
2. National Archives of New Zealand, Auckland (NANZ), YCAA 1048/10 17, patient 2910, 27 November 1903.
3. Stephen Garton, *Out of Luck: Poor Australians and Social Welfare*, The Australian Experience (Sydney: Allen & Unwin, 1990); Margaret Tennant, *Paupers and Providers: Charitable Aid in New Zealand* (Wellington: Allen & Unwin/Historical Branch, 1990); Richard Kennedy, *Charity Warfare: The Charity Organisation Society in Colonial Melbourne* (Melbourne: Hyland House, 1985), p. 32; Christina Twomey, *Deserted and Destitute: Motherhood, Wife Desertion and Colonial Welfare* (Melbourne: Australian Scholarly Publishing, 2002), p. 34.
4. Margaret Tennant, *The Fabric of Welfare: Voluntary Organisations, Government and Welfare in New Zealand, 1840–2005* (Wellington: Bridget Williams Books, 2007).
5. Tennant, *The Fabric of Welfare*, p. 59.
6. Tennant, *The Fabric of Welfare*, pp. 59, 61; see also Christina Twomey, 'Courting men: Mothers, magistrates and welfare in the Australian colonies', *Women's History Review*, 8:2 (1999), pp. 235–6.
7. Tennant, *The Fabric of Welfare*, p. 63.
8. *Annual Report on Lunatic Asylums of New Zealand*, *AJHR*, H-13 (1881), p. 1.
9. Alan Atkinson, *The Europeans in Australia*, Vol. 2: *Democracy* (Melbourne and New York: Oxford University Press, 2004), p. 281.
10. Michael Cannon, *Melbourne After the Gold Rush* (Main Ridge: Loch Haven Books, 1993), pp. 414–22. For a history of the Melbourne City Mission, see Catherine Waterhouse, *Going Forward in Faith: A History of the Melbourne Citymission* (Fitzroy: Melbourne Citymission, 1999).
11. Cannon, *Melbourne After the Gold Rush*, p. 415.
12. For example, Margaret Mutch writes about the Costley Home in Auckland from this point of view, especially when seeing the Home through the eyes of contemporary commentators; see Mutch, 'Aspects of the Social and Economic History of Auckland, 1890–1896', unpublished Masters thesis, University of Auckland, 1968, p. 127.
13. Mutch, 'Aspects of the Social', p. 215.
14. Tennant, *The Fabric of Welfare*, p. 62.
15. For more on the Immigrants' Aid Society, see Shurlee Swain, 'Immigrants home', in *eMelbourne: The City Past and Present*, Encyclopedia of Melbourne online, University of Melbourne, www.egold.net.au/biogs/EG00090b.htm, accessed 1 August 2011; Jean Uhl, *Mount Royal Hospital: A Social History* (Parkville: Mount Royal Hospital, 1981).
16. Tennant, *Paupers and Providers*, p. 14.
17. Tennant, *Paupers and Providers*, p. 18.
18. John Murray Moore suggested that there was a need for a home for 'tramps' among the existing establishments; see Moore, *New Zealand for the Emigrant, Invalid, and Tourist* (London: Sampson Low, Marston, Searle and Rivington, 1890), p. 166. For a discussion of the 'fabric' of welfare and charitable aid in New Zealand, see Tennant, *The Fabric of Welfare*.

19 See John Hunter Kerr [attrib.], *Glimpses of Life in Victoria, by 'A Resident'* (Melbourne: Melbourne University Press, 1996 [1876]), p. 273.
20 See Catharine Coleborne, *Reading 'Madness': Gender and Difference in the Colonial Asylum in Victoria, Australia, 1848–1888* (Perth: Network Books, Australian Public Intellectual Network, 2007), p. 127; Coleborne, *Madness in the Family: Insanity and Institutions in the Australasian Colonial World, 1860–1914* (Basingstoke and New York: Palgrave Macmillan, 2010), p. 63.
21 *Report of the Inspector of Asylums on the Hospitals for the Insane for the Year 1870* (Melbourne: John Ferres, Government Printer, 1871), in VPP, pp. 3–4.
22 See the numbers provided by Richard Broome in *The Victorians Arriving* (Sydney: Fairfax, Syme and Weldon, 1984), p. 98.
23 Dr James Saunders Greig, 26 August 1870, Royal Commission into Charitable Institutions, VPP Session/vol. 2, 1871, pp. 26–7.
24 Greig, 26 August 1870, Royal Commission.
25 Dr James Saunders Greig, 22 August 1890, *Royal Commission on Charitable Institutions, Synopsis, Minutes of Evidence and Appendix* (Melbourne: Robert S. Brain, Government Printer, 1892), pp. 372–3.
26 Dr Walter Balls-Headley, 20 June 1890, *Royal Commission on Charitable Institutions, Synopsis, Minutes of Evidence and Appendix* (Melbourne: Robert S. Brain, Government Printer, 1892), p. 191.
27 Uhl, *Mount Royal Hospital*, p. 9.
28 Duncan MacGregor, 'The problem of poverty in New Zealand', Part I, *New Zealand Magazine* (January 1876), pp. 60–75; (April 1876), pp. 207–16; (July 1876), pp. 311–21. For commentary on these essays see also Tennant, *Paupers and Providers*, pp. 44–6. Tennant contextualises MacGregor's interest in the question of poverty as being formed through his Scottish heritage and experience, his travel to Australia, his interactions with notable welfare champion, Grace Neill – who was the first female inspector of hospitals, asylums and charitable aid – and his work in the Otago Lunatic Asylum. These were all experiences which afforded him greater interaction with and awareness of poverty and need than many people of his social and professional status. He was, perhaps, as Tennant claims, New Zealand's earliest 'social researcher'. See Penny Ehrhardt, with Ann Beaglehole, *Women and Welfare Work, 1893–1993* (Wellington: Department of Social Welfare/Historical Branch, 1993), pp. 9–13.
29 Quoted and described in Tennant, *Paupers and Providers*, pp. 45–6.
30 Mutch, 'Aspects of the Social', p. 124.
31 Birthplaces were not always listed, also suggesting that some institutional inmates had few family contacts in the colonies, or that information could not be deduced at committal.
32 For example, the database shows that at the Yarra Bend, 209 men were from Ireland, 303 from England, eighty-seven from Scotland, and thirty-nine from Germany. At Auckland, fifty-five were from Ireland, 126 from England, twenty-five from Scotland, and four from Germany.
33 See for instance discussion about official reporting in Coleborne, *Madness in the Family*, pp. 36–41.
34 *AJHR*, 1872 Session I, D-16a, pp. 3–4.
35 Hammerton also briefly inserts the risk of mental breakdown following emigration as a topic worthy of more study, also citing Jan Gothard's *Blue China: Single Female Migration to Colonial Australia* (Melbourne: Melbourne University Publishing, 2001); see Hammerton, 'Gender and migration', in Philippa Levine (ed.), *Gender and Empire*, Oxford History of the British Empire (Oxford: Oxford University Press, 2004), pp. 167–8. Tropical climates were linked in the late nineteenth century to mental breakdown, especially among white men; see Warwick Anderson, *Colonial Pathologies: American Tropical Medicine, Race, and Hygiene in the Philippines* (Durham, INC, and London: Duke University Press, 2006), pp. 134–5.
36 Arguably, such strangers were, as Georg Simmel suggests of 'foreigners' more generally in his essay 'The stranger', a potential threat as they promised unknown

capacity to belong; see Kurt H. Wolff, *The Sociology of Georg Simmel* (New York: Free Press, 1950), p. 402.
37 Christina Twomey, '"Without Natural Protectors": Histories of Deserted and Destitute Colonial Women in Victoria 1850–1865', unpublished Ph.D. thesis, University of Melbourne, 1995, p. 73.
38 Graeme Davison, David Dunstan and Chris McConville (eds), *The Outcasts of Melbourne: Essays in Social History* (Sydney, London and Boston: Allen & Unwin, 1985), p. 19.
39 Richard Broome, *The Victorians Arriving* (Sydney: Fairfax, Syme and Weldon, 1984), p. 76. Broome describes how in November of 1852, the Immigrants' Home at Princes Bridge could accommodate 240 people. An unused abattoir at Batman's Hill was also converted for this use, while the Immigrants' Home at South Yarra housed 600, and a Wesleyan House in Drummond Street in Carlton also housed several hundred, meaning that overall, temporary shelter was available for around 1,420 immigrants.
40 Broome, *The Victorians Arriving*, p. 77.
41 *Traveller Under Concern: The Quaker Journals of Frederick Mackie on his Tour of the Australasian Colonies, 1852–1855*, ed. with an Introduction by Mary Nicholls (Launceston: Foot and Playsted, 1973), p. 181.
42 Nicholls, *Traveller Under Concern*, p. 182; p. 181.
43 Nicholls, *Traveller Under Concern*, p. 184.
44 Nicholls, *Traveller Under Concern*, pp. 182, 197.
45 University of Melbourne Archives (hereafter UMA), Melbourne City Mission 1856–1899, 89/90 Melbourne and Suburban City Mission Journal, Thomas Murray, Missionary, Hotham District, 1877–1881, 15/13, p. 30; p. 43; p. 62; p. 67; p. 70.
46 See Lynne Strahan, *Out of the Silence: A Study of a Religious Community for Women: The Community of the Holy Name* (Melbourne: Oxford University Press, 1988).
47 UMA, Melbourne City Mission, 89/90, Percival Dale, 9/2 (c. 1962), Colonel Percival Dale, *Loving Service in our Community 1855–1962, Being the Story of the Work of the Melbourne City Mission*, p. 8.
48 UMA, Melbourne City Mission, 89/90, pp. 7–8.
49 Davison, Dunstan and McConville (eds), *The Outcasts of Melbourne*, pp. 7–8; p. 15; Andrew Brown-May, *Melbourne Street Life: The Itinerary of Our Days* (Melbourne: Australian Scholarly Press/Arcadia and Museum Victoria, 1998), pp. 121–2.
50 Shurlee Swain, 'The poor people of Melbourne', in Davison, Dunstan and McConville (eds), *The Outcasts of Melbourne*, pp. 99, 101.
51 Susanne Davies, '"Ragged, dirty ... infamous and obscene": The "vagrant" in late-nineteenth-century Melbourne', in David Philips and Susanne Davies (eds), *A Nation of Rogues? Crime, Law and Punishment in Colonial Australia* (Parkville: Melbourne University Press, 1994), pp. 156, 162.
52 *Illustrated Australian News* (18 July 1868), pp. 4–5.
53 *Illustrated Australian News* (18 July 1868), p. 4.
54 John Stanley James, *The Vagabond Papers*, edited by Michael Cannon, abridged edn (Melbourne: Melbourne University Press, 1969), p. 146.
55 *Twenty-first Annual Report of the Immigrants Aid Society* (Flinders Lane West: Mason, Firth & McCutcheon, General Printers, 1874), p. 3.
56 Catharine Coleborne, '"His brain was wrong, his mind astray": Families and the language of insanity in New South Wales, Queensland and New Zealand, 1880s–1910', *Journal of Family History*, 31:1 (2006), pp. 45–65.
57 Dr H. Earley, *Hints Upon Health, Addressed to Newly Arrived Immigrants* (Melbourne: B. Lucas, Collins Street, 1853), p. 1.
58 Reverend William Jarritt, *Hints to Immigrants Upon Colonial Life and Its Requirements* (Melbourne: Argus, Collins Street, 1853), pp. 3–4.
59 Ken Buckley and Ted Wheelwright, *No Paradise for Workers: Capitalism and the Common People in Australia, 1788–1914* (Oxford: Oxford University Press, 1988).

60 Milton Lewis and Roy MacLeod, 'A workingman's paradise? Reflections on urban mortality in colonial Australia 1860–1900', *Medical History*, 31 (1987), p. 402.
61 F. Norton Manning, *Ten Years at Gladesville* (Sydney: Thomas Richards, Government Printer, 1880), p. 3.
62 Manning, *Ten Years at Gladesville*, p.3.
63 Annabel Cooper, 'Poor men in the land of promises: Settler masculinity and the male breadwinner economy in late nineteenth-century New Zealand', *Australian Historical Studies*, 39:2 (2008), p. 258.
64 William Howitt, *Land, Labour, and Gold, or, Two Years in Victoria with Visits to Sydney and Van Diemen's Land*, Vol. 1 (Sydney: Sydney University Press, 1972 [1855]), p. 279.
65 Howitt, *Land, Labour, and Gold*, p. 289.
66 Kerr, *Glimpses of Life in Victoria*, p. 273.
67 *Report of Sub-Committee of the IAS, Appointed on the 6th of June, 1873, to Examine into the Condition and Prospects of the Inmates – Male and Female – at Present Resident in the Immigrants' Home, Princes Bridge* (Flinders Lane West: Mason, Firth, & McCutcheon, General Printers, 1873), p. 3.
68 A point supported by Jean Uhl's account of the way hospitals, benevolent asylums and the IAS interacted in the nineteenth century; see Uhl, *Mount Royal Hospital*, p. 13.
69 N. W. Pollard, *Homes in Victoria, or, The British Emigrant's Guide to Victoria, To Accompany Passage Warrants*, Vol. 1, Victorian Institutions and Establishments (Melbourne: Walker, May and Co., 1861), p. 20.
70 Pollard, *Homes in Victoria*, p. 18.
71 Pollard, *Homes in Victoria*, p. 19.
72 Kerr, *Glimpses of Life in Victoria*, p. 287.
73 *Twenty-First Annual Report of the Immigrants Aid Society* (Flinders Lane West: Mason, Firth, & McCutcheon, General Printers, 1874), p. 6.
74 'The Immigrants' home', *Illustrated Australian News* (18 July 1868), pp. 4–5.
75 State Library of Victoria (SLV), Immigrants' Aid Society (IAS) Pamphlet, LT YA362.6 V66. This pamphlet reproduced the *Argus* article of 1869 in its entirety.
76 See the annual reports produced by the IAS. See also Dr H. Earley, *Hints upon Health*, and Reverend William Jarritt, *Hints to Immigrants Upon Colonial Life and its Requirements*.
77 See Royal Melbourne Hospital Archives, Parkville, Melbourne (RMH Archives), Minute of the IAS, 1869–1871.
78 *Twenty-First Annual Report of the Immigrants' Aid Society* (Flinders Lane West: Mason, Firth, & McCutcheon, General Printers, 1874), p. 4.
79 PROV, VPRS 7400/P1, unit 5, folio 128, 25 April 1873.
80 PROV, VPRS 7400/P1, unit 10, folio 333, 12 March 1894.
81 PROV, VPRS 7400/P1, unit 13, folio 302, 17 February 1903.
82 This type of comment was a constant refrain, repeated in different ways, including by 1880: see *Twenty-Seventh Annual Report of the Immigrants' Aid Society*, pp. 5–6.
83 PROV, VPRS 7400/P1, unit 6, folio 37, 12 July 1879.
84 PROV, VPRS 7400/P1, unit 6, folio 36, 12 July 1879; VPRS 7400/P1, unit 6, folio 64, 26 September 1879; VPRS 7400/P1, unit 6, folio 76, 21 October 1879; VPRS 7400/P1, unit 10, folio 59, 7 May 1891.
85 PROV, VPRS 7400/P1, unit 11, folio 37, 31 October 1894.
86 PROV, VPRS 7400/P1, unit 8, folio 134, 27 November 1885.
87 PROV, VPRS 7400/P1, unit 12, folio 48, 21 September 1897.
88 *Report of Sub-Committee of the Immigrants' Aid Society*, p. 4.
89 A. James Hammerton argues that historians have not always been aware of the gendered aspect to migration histories. See A. James Hammerton, 'Gender and migration', in Philippa Levine (ed.), *Gender and Empire*, Oxford History of the British Empire (Oxford: Oxford University Press, 2004), p. 156. However, feminist historians have indeed tackled the subject of gender and migration: see for

example Charlotte Macdonald, 'The "social evil": Prostitution and the passage of the Contagious Diseases Act (1869)', in Barbara Brookes, Charlotte Macdonald and Margaret Tennant (eds), *Women in History: Essays on European Women in New Zealand* (Sydney: George Allen & Unwin, 1986), pp. 13–33. The notion of making migrants visible or invisible is borrowed here from Laura Tabili, 'A homogeneous society? Britain's internal "others", 1800–present', in Catherine Hall and Sonya O. Rose (eds), *At Home with the Empire: Metropolitan Culture and the Imperial World* (Cambridge: Cambridge University Press, 2006), p. 72.
90 Uhl, *Mount Royal Hospital*, p. 42.
91 M. J. Kernot, *Reminiscences of the Carlton Refuge, 1854 to 1919* (Melbourne: Carlton Refuge/ Ford & Son, 1919), p. 3.
92 This is a phrase used by Kathryn Cronin to explain the sometimes sad histories of the Chinese in colonial Australia; see Cronin, *Colonial Casualties: Chinese in Early Victoria* (Melbourne: Melbourne University Press, 1983).
93 David Goodman, *Gold Seeking: Victoria and California in the 1850s* (Sydney: Allen & Unwin, 1994), p. 200.
94 Goodman, *Gold Seeking*, p. 197.
95 Miles Fairburn, 'Vagrants, "folk devils" and nineteenth-century New Zealand as a bondless society', *Australian Historical Studies*, 21:85 (1985), pp. 495–514.
96 PROV, VPRS 7399/P1, unit 2, folio 199, 1873.
97 Coleborne, *Madness in the Family*.
98 *Annual Asylum Report*, 1891.
99 Uhl, *Mount Royal Hospital*, pp. 42–3.
100 *Nineteenth Annual Report of the Immigrants' Aid Society* (Finders Lane West: Mason, Firth & McCutcheon, General Printers, 1872), p. 6.
101 *Annual Report of Asylum Inspector*, VPP, 1891, p. 35.
102 UMA, Melbourne, Melbourne City Mission 1903–1936, 5/1, Annual Reports, *Forty-Seventh Annual Report of the Committee of the Melbourne City Mission or the Year ending 20th June 1903*, 89/90, p. 17.
103 John Singleton, *A Narrative of Incidents in the Eventful Life of a Physician* (Melbourne: M. L. Hutchinson, 1891), p. 117.
104 Cited by Judith Elphick, 'Auckland 1870–74: A Social Portrait', unpublished Masters thesis, University of Auckland, 1974, p. 34. Philson's Annual Report of 1874 was published in the Auckland Provincial Government Gazette of 1875, p. 34.
105 Elphick, 'Auckland 1870–74', p. 34.
106 Terence Hodgson, *The Heart of Colonial Auckland, 1865–1910* (Auckland: Random Century, 1992), pp. 75–81.
107 Tennant, *Paupers and Providers*, p. 15.
108 Elphick, 'Auckland 1870–74', p. 164.
109 Tennant, *Paupers and Providers*, p. 22.
110 Moore, *New Zealand for the Emigrant*, pp. 166–8.
111 Moore, *New Zealand for the Emigrant*, p. 241.
112 Tennant, *The Fabric of Welfare*, p. 63.
113 Margaret Tennant, 'Elderly indigents and old men's homes 1880–1920', *New Zealand Journal of History*, 17:1 (1983), p. 16.
114 Andrew Garran (ed.), *Picturesque Atlas of Australasia*, Vol. 3 (Sydney, Melbourne and London: The Picturesque Atlas Publishing Company, 1980 [1886]), p. 60.
115 *Auckland Illustrated: 53 Views of City and Suburbs*, Gold Medal Series (Auckland, Christchurch, Sydney and London: Fergusson, c. 1910).
116 Harold Archibald Sommerville, *Auckland Hospital and Charitable Aid Board: A History of its Buildings and Endowments* (Auckland: Whitcombe & Tombs, 1919), p. 47.
117 *Auckland Industrial and Mining Exhibition, Official Handbook and Catalogue* (Auckland: Geddis and Blomfield, Observer Office, 1898), pp. 21–3.
118 In 1898 there were allegations of cruelty and abuse at the home investigated by a government Commission. See: *Report of Commission on the Costley Home*, New

Zealand, H-26, 1904, *AJHR, 1858–1999* AtoJsOnline, National Library of New Zealand/Te Puna Mātauranga o Aotearoa, http://atojs.natlib.govt.nz, accessed 1 August 2014. Auckland War Memorial Museum Library Auckland Hospital and Charitable Aid Board, MS 287, 91/40, F1: 1898, Costley Home Commission Evidence; newspaper cutting, *The Auckland Star* (December 1903). See also Tennant, *Paupers and Providers*, p. 47.

119 Tennant, *Paupers and Providers*, p. 23.
120 Jenny Coleman, 'Reframing benevolence: from palliative charity to social reform in early 1870s Auckland', unpublished paper presented at the Australasian Welfare History Workshop, 15–16 November 2011, Massey University (Palmerston North) and University of Waikato (Hamilton). Thank you to Jenny Coleman for sharing this paper with me.
121 Mutch, 'Aspects of the social', pp. 124–5.
122 See the descriptions of a variety of inquiries into asylum care and management in colonial Victoria in Catharine Coleborne, *Reading 'Madness': Gender and Difference in the Colonial Asylum in Victoria, Australia, 1848–1888* (Perth: Network Books, Australian Public Intellectual Network, 2007); see also Lee-Ann Monk, *Attending Madness: At Work in the Australian Colonial Asylum*, Clio Medica 84: The Wellcome Series in the History of Medicine (Amsterdam and New York: Rodopi, 2008).
123 Auckland War Memorial Museum Library, Auckland Hospital and Charitable Aid Board, Evidence from Frederick William King before the Commission of Inquiry into the Costley Home, Auckland, 12 November 1903, MS 287, 91/40, F1, p. 13. See also Monk, *Attending Madness*, p. 76.
124 Margaret Tennant, *The Fabric of Welfare*, p. 61.
125 Mutch, 'Aspects of the social', p. 38.
126 Mutch, 'Aspects of the social', p. 60.
127 Erik Olssen, 'Towards a new society', in Geoffrey W. Rice (ed.), *The Oxford History of New Zealand*, 2nd edn (Auckland: Oxford University Press, 1992), p. 257.
128 Margaret Tennant, 'Elderly indigents', pp. 3–20; see Table 1 on p. 6; see p. 20.
129 William Pember Reeves, *State Experiments in Australia and New Zealand*, Vol. 2 (South Melbourne: Macmillan of Australia, 1969 [1902]).
130 'The Costley Home, Epsom', *Auckland Star*, 1 December 1898, p. 7.
131 NANZ, YCAA 1048/9 381, patient 2877, 28 August 1903.
132 NANZ, YCAA 1048/5 619, patient 1715, 6 August 1891.
133 NANZ, YCAA 1048/10 25, patient 2918, 1 December 1903.
134 *Report of Commission on the Costley Home*, New Zealand, H-26, 1904, p. 3. *AJHR*, AtoJsOnline, National Library of New Zealand/Te Puna Mātauranga o Aotearoa, http://atojs.natlib.govt.nz, accessed 1 August 2014.
135 *Report of the Inspector-General of Hospitals and Charitable Aid in the Dominion*, H-22, 1909, p. 49. *AJHR*, AtoJsOnline, National Library of New Zealand/Te Puna Ma̅tauranga o Aotearoa, http://atojs.natlib.govt.nz, accessed 1 August 2014.
136 John Kousgård Sørensen, 'Ingeborg Stuckenberg in New Zealand', in Henning Bender and Birgit Larsen (eds), *Danish Emigration to New Zealand*, trans. by Karen Veien (Denmark: Danes Worldwide Archives, 1990), pp. 50–1.
137 Margaret McClure, *Saving the City: The History of the Order of the Good Shepherd and the Community of the Holy Name in Auckland, 1894–2000* (Auckland: Hostel Advisory Group/David Ling Publishing Ltd, 2002), pp. 9–10.
138 McClure, *Saving the City*, pp. 17–19.
139 No further details are discernible in the brief note about this case. See Royal Melbourne Hospital Archives, Parkville, Melbourne (RMH Archives), Minute Books of the Immigrants' Aid Society (IAS), 1869–1871, p. 118.
140 See Coleborne, 'Making "mad" populations in settler colonies: The work of law and medicine in the creation of the colonial asylum', in Diane Kirkby and Catharine Coleborne (eds), *Law, History, Colonialism: The Reach of Empire*, Studies in Imperialism (Manchester: Manchester University Press, 2001), pp. 106–22.

141 See also Richard Broome, *Aboriginal Australians: Black Responses to White Dominance 1788–2001*, 3rd edn (Crows Nest: Allen & Unwin, 2001), pp. 56–72; pp. 74–90.
142 Lorelle Barry and Catharine Coleborne, 'Insanity and ethnicity in New Zealand: Māori encounters with the Auckland Mental Hospital, 1860–1900', *History of Psychiatry*, 22:3 (2011), pp. 285–301.
143 Coleborne, 'Making "mad" populations in settler colonies', p. 114.
144 NANZ, YCAA 1048/8 309, patient 2459, 10 January 1900. See Bronwyn Labrum, who writes about patient delusions where European patients referred to the conditions and experiences of Māori: 'The boundaries of femininity: Madness and gender in New Zealand, 1870–1910', in Wendy Chan, Dorothy E. Chunn, and Robert Menzies (eds), *Women, Madness and the Law: A Feminist Reader* (London, Portland, OR, and Coogee: GlassHouse Press, 2005).
145 Helen Gilbert and Anna Johnston (eds), *In Transit: Travel, Text, Empire* (New York: Peter Lang, 2002), pp. 2, 12.
146 Anthony Trollope, *Australia and New Zealand*, Vol. 1 (Victoria and London: Dawsons of Pall Mall, 1873), pp. 395–6.
147 Tennant, *The Fabric of Welfare*, p. 62.
148 Catharine Coleborne, 'Regulating "mobility" and masculinity through institutions in colonial Victoria, 1870s–1890s', *Law Text Culture*, 15 (2011), pp. 45–71.
149 Shurlee Swain, 'Writing the history of women and welfare', *Australian Feminist Studies*, 22: 52 (2007), p. 43.
150 Kay Daniels, 'Introduction', in Kay Daniels, Mary Murnane and Anne Picot (eds), *Women in Australia: An Annotated Guide to Records*, Vol. 1 (Canberra: Australian Government Publishing Service, 1977), p. xiii. See also Christina Twomey, *Deserted and Destitute: Motherhood, Wife Desertion and Colonial Welfare* (Melbourne: Australian Scholarly Publishing, 2002).
151 Tabili, 'A homogeneous society?', p. 54.

CHAPTER THREE

Passing through: narrating patient identities in the colonial hospitals for the insane, 1873–1910

When Peter Jamieson was admitted by police to the Yarra Bend Hospital for the Insane in 1891, he had no idea where he was. Aged thirty-two and originally from England, Jamieson was a single man who had been working as a labourer in colonial Victoria. By 1916, he had died in the institution, having been diagnosed as suffering from dementia, aged fifty-seven. The notes in his case read, 'Does not know where he is ... thinks he is in ... England, or has just come off a man of war there'.[1] Apprehended by police in the inner-city district of Hotham in Melbourne, Jamieson was likely to have been found in a confused state, as others were, and deemed incapable of caring for himself. Although we cannot know exactly how long he had been in the colony – the records of the Yarra Bend, unlike some other colonial institutions elsewhere, did not state length of time since immigrants first arrived in the colony, or the name and date of their ship – we can assume he had come as a single man to the colony in the previous decade.[2] He had possibly, like so many men and women who ended their days inside institutions, been passing through the colony in search of a life of opportunity, adventure and eventually perhaps, a settled existence. Instead, a chance glimpse of his life and circumstances appears in the patient case records of the hospital for the insane, the details of his person passed through a checklist pro forma of institutional categories required under contemporary law to be annotated by institutional authorities.

This chapter examines these mobile peoples of the colonial worlds they passed through by surveying the different ways these people were reflected upon, counted, described, understood and made into categories inside institutions, how their very identities were the result of a winnowing process of detailed case-making inside institutions in the period, and were then framed inside narratives of insanity. There were multiple 'narratives' being formed here: the relatively under-examined narrative of the inmate or patient, most often silent; the narratives of family and friends, and police, told in more depth in other studies; the narrative trajectory of the 'case' itself; and for the purposes of this study, a fractured and sometimes blurred meta-narrative of the institutionalised peoples of the colonies who were previously mobile, often migrants, and part of a larger story of settlement and unsettlement. The various aspects of these different narratives make their way into this chapter, but it places more emphasis on the ways in which institutional records provide historians with the substance of stories about people, and also how they retained and constrained individuals through the collection of data.

Institutional records were designed to classify individuals who were passed through a range of categories which acted to retain the lumpier information about them: the known facts about individuals admitted to institutions became the substance of their institutional identities. Although these details prove useful in provisionally outlining a 'patient demographic profile', as previous researchers have done in many similar studies of the institutionalised insane, it is also important to critically assess the categories used to define and interpret inmates. The 'interpretative gestures' made inside the clinical cases collated by these institutions have formed the basis for previous studies of colonial insane in many contexts, as this chapter also reiterates.[3] Colonial archival textual productions might be seen, in the words of Ann Laura Stoler, as 'documents of exclusion', and they also arguably organised and produced forms of colonial identity.[4] This chapter therefore also examines the production and codification of meanings about the insane populations contained inside institutions, and at the same time it provides something of an overview of the colonial populations of the insane as a foundation for the later chapters of this book.

The data presented here is derived from a database which itself arranges and organises inmates into groups for counting and analysis, adding another layer to the categorising of individuals and social groups.[5] Here, I aim to destabilise a reading of the labels and categories applied in the colonial record at the same time as I seek to show how these were deployed. In addition, the very specific impact of the application of such 'categories' on some individuals, and groups, including Māori and Indigenous Australian inmates, features as an aspect of this discussion. Although the previous chapter alluded to other social institutions which also took details about individuals, including the Immigrants' Homes in Victoria and other welfare institutions of the period, the records of those institutions are more limited than those of the hospitals of the insane featured in this chapter.[6]

Moreover, the clinical case files and case records of the hospitals for the insane offer more specific examples of how 'certain populations became subject to the institutional power of medicine'.[7] The obvious markers of 'identity' being mobilised by institutions were collected during the admission process. These included the notation of basic details about sex and age, as well as other socially marked and filtered aspects of the individual's identity, including place of birth, marital status, occupation, religious observance and so on. Photographs of inmates were also taken at the time of admission, more often in the first decade of the twentieth century in the case of both the Yarra Bend Asylum and the Auckland Asylum, with the practice of photographing patients noticeably more common at Auckland in the 1890s.[8] Barbara Brookes examines these photographic practices for other institutions, including Dunedin's public asylum, Seacliff Asylum, and also comments on the almost 'routine' practice of photographing inmates from the mid-1890s.[9] Examples of patients resisting this practice indicate ways in which attempts to physically subject individuals to such objectifying modes of institutional surveillance were sometimes met with extreme reactions and assertions of identity.

All of these markers of difference were part of the work of 'empire'. Catherine Hall's argument that the 'time of empire was the time when anatomies of difference were being elaborated, across the axes of class, race and gender' can be used to justify this approach to the institutional records.[10] Hall is talking about discursive categories which were, she says, 'the work of culture', and were historically bound and contingent. Inside the institutional records used here, the categories were used to highlight patterns across the colonial institutional population. This was the work of empire, a form of governmentality with 'the regulatory machinery' of institutions and their reports providing the 'foundational structures on which psychiatry was built'.[11] But these categories were also reminders of imperial and colonial identities, particularly when they were deployed to help define the characteristics of individuals and groups. Both class and gender emerged in the period as a distinctive feature of a changing industrialising world, and spoke to sex roles and prescriptions for behaviour, spatial arrangements and codes for public and private life. Meanwhile, colonial encounters highlighted racial differences and distinctions and therefore hierarchies.[12] Inside the colonial institutions, such encounters between peoples served to draw attention to a broad array of possible colonial identities and subjects, given the ethnic mix of the public institutions and of colonial society more generally. Public asylums were places where 'everyone' admitted was deemed 'mad', so there is also a sense in which these institutions collapsed differences between people, herding them into state care and confinement. However, the fine calibration of 'difference' announced by the format of patient cases suggests that difference was important.

Sex difference, now more often coded as 'gender', was a major marker of difference inside social and medical institutions. For men and women to occupy the 'same' institutional space actually meant separate wards and distinct record-keeping practices in the form of separate casebooks, so gender was a category which created a spatial segregation. Fences, walls, boundaries and demarcations of most asylums in the period were also used to manage the gendered bodies of inmates in institutional space: this also required specific spaces to be set aside for men and women, and gendered staffing regimes.[13] More than this, though, gendered divisions emerge in the contents of records in relation to diagnoses, the attributed causes of mental illness, and in treatments.[14] There was only patchy institutional recording of information about birth, nationality and the even more explicit, though anachronistic, category of 'ethnicity'. Yet traces of ethnic identification, and racial ascription, do exist in these records.[15] An important distinction for contemporaries was 'colonial born' versus 'foreign born' among the institutional inmates they surveyed. More specific still was the finer calibration of 'native person' versus 'colonial born' Europeans.

Class differences are only partly discernible in occupational categories collected by institutions, but they played a role in producing certain theories about insanity in colonial worlds. For example, this chapter and subsequent chapters reflect on gendered occupational categories including 'labourer' and 'domestic servant'. In both examples, contemporaries held beliefs about the impact of a lonely life upon single, peripatetic male labourers or miners who were often found insane in more remote areas of colonial places and brought to the colonial metropolitan institutions; or similarly, about the situations of many women working in domestic service who were brought to the asylum by employers or older men, their stories viewed and narrated through the prism of nineteenth-century institutional ideas about gender and femininity. Religion is another category which can amplify the meanings of 'place of birth', and which solidified existing contemporary prejudices about aspects of a person's identity, as in the case of Chinese inmates categorised as 'pagan', or Irish Roman Catholics. Religion was also cited as a cause of mental disturbance, though religious belief and worship among patients could be interpreted as a form of patient identity and the exercising of patient agency.[16] There are, then, also ways to locate the expressions of identities, indeed, the very patient utterances of identity in its varied forms, as a counter-argument to the notion that patients were merely all victims of a textual control through the recording of details about them, as parts of this chapter also show. Yet some categories were actively investigated while others were not.

In addition, the 'unmarked' categories inside institutional records require some elaboration and interrogation to make sense of the production of meanings inside these texts, which were then also used beyond their immediate purpose as legal documents of admission, and were assessed as the major source of statistical information for reporting institutional outcomes over time in the colonial period and beyond. Interested in the differences between groups of 'races', the nineteenth-century imperial recorders tended to mark out differences between similar ethnic groups to some extent, such as making distinctions between forms of 'white' ethnic identification when collecting data about Welsh, Scottish and English. In terms of an ethnic identification, 'whiteness' itself remains less visible, while at the same time it was becoming more explicit in wider society. Yet in official reports, which contained written summaries of the supposed causes of insanity and 'racial' difference, the Irish tended to be separated out among the Anglo-Celtic populations, receiving greater attention in terms of the discussion about insanity and birthplace. Other groups, including Aboriginal Australians, are more or less absent for different historical reasons, and the issue of their invisibility can also shed light on the very visible categories remaining and dominating the colonial record, and also tell us much about imperial identities inside these specific forms of social institution.

Identities were created in the act of inscribing the categories which meant so much to contemporary observers, medical writers and institutional authorities, as in the example of Peter Jamieson which opened this chapter. As another example, in the asylum inspectors' reports in Victoria in the 1880s, the category of 'Chinese' appears in a list of overall totals of 'types' of inmate, along with curable, epileptic, harmless imbeciles, adult idiots and various forms of admission for general inmates deemed 'lunatics' (such as police admission family admission or institutional transfers).[17] This suggests that the Chinese were not necessarily viewed as inherently 'mad', but viewed rather as inscrutable, and as a category of inmate whose numbers needed to be monitored, given debates and fears about the presence of Chinese inside asylums in the 1870s.[18] These tables show that contemporaries also tried to look at their data from different angles in their search for pathological assemblages, aware of the range of inmates in these institutions, and these should also be read and understood in the context of nineteenth-century discussions about who belonged inside institutions and who did not.

Institutions undertook to represent diagnoses inside the patient case notes, and also the possible causes of mental breakdown or related and possibly contributing factors. The circumstances of committal – whether through family or police – and discharge; the instances of trial leave and readmission; the frequency of death inside institutions, and length of stay, as well as other details about the patient population, are all relevant to this discussion about the role and function of the patient case notes and their production of meanings about the colonial insane and their identities over time.

'Documents of exclusion': Institutional case records, 1873–1910

By the mid-1870s, the system of colonial psychiatric institutions in the Australian colonies and in New Zealand had been in existence for almost two decades. In Victoria, the Lunatics Act (1867) determined that institutions would collect specific information about persons admitted under the act, and that this information would be kept and collated for the purposes of regular reporting. Similarly, in New Zealand, the Lunacy Act (1868) required asylum record-keeping for colonial statistical reports. In both cases the colony made frequent use of the collated data about institutionalised persons, with public debate about the cost of institutional care and the management of the insane a regular feature of newspapers of the day, a curiosity driven by the need to know about the people behind the walls of the institutions, and the costs they incurred, as well as about legal issues relating to the confinement of the insane.[19] Over time, with subsequent statutes and amendments, new legislative requirements served to tighten such requirements for reporting, and by the end of the period examined here, the institutional reporting of asylums, later hospitals for the insane, was widely known, and a regular element in the production of colonial statistics, along with other forms of social reporting.

From the earliest years of the official reporting of the asylum populations in the colonies, conducted annually and reported to the parliament in the form of written and tabled papers with extensive appendices, these records provided inspectors with the substance of their statistical overviews and summaries. A survey of all of the annual asylum inspectors' reports across Victoria and New Zealand from the 1870s until the end of the first decade of the twentieth century indicates a slight, but significant change in emphasis of interest in specific categories of inmate, and in aspects of patient demographic patterns. For example, in the 1877s, the majority of the Auckland institutional population was born overseas, with only eleven of 219 born in New Zealand and only ten listed as Māori; by 1900, a mere 28 per cent of patients was born overseas.[20]

In this sense, institutional case records become documents of inclusion for historians – the evidence of peoples in the past occupying social spaces, living their lives, and being noticed by colonial authorities. Yet separated from the rest of the colonial world through legal mechanisms and by actual physical walls, these were typically documents of exclusion, preventing freedoms of movement and demonstrating the power of law over individuals in the period. These are 'lost lives': often partial, and providing only fleeting glimpses of the presence of past people, they present paradoxical challenges to users of institutional archives, and especially to historians forming narratives of mental breakdown and institutional confinement.[21]

As well as providing the content for inspectors and their reports, patient case records held descriptive power and produced social differences. The form and function of institutional records is a popular subject for historians of psychiatry and its institutions. Scholars tend to agree that case notes contained in patient casebooks, or the case files kept in addition to casebooks in some institutions, present difficulties of interpretation. In the course of providing an argument about their uses in the Scottish context, including their value for annual reporting, the role of case histories in teaching and educating, and in creating a wider knowledge of mental breakdown, Jonathan Andrews draws attention to their 'deficiencies' including gaps in the record, 'inter-textual inconsistencies and sins of omission', as well as silences due to censored records.[22] Having accepted or put aside this set of problems, other scholars have tackled casebooks on a large scale, amassing data with a view to using it to find out about epidemiological aspects of insanity in various sites.

The very form of casebooks makes this possible. They were presented most often after the 1870s as a form with specific categories for the institution's scribe, doctor or attendant to fill in. Changing conventions in the pro forma pages of the Yarra Bend Asylum over the course of the 1860s to the 1880s show that after 1867 legislation produced specific outcomes in terms of textual representations of patients.[23] Case notes after this date were focused on the collation of specific detail about inmates: whether they had been 'disordered before', the length of time, whether doctors considered the condition to be hereditary, and also asked for details about the 'bodily conformation' of patients including bodily marks or deformities.[24] In addition, the casebook pro forma set out specific spaces for brief details to be amassed, limited the extent to which recorders could overlay the 'facts' with narratives of their own, but also introducing the specificity of inquiry which forced those being admitted into categories. The social aspects of their lives – 'habits of life', occupation, family background and so on – intertwined with the information about the organic nature of their disease where relevant. The various different institutional conventions of recording details in the case notes of colonial institutions still requires more scholarly attention, in part to shed light on the specific part played by institutions in the management of health populations over time.

Producing social differences in the institution

The very production of social difference in the form of sex/gender, racial, class, or other difference inside institutions, carried with it burdens of meaning yet to be fully explicated in settler-colonial worlds. The discussion below sets out some ways of understanding the patient populations at the Yarra Bend and Auckland asylums in basic terms by drawing both on the official statistics, and on the data collated for this study.[25] It shows that there were some consistent patterns of committal along the lines of sex/gender, age, marital status, ethnicity, religious affiliation and occupational categories, before considering how other forms of 'identity' – including emerging occupational categories, appearing and disappearing identities, and questions of 'colonial identity' – might be revealed in the same records. The discussion here is selective, taking specific examples of useful 'categories' to unpick and examine the many at work inside institutions in the period.

Sex/gender

In the institutions of the period, more men than women were committed, which, as historians can show, indicates both that the asylum populations reflected the demographic profile of the society from which they drew, but also that men, being more numerous in colonial societies, were also more often unmarried, itinerant and vulnerable to arrest and institutionalisation. The category of sex was most often filled out for all patients, and, aside from one or two infamous cases of women 'passing' as men that exist in the historical record, it was clearly accurate, even if it did not account for variances in sexuality or gendered behaviours much of the time.[26] Official statistics show a consistently larger number of men than women at both institutions in the period under examination. This study's samples of patients for the Yarra Bend and Auckland are summarised below in Table 3.1, which compares sex and marital status across the two institutional sites.

Of the 1,747 men in the Yarra Bend sample, 547 were married and 931 were single, reinforcing the idea that single men were slightly more likely to be confined than married men. The Auckland cases reveal a similar pattern in the sample, with more single men than women confined, though not such a large difference between men and women. Overall, single men represent 31 per cent of the total sample of patients, as opposed to 15 per cent of women. The total number of 1,115 married patients over this period, where this information was

Table 3.1 Marital status of inmates in the sampled data

Institution/group	No.	Married	Single	Widowed	Divorced/separated
YBA women	1321	568	497	207	1
YBA men	1747	547	931	111	4
AA women	310	146	113	43	2
AA men	558	167	317	39	2
Total	3936	1428	1858	400	9

Source:
Database of all patients sampled for every three years from patient casebooks from the Yarra Bend Asylum (YBA) and the Auckland Asylum (AA), 1873–1910, showing sex and marital status, for all patients, where information was recorded.

known, includes roughly equal number of men and women, meaning that married men and married women both constitute 18 per cent of the total of sampled patients. Interestingly, more men than women in the Yarra Bend group – sixty-two as opposed to fifteen – presented cases with missing information as to their marital status, suggesting that the social connections provided by wives and families, or other social contacts, were possibly important also to the gathering of personal details for men. Very few of the Yarra Bend or Auckland patients were separated or divorced, highlighting the fact that although divorce was legally possible from the 1860s in the colonies, it was difficult to obtain a divorce for social, cultural and financial reasons.[27]

Widows and widowers comprised another group of patients, with double the number of widowed women at the Yarra Bend. Of the 318 widowed men and women, only sixteen reported the cause of their mental illness to be 'grief', 'loss' or 'bereavement'. Yet in many other instances, old age, living alone, poverty and alcoholism featured, perhaps all realistic aspects of widowed life which were not attributed as such. The ages, too, of institutionalised people followed the pattern expected by authorities: most inmates were in the middle stages of life when organic disease, and social pressures, tended to take their toll; older members of the population became more vulnerable to illness, dementia and brain disease and diseases caused by poverty and destitution.

A less obvious aspect of the category of 'sex', as stated above, is the question of sexuality. Later chapters of this book examine this theme more carefully with a view to situating colonial identities as ones also formed through sex, gender and sexuality, which is somewhat difficult at time due to the relatively sparse records in most cases. However, mostly hidden inside institutional statistics, the discussions about sexual behaviours reveal other aspects of colonial identities.

Ethnicities

The collation of data about inmates' backgrounds was not benign. The commentaries about the presence of 'foreigners' in Victoria in Census reports (see for instance the 1881 Census for Victoria) shows that there was a keenness to 'know' the population and its character, something which colonial social institutions replicated in their own reporting. In the previous chapter, Table 3.1 described the general overview of the colonial-born and foreign-born populations captured by the study's sample. Table 3.2 breaks this information from the sample down even further in a simple representation of birthplaces. Birthplaces can stand in for 'ethnicity', as argued elsewhere, but are not the only measure of ethnic identities inside institutions. Angela McCarthy shows a range of ways that institutional records evince information about ethnicity and identity, including language, accent, references to ethnicity and nationality, among other themes.[28] To locate ethnicity inside institutional data, historians need to look carefully at a range of representations of inmates, from birthplaces or places of origin to representations of bodily identity, and including names, sounds and gestures, as well as the content of delusions.[29]

Table 3.2, though, sets out the main birthplaces simply grouped to provide an overview of the dominant populations of the two institutions in this study. That the institutions were primarily housing white, English- and Irish-born, should not be surprising. The higher number of contintental 'European' inmates at the Yarra Bend, particularly among the men, reflects the men travelling to become miners or to seek work as labourers after the great population growth of the Victorian colony in the middle of the century. The official asylum reports also noted these trends and percentages of inmates born in the different places listed. The dominance of the white 'British' inmates preoccupied contemporary commentators in the sense that they endeavoured to sort

Table 3.2 Birthplaces

Institution/group	No.	England	Ireland	Scotland	Wales	Europe	China	Other
YBA women	1321	121	176	56	6	26	0	9
YBA men	1747	306	209	87	11	103	30	27
AA women	310	67	33	13	1	3	0	2
AA men	558	127	55	25	5	28	1	10
Total	3936	621	473	181	23	160	31	48

Source:
Database of all patients sampled for every three years from patient casebooks from the Yarra Bend Asylum (YBA) and the Auckland Asylum (AA), 1873–1910, showing places of birth for all patients where information was recorded.

out why mental illness continued in the colonies, and whether it was imported.

Among the 'others' born outside of the places listed in Table 3.2 and inmates at the Yarra Bend were two men: Moses Maroon and Hamid Hamese. Maroon, born in Syria, was a street hawker. He was taken to the asylum in 1894, unable to speak much English, and suffering from delusions. Hamese, taken to the institution in 1906, was also a hawker, and listed as 'Mahometan', and without a fixed address.[30] Their fates as men vulnerable to institutional committal signal the relevance of ethnicity, and even while non-Anglo men and women were in a minority, their situations highlighted the plight of people who were culturally and socially adrift in the predominantly 'British' colonies.

Several inmates were 'colonial born' but had moved between colonial sites. Their internal migrations tell us something too about the colonial identities belonging to places and then understood as 'identities' in the official records. At Auckland, seventeen patients were described as being born in 'Colony' or 'colonial', terms not used as a place of birth in the records of the Yarra Bend. Both terms indicated that these inmate identities were firmly 'colonial', or at least assumed to be so; most were born in the 1860s, with one born in the 1850s.

Religious affiliation

Reflecting the dominant European heritage of the institutional population, most patients were Christians, where a religious denomination was noted in the record. A variety of Christian faiths are listed in the patient case notes: Bible Christian, Church of Christ, Free Church of Scotland, Baptist, Congregationalist, Presbyterian, Church of England, Protestant, Lutheran, Catholic, Wesleyan, to name a few, but were often reduced to a smaller list in the official reports of the period. The intersections between ethnic groups and religious affiliation is in some instances clear, such as the group of Irish Catholics at the Yarra Bend Asylum (285 of the total Catholic population in Table 3.3), or Lutheran worshippers from Germany. In other cases, there is no link between religious faith and ethnicity, but what is striking is the difference between the population in Victoria's institution when compared with New Zealand's institution at Auckland: while the Yarra Bend and Auckland have roughly equal percentages of protestant, Church of England believers, at 34 per cent and 36 per cent respectively, far more Catholics were housed at the Yarra Bend: 29 per cent, compared with only 18 per cent at Auckland. This reflects the differing populations of Irish, Italian and continental Europeans coming to colonial Victoria, rather than suggesting that Catholics were more susceptible to committal in the Victorian context.

Table 3.3 Religious affiliations

Institution/group	No.	Church of England/ Protestant	Roman Catholic	Presbyterian	Wesleyan	Lutheran	Jewish	Other
YBA women	1321	440	410	125	75	11	10	79
YBA men	1747	630	485	180	79	44	19	127[a]
AA women	310	118	52	18	20	2	2	18
AA men	558	201	108	58	30	6	3	29[b]
Total	3936	1389	1055	381	204	63	34	253

Notes:
[a] The number of 'other' faiths listed here includes ten men described as 'pagan', 'heathen', and 'Confucian'; a variety of Christian beliefs are also represented.
[b] This number includes Hauhauism, among other beliefs.

Source:
Database of all patients sampled for every three years from patient casebooks from the Yarra Bend Asylum (YBA) and the Auckland Asylum (AA), 1873–1910, showing religious affiliation for all patients where information was recorded.

Table 3.3 lists the major religious affiliations, and generalises some of those faiths named above under 'other'. Interestingly, read in the light of Table 3.2, more detail was gathered about religious belief than about birthplaces of inmates, at least in the data collected for this study.

'Jewish' was one label used to describe both the religious beliefs held by an inmate, and also an 'ethnic' identification, with 'Jew', 'Jewish', 'Jewish persuasion', 'Hebrew' and the more querulous 'Jew?' evident in the institutional records of the Yarra Bend from the early 1870s to 1909. In an institutional minority, the visibility of Jewish inmates, or those 'suspected' of being Jewish, is interesting. Leonard Smith's important work about Jewish inmates in the industrial cities of England in the middle of the nineteenth century suggests that at that time, the Jewish community was itself concerned about mental illness and the confinement of Jews. Many of the new Jews entering English communities with an established middle-class Jewry were poor immigrants and more likely to exhibit social dislocation and mental disorder.[31] Looking at a selection of cases as vignettes, Smith wondered about the meanings attached to aspects of Jewish inmates' behaviours. Ann Goldberg also examines the presence of a small group of patients described as Jewish in a German asylum, Eberbach, in an earlier period.[32] Goldberg suggests that although there are limits to the 'medicalization' thesis, in which scholars contend that some social groups are more readily confined inside medical and carceral institutions in this period, she does find that Jewish patients tend to be very explicitly labelled, and were also treated more harshly in that context.[33] Only twenty-nine of the total sample of inmates for the Yarra Bend were accorded Jewish status, with fewer still at Auckland, just five of the total sample. 'Jewess-housewife' was also recorded as an occupational category in one instance at the Yarra Bend, reinforcing Goldberg's notion of the 'explicit' nature of the Jewish label.

However, in this early period, Jewishness was not yet 'an accepted category of science and medicine'. Instead, it referred to '"national" and religious characteristics'.[34] Although Goldberg shies away from an interpretation of the biological meanings of 'Jew' at work in the asylum, she does comment in some detail about how the label functioned as a reminder of social exclusion and the anti-semitism which pervaded the society she examines, arguing that being Jewish may have interfered with proper medical treatment.[35]

In the colonial asylums, the labels used to refer to Jews also hinted at migrant identities. By 1881, there were over 4,000 Jewish people living in the colony of Victoria, with the vast majority living in Melbourne and its suburbs.[36] Jewish peoples migrating to Victoria were not restricted from participating in any professions or social roles in colonial Victoria, unlike in England, the point of origin for most Jewish immigrants who arrived in Victoria to start a new life in the colonies. Their presence in institutions, then, does not necessarily signal their marginalisation as Jewish people in the same way that it may have done in European or English institutional contexts.[37] Allied to the Irish insane by Elizabeth Malcolm in her study of the Irish in English institutions, Jewish people in England seemed to be regarded differently inside institutions, suggesting that colonial institutional authorities, most of whom trained in England and Scotland, may have harboured similar views about such minority groups; these were institutions in the imperial model, and run by agents of imperial medicine. Yet the presence of Jewish people might also simply serve to remind us of the ethnic diversity of early Melbourne. Similarly, the identification of the 'Mahomedan' inmates at the Yarra Bend reminds us of the relative religious and ethnic diversity of Victorians in this period.

Chinese inmates – who were more numerous at the Yarra Bend than at Auckland in this period, and who were drawn to the Victorian goldfields, and later to the Otago fields in the New Zealand's South Island – are often described as 'pagan', or 'heathen', designations which made them decidedly non-Christian in the dominant white Christian world of the institutions. Their identities, discussed more fully in the final chapter of this book, shed light on the way 'others' in the institutions helped authorities to define and create 'ideal' identities for the colonial insane population. At the Auckland Asylum, several Māori patients were identified as belonging to the Hauhau faith. Hauhauism was practised by the followers of one of several Māori religious sects of the period and was the faith of the Paimārire Church.[38]

Occupations

Historians have provided much in the way of demographic analysis of occupational categories and structures in different contexts, linking population and work.[39] Much is known about the 'occupational geography' of Britain between 1851 and 1911, a geography which most certainly shaped colonial patterns of work and settlement.[40] Census data collated in Victoria and New Zealand also reveals the types of work men and women engaged in over the period. Institutional reports also show an attention to the significance of occupational categories in determining the status or walk of life for inmates. Over the second half of the nineteenth century, the official asylum inspectors' reports in both Victoria and New Zealand prescribe a far wider range of occupational categories for men than for women. For example, the Annual Report on Lunatic Asylums for 1881 in New Zealand listed just ten occupational types for women, but fifty-three for men, including 'vagrant'.[41] By counting 'the station or occupation of patients admitted' during each year, these reports offered some basic notions of the economic class or social status of inmates, given these were public institutions which took men and women from all walks of life.[42]

Reflecting the wider labour force choices for men, the lists of occupational categories for each year also highlight some trends, not only in the dominant workforce roles for both men and women, but also in their signalling of social status based on marital status: sometimes being the wife of a professional man, or a settler or farmer, for example, allowed an otherwise invisible social status to emerge. Just as there was a wide range of forms of domesticity for women in employment – including domestic work outside and inside the home, for an employer or within a familial setting – so too were men occupied across all forms of outdoor labour beyond the simple category of 'labourer'. Men were also engaged in a variety of trades and crafts as well as less skilled physical labour. Miners, sailors, gum diggers and hawkers, all mobile men, move in and out of the annual report lists. Colonial meanings of 'skilled' and 'unskilled' had surely shifted from their more fixed understandings in the metropole.[43] Just how working-class men suffered and endured mental illness, and how this took specific forms in the colonial world, is discussed further in the following chapter. Akihito Suzuki's suggestion that 'the madness of working-class men was much more nuanced than, and sometimes significantly different from, that conceived by middle-class commentators' is a useful one, given the broad range of working roles men had.[44]

Similarly, not all women were middle-class hysterics; as well as their own complex and variegated domestic employment, women were sometimes vagrant, prostitutes or barmaids, in small numbers, but nonetheless signifying particularly mobile identities. The governess, too, already the subject of some historical attention, appears in the records of the institutions in small numbers, and a small number of women were school teachers or employed in other professional work.[45]

The samples for this study provide too many occupational titles and names to reproduce in their entirety as a table, but the major categories are summarised broadly in Table 3.4. This means that the many different forms of male labour, for example, or of female domestic work, have necessarily been subsumed within their broader categories. Among the listed occupations counted as 'domestic' for men housed at the Yarra Bend, for example, are 'cook', 'servant', 'waiter' and 'home cleaner'. Interestingly, of the twenty-seven men listed as doing this type of domestic work in Melbourne's asylum, a number were born in China, India, Mauritius or Ireland, suggesting that domestic work for men was given to men of a somewhat 'inferior' status in the colonial setting. Among the labourers, too, were farmers, farm hands and those working

Table 3.4 Occupations

Institution/group	No.	Domestic	Labourer	Clerical	Education/religious	Other
YBA women	1321	570	0	5	35	100
YBA men	1747	27	488	46	23	956
AA women	310	202	2	0	8	22
AA men	558	19	319	29	15	114
Total	3936	818	809	80	81	1192

Source:
Database of all patients sampled for every three years from patient casebooks from the Yarra Bend Asylum (YBA) and the Auckland Asylum (AA), 1873–1910, showing major occupational categories for all patients where information was recorded.

on the land or with animals. Women worked as milliners, dressmakers, seamstresses (all listed under 'other' in Table 3.4) which was more skilled work. Teachers and governesses account for the women listed below as being involved in education; some women inmates were members of religious orders.

The newer category of 'pensioner' appears in institutional records from the 1880s. Pensioners became a newer category of colonial identity, I suggest, as the population aged and came to comprise older members of both those with families and those without, meaning that some older people who had come to the colonies many years before were now in need of both familial and institutional support, as Margaret Tennant also shows for the elderly in New Zealand who were increasingly housed in homes for the aged poor.[46] The numbers of inmates whose age had left them vulnerable to mental illness, disorder or conditions related to ageing create an impression of a class of people left to fend for themselves. The official pension for aged persons was available in Victoria by the turn of the century in a move that followed the earlier passage of laws for pensions in New Zealand in 1898. Between the 1890s and 1901 in the Australian colonies, the numbers of people aged sixty-five and over had risen by some 60 per cent. The stories of the eleven 'official' pensioners recorded in the cases of the Yarra Bend sample show that most were brought to the institution in the early 1900s aged in their sixties and seventies, with one man, Thomas Stevens, aged ninety-three at the time of his admission. Two were younger men retired from their civil service jobs, and one man had been separated from his wife for over sixteen years, showing how marital discord could also leave men and women vulnerable to illness and institutional committal.

In a small though significant set of cases in both institutions, the patient's record also includes information about the father's occupation. At the Yarra Bend, there were twenty-four cases which included this information for mostly male patients (only four were women). These cases most likely set out the male parent's position in life for two reasons: most of these patients were aged under thirty, with most in their twenties (with one aged forty-two); second, although not all of these patients are given a formal diagnosis, most seem to hint at or state the presence of some form of congenital disease such as idiocy, imbecility or dementia, indicating their general dependence on family. A similar pattern is in evidence at Auckland, although among the five patients, the majority were slightly older women who were also in situations of dependency on fathers and parents.

Appearing and disappearing categories: mobility and institutionalisation

The poverty and deprivation experienced by many institutional inmates reminds us of the loose and somewhat malleable constructions of colonial identity being deployed in the institutional records, as well as the difficultly contemporary institutions had in obtaining information about asylum inmates, even at the time of committal.[47] 'Very poor circumstances' was cited as an 'occupation' in a few instances. Mobile and itinerant people had no fixed addresses, and were unlikely to have been in contact with family members. Their mobility fed into anxieties about how to define them, and certainly about where they belonged in the social institutional spaces of the period. As the previous discussion of occupational categories also shows, some degree of colonial mobility among miners, labourers and other employed men was more or less accepted and understood, but the urban mobility and poverty of the vagrant population was not. Angela Hawk also suggests that vagrancy laws, alongside lunacy legislation, provided police with an opportunity to police mobility during the goldrush era, as well as emanating from the earlier convict era and the need for the tracing of convicts and ticket-of-leave men and women.[48]

The broadly defined colonial vagrancy laws of the nineteenth-century places mentioned here echoed the expectations of imperial society, as I argue elsewhere in more depth.[49] Vagrancy was an offence in Victoria and New Zealand, with the specific colonial laws, An Act for the Better Prevention of Vagrancy and Other Offences (Victoria) enacted in 1852, and the Vagrant Act (New Zealand) in 1866. Regarded by scholars and by contemporary commentators alike as very broad laws designed to sweep up people who loitered, consorted, looked predatory, or who solicited for acts of prostitution, begged, or who simply wandered around without much purpose, the vagrancy laws in colonial society extended the imperial vagrancy law of the early nineteenth century in that they further characterised and defined the anxieties of colonial conditions.[50] Both acts included a provision which singled out Europeans who associated with Aboriginal or Māori, or 'Aboriginal natives': both acts, therefore, turned on a colonial preoccupation. Studying rates and types of violent offences in nineteenth-century Auckland, Dean Wilson deduced that those policed under the Vagrant Act of 1866 and appearing before the courts were 'most certainly there to be disciplined by their social superiors', with drunk and abusive prisoners very loud about their 'disdain' of court proceedings.[51] Vagrancy, then, was a charge used to contain the mobility of some colonial citizens, but it was often a short-term fix and offenders tended to be recidivists. David Goodman suggests that the colonial vagrancy law was particularly important in establishing forms of 'order' in the colony of Victoria.[52] Colonial societies of different kinds reshaped the mobility of Indigenous peoples, and even wilfully misunderstood the travelling and movement of Indigenous populations. In white settler colonies, this type of settler mentality, with its emphasis on the settling down of peoples who had been on the move, also found expression in the suspicion of those white Europeans who travelled without 'good' cause, and non-whites, including hawkers, drawing on imperial models for law-making around vagrancy.

Vagrants also ended up inside the hospitals for the insane where their mobility was addressed more directly. Some colonial laws dealing with insanity explicitly mentioned vagrants and paupers as appropriate populations to 'control', such as a Western Australian law of 1871,[53] but over time in Victoria there were debates about the problematic expansion of the institutional populations which hinted at such practices of confinement being highly inappropriate for the colonies. Significantly, as parts of this book explain in more detail, the hospitalisation of vagrants tends to follow their stints in other social welfare institutions in the colonies, including Melbourne's Benevolent Asylum, the Salvation Army Home, or a lodging house, all sites where the mobile come into contact with others who wished to confine them or to monitor their behaviour. Cases of vagrants hospitalised at Auckland Asylum, including one described as a 'beggar', were transferred from the prison at Mount Eden, with one transferred from a refuge.

Inside institutions, the terms 'tramp' and 'traveller', tended to be male, but among the institutionalised number there were some transient women. The gendered category of 'the vagrant' itself demands more discussion: Chapters 4 and 5 include reflections on these aspects of the gendered patient identity. Nineteenth-century observers may not have readily identified the woman 'vagrant' or 'tramp'. This may have been an 'impossible category' at a time when women were viewed as victims of circumstance rather than as actively seeking lives as tramps or travellers, as Tim Cresswell shows in his work on female tramps and hobos in the American context.[54]

Historians have noted an attention to the wanderers and persistently mobile populations in other colonial institutions for the insane.[55] Their work has often singled out European attempts to control the wandering of Indigenous peoples, as in the case of Aboriginal peoples around early Melbourne.[56] Among the very few Aboriginal and Māori inmates confined in the Australasian colonies, references to 'wandering' are few. However, two Indigenous inmates at the Yarra Bend had seemingly wandered away from Aboriginal missions, one at Coranderrk and the other at Lake Condah. Their status as inmates caught in the institution signalled their being out of place, at least in terms of dominant European constructions and occupation of colonial space.[57]

There were other ways in which identity was more difficult to fix. Wandering could also be a symptom of dementia or memory loss, as many records reveal, rather than a sign of wanton disregard for settling down. At the Yarra Bend, thirty-nine cases of men and women wandering reveal a multiplicity of reasons or causes for their movement, including dementia, anxiety and vagrancy. Wandering was described in several cases as a 'habit of life' and as something these individuals had done for some time, or were known to do: 'wanders around aimlessly'; 'wanders and gets lost'; 'is apt to wander away from home'; 'wanders about by himself'; 'husband states that she wanders from home'; and finally, 'wanders about in nightclothes', suggesting a tendency to sleepwalking.

In Victoria and New Zealand, the practice of going by more than one name was prevalent among men and women arrested on vagrancy charges, as the colonial *Police Gazettes* show. This has a bearing on institutional records, too. A number of the institutionalised people at the Yarra Bend and Auckland asylums used aliases. Mrs Janice Gibson, aged forty-eight, was arrested by police in September of 1873 in Collingwood, Melbourne and taken to the Yarra Bend where it was noted that she went by an alias.[58] Aged forty-five, Mrs Elizabeth Rich's alias of 'O'Toole' was perhaps explicable considering she had been treated at both the Melbourne and Women's Hospitals and was known to staff as an alcoholic. Marked with tattoos on her arm, charwoman Elizabeth had also been at the Yarra Bend twenty years earlier before her admission by police, suffering from delusions, in 1900.[59] Wah Yee went to the Yarra Bend in 1894 carrying a letter from a doctor addressed to a 'William Brady', further confusing his identity or perhaps suggesting the use of a European alias.[60] Several other inmates used aliases and some more than one. At Auckland, inmate John Thompson, a gum digger and engineer aged twenty-nine, was also known as William Hallows.[61] Aside from the likelihood that some people were confused about their identities during bouts of mental disturbance, the use of alternative identities could suggest that people were escaping detection or seeking shelter in some instances. This was more usual, perhaps, in welfare institutions: the case of John Beecroft, an 'imposter' at the Melbourne Immigrants' Home, attracted the ire of the authorities in 1870 and he was handed over to the police for 'imposing' on the burdened institution.[62] The use of disguises in the period perhaps echoed forms of 'imperial adventure', and hint at what Kirsten McKenzie characterises as opportunities for reinvention in this 'changing world'.[63] Using clothing, disguises and 'passing' as others was a common trope of imperial literature and seeped into everyday practices.[64] Although scholars have tended to look at imposters and opportunists of the wealthier set, the evidence suggests such practices of identity fashioning were more common among women and men of the poor classes of the colonies.[65]

The very lack of certainty over the identities of many inmates, many of whom had no family support, shows that processes of institutional record-keeping had limitations and weaknesses, yet it also yields more clues about the importance and relevance of 'identifying' colonial peoples in place. Policing in Victoria developed along the lines of both the London Metropolitan police, and the Irish constabulary. These two models reflected urban and rural populations and differences between the modes of policing required in those spaces, as Goodman points out.[66] The *Police Gazettes* in Victoria and New Zealand practised techniques for police to trace and search for people on the move who were wanted for criminal activity, or were arrested under the vagrancy laws, or who were missing persons, including escaped asylum inmates. The descriptions of individuals were full and detailed. In Victoria, the *Victoria Police Gazette* was published weekly from 1853.[67] The *New Zealand Police Gazettes* were published weekly from 1861, but photographs of wanted persons did not appear until 1908, making linguistic portraits of missing persons or offenders very valuable.[68]

People admitted to both institutions also suffered from delusions of identity. In many cases, delusional identities reveal patterns in the historical constructions of powerful social and political identities. For a labouring man to imagine himself a duke, or a miner to believe he owned a rich gold mine and employed thousands of men, are both explicable given the historical context: identifications with the socially powerful at a time of personal stress and confinement points to concerns over identity in any age. Given the imperial context, it should not be surprising that patients often imagined themselves as royalty or related to royalty. European patients tended to locate their delusional identities as queens, kings and princes of the day, while a few Chinese delusional patients believed themselves to be Chinese emperors.

Diagnoses

Medical institutions were ultimately concerned with the question of what was wrong with a person admitted to the asylum, and in the likely causes of the illness. More detailed interpretations of specific, gendered diagnoses for colonial institutional inmates appears in subsequent chapters, but here, the general patterns of diagnosis are described across the two institutions to show how dominant medical diagnoses emerged to pattern understandings of colonial mental disease for men and women. At the time of committal, the description of symptoms for men and women indicate that families, employers, police and other social contacts noted differing aspects of male and female behaviour, and that this in itself tended to reflect gender norms. Historians show that both men and women tended to fall into specific diagnostic categories for nineteenth-century mental disorders, with some differences in the presentation and articulation of symptoms, and more men diagnosed with GPI.[69] Table 3.5 describes the major medical diagnoses for men and women, but excludes the vast array of cited 'causes', the language around which is discussed elsewhere. The reputed causes for insanity were often complicated with the diagnosis itself, depending

Table 3.5 Medical diagnoses

Institution/ group	No.	Mania	Melancholia	PI[a]	GPI[b]	Dementia	CI[c]
YBA women	1321	378	183	40	15	179	46
YBA men	1747	236	174	0	149	283	57
AA women	310	54	47	21	0[d]	20	18
AA men	558	80	66	0	22	44	27
Totals	3936	748	470	61	186	526	148

Notes:
[a] PI (Puerperal Insanity)
[b] GPI (General Paralysis of the Insane)
[c] CI (Congenital imbecile/idiocy)
[d] Women at Auckland Asylum did receive the GPI diagnosis; there are none in this current sampled data.

Source:
Database of all patients sampled for every three years from patient casebooks from the Yarra Bend Asylum (YBA) and the Auckland Asylum (AA), 1873–1910, showing major diagnoses for all patients where information was recorded.

Table 3.6 Patient outcomes

Institution/group	No.	Discharged	Death	Leave/trial absence
YBA women	1321	502	270	79
YBA men	1747	396	526	95
AA women	310	156	71	61
AA men	558	246	196	51
Total	3936	1300	1063	286

Source:
Database of all patients sampled for every three years from patient casebooks from the Yarra Bend Asylum (YBA) and the Auckland Asylum (AA), 1873–1910, showing outcomes for all patients where information was recorded.

on the record-keeper of the day, making a completely accurate count of this data almost impossible.[70]

This data shows that mania, melancholia – and more rarely, 'depression' – dementia, and other diagnostic categories were used for both men and women inside the institutions for the insane. Delusions could accompany any form of insanity and complicated each of these categories, and have not been counted separately in Table 3.5. Their frequency and content can provide more information about gender and behaviour, along with ideas about colonial life.

Finally, the stories of patient committals and outcomes can tell us a little more about patient identities and attitudes to specific patients, as the various threads of later chapters show. The outcomes for patients need to be understood and read against gender, age, marital status and other aspects of their patient 'identities', including familial connections in the colonies. The figures in Table 3.6 are based on the data where it was recorded, meaning that it is likely to be incomplete, and is not checked against all other forms of register for trial leave and so on, partly because the records across the two institutions are not the same, or are not extant. Table 3.6 does tell us, though, that one-third of patients died inside the institutions, and relatively few were allowed out on periods of trial leave or absence.

Bodies and identities

Historians agree that the body was a 'central trope of colonial discourse'.[71] This argument has been more readily applied to institutions for the insane in colonised countries with separate institutions for non-white 'native' inmates, including India.[72] But in white settler colonies, too, institutions had made practices and rules for the management of bodies in spaces, herding large numbers of sometimes physically unruly people into dining halls, schools, dormitories and yards. Other bodies were silent, unresponsive and even catatonic. Some had to be secluded and restrained, others, force-fed. Working bodies were able to move more freely between outdoor and indoor spaces, farming and labouring, or gardening, cooking, sewing and laundering clothes. The bodies of some were physically strong, violent and could make their escapes. But many more were weak, emaciated, malnourished, injured and sick. In other words, there were multiple bodily identities inside institutions. What institutional authorities made of the bodies themselves and their skin, size, shape, their very forms, can tell us more about the role of the physical body in the creation of institutional identities.

Tattoos were relatively rare among institutional inmates, and surprisingly, are not noted often among Māori in the sample, although most Māori women probably wore the moko as a lip tattoo from the late nineteenth century.[73] Two Māori women came to Te Whau with tattoos: Nga Kina, who was admitted in March 1894, was described as a 'Widow – Aboriginal native from Kaipara', and the following day was described as 'A Maori. Eyes brown hair black. Lips tattooed. Bridge of nose low. Molars prominent, forehead somewhat narrow and light.'[74] Pare Te Aho, admitted at age thirty-six, was a married woman admitted in October 1903. Her case note mentioned 'Maori tattoo marks on mouth and chin'. However, these tattoo marks are not visible in the photograph of Pare in her record.[75] Given the habit among colonial populations of taking an alias, perhaps to avoid police detection, a tattoo could act as an identifying mark for colonial institutional authorities, as could the numerous rashes, bruises and scars noticed on the bodies of inmates. Such marks also functioned as a means of understanding illness, or the violent lives some inmates led outside the institution.

One specific technology of the institution, the practice of photographing inmates at the time of their admission to the asylum, provides another opportunity to examine patient identities and their representation inside the casebooks. It was easier for institutions to photograph inmates than it was for police to use photographic materials to identify criminal, missing or vagrant people. Institutions, then, surely contributed to a new state surveillance of individual subjects.[76] Although it may not have captured all of the marks on the unclothed bodies examined during the admission process, photography did act to capture images of people's skin, clothing, hair, stance, eyes and face, and sometimes their physical movements. The technology of photography inside the asylum provided doctors and institutional authorities with new ways of presenting both individual 'cases', and also pictorial accounts of the institution itself to outside observers.[77] When descriptions of the patient accompanied these images and noted patients' complexions or skin tone, it is easy to see that the untidy appearance and sometimes dirty skin of unwell and unwashed people was confused with racial difference, as in the case of young Joseph Vogt, who was described as 'dusky' in Melbourne in 1885.[78] The practice of photographing inmates also emanated from the European science of patient classification, or the diagnosis of patients into illness typologies.[79]

Photographs of inmates tend to graphically remind readers of case notes of the various struggles over institutional confinement. Patients being photographed resisted, or were, in Brookes' estimation, 'less passive subjects of the powerful doctor's gaze than we might imagine'.[80] Bodies were also recalcitrant. The institution was 'unable to photograph' at least one woman, 82-year-old Miss Sarah Brookes, at the Yarra Bend in 1906 because of her advanced senility.[81] Several others refused to be photographed.

Conclusions: the production of meaning in casebook texts

The clinical case notes at both the Yarra Bend and Auckland, as in other institutional settings in this period, were iterative and repetitive documents which ultimately codified information about individuals. Moving through the institution during their medical inspection rounds, doctors would often add little to the initial pages of a patient's case, especially if there was no real change observed in the condition of the person. Therefore, the data collected at the time of admission, which tended to 'capture' inmates in words and on paper, remains the significant document for historical inquiry, especially for studies – such as the present one – which take large samples of data.

Clinical cases were more than documents of knowledge about individuals, their diagnoses and the outcomes of their institutional treatments. They were also social documents which inscribed and ascribed institutional identities to both individuals and social groups. They were and are representations which attached meanings to bodies.[82] These representations were historically and geographically specific, and drew on their social, cultural and political contexts, as well as reflecting changes in medical knowledge and approaches over time.[83] In some instances the ways that such identities inside medical, clinical settings had direct and often deleterious effects on inmates, making them subject to experimental treatments or horrifying neglect.[84] In other examples, positive outcomes for specific groups also signify the power of institutional classifications.[85] In the contexts examined in this study, the effects and outcomes of institutional categorising are more subtle, and perhaps less obvious, but are nonetheless significant in terms of the meanings of institutional cases and their interpretation, and provide instructive examples of the ways meanings can be made from settler-colonial institutional discourses.

The arguments in this discussion are also of wider significance in the field of mental health history, as historians continue to grapple with ideas about how to adequately write about 'patients' in the past. The tendency to perpetuate practices of labelling and ascribing identities to 'the mentally ill' has been difficult to avoid. Clinical case records are also highly repetitive and share characteristics. That they then tend to solidify categories of inmate and person – especially when assessed using large samples of historical data – is unsurprising.

Institutional populations of the insane, and indeed, the very problem of insanity itself, are often left out of accounts of imperial mobility. Despite their relative invisibility before, for example, the subjects given new biographical power by the contributors to the collection *Transnational Lives* have in common their potential for individuation in historical narratives.[86] Unlike those people, asylum inmates tended to be grouped together and collectively examined, studied and understood as 'the mad'. These inmates all passed through the institutions during the period of this study, and the ink which recorded their presence marked it inside the more permanent artefacts accessed for this study. Their often scant and very partial records nonetheless present opportunities for interpretation, both of the overall institutional population, and of the ways in which the institutional authorities sought to understand it. How their cases were narrated inside the pages of the casebooks and case files depended upon the bones of the information known about them. In some instances, the outcomes of their institutional confinement also depended upon knowing more rather than less about their circumstances, as other studies also show.[87]

Casebook narratives of the insane, as I argue elsewhere, were narratives of 'shifting subjects', with little or no resolution of the problem, or cure for mental illness, in most cases.[88] The formation of the gendered clinical narrative was one of a series of textual representations of the female patient in colonial society.[89] It was the patient casebook narratives and their tropes which drove the analysis. This chapter has extended these arguments and offers some new insights into the production of meaning inside clinical texts, taking further ideas about the ways in which colonial institutions created cases, formed an institutional language and asserted versions of colonial identity. In the following chapters, I examine the different forms of colonial masculinity and femininity contained in patient case notes and in wider discussions about institutional inmates.

PASSING THROUGH: PATIENT IDENTITIES, HOSPITALS

Notes

1 PROV, VPRS 7399/P1, unit 9, folio 9, 9 April 1891.
2 Angela McCarthy's research shows that records from Dunedin asylums noted immigrant inmates' ships of arrival in some cases; see McCarthy, 'Migration and madness in New Zealand's asylums, 1863–1910', in *Migration, Ethnicity, and Mental Health: International Perspectives, 1840–2010*, Routledge Studies in Cultural History (New York and Abingdon: Routledge, 2012), pp. 55–72.
3 See Catharine Coleborne, *Reading 'Madness': Gender and Difference in the Colonial Asylum in Victoria, Australia, 1848–1888* (Perth: Network Books, Australian Public Intellectual Network, 2007), p. 58. Here, I cite from Jann Matlock, *Scenes of Seduction: Prostitution, Hysteria, and Reading Difference in Nineteenth-Century France* (New York: Columbia University Press, 1994), pp. 140–1.
4 Ann Laura Stoler, 'Colonial archives and the arts of governance: On the content in the form', in Carolyn Hamilton, Verne Harris, Jane Taylor, Michele Pickover, Graeme Reid and Razia Saleh (eds), *Refiguring the Archive* (Dordrecht, Boston and London: Kluwer Academic Publishers, 2002), p. 89.
5 See my argument in Catharine Coleborne, 'Locating ethnicity in the hospitals for the insane: Revisiting case books as sites of knowledge production about colonial identities in Victoria, Australia, 1873–1910', in McCarthy and Coleborne (eds), *Migration, Ethnicity, and Mental Health*, p. 86.
6 The previous chapter described the transfers between social welfare institutions and the asylums, drawing mainly on the records of the hospitals for the insane. The records of the Victorian Immigrants' Home contain little useful information, and even when cross-checked against individuals said to have been transferred between sites, these yielded very little worthwhile data and added little to the discussion. This does not detract from the points made, however, of the relevance of the network of social and welfare institutions; it simply reinforces the points made in this chapter about the volume of data produced by the hospitals for the insane.
7 Franca Iacovetta and Wendy Mitchinson (eds), *On the Case: Explorations in Social History* (Toronto, Buffalo and London: University of Toronto Press, 1998), p. 6.
8 The database records that 286 of the total Auckland sample of 868 patients were photographed, while only 100 of the total of the Yarra Bend sample of 3,102 patients were photographed. I suggest that the larger numbers of admissions at the Yarra Bend made the task of photographing inmates more onerous. For more information about this era in mental health institutions in Victoria, see Belinda Robson, 'The Construction and Experience of Female Mental Illness in Melbourne, 1906–1909', unpublished Honours thesis, University of Melbourne, 1988.
9 See also Barbara Brookes, 'Pictures of people, pictures of places: Photography and the asylum', in Catharine Coleborne and Dolly MacKinnon (eds), *Exhibiting Madness in Museums: Remembering Psychiatry through Museums and Display*, Routledge Research in Museum Studies (New York and London: Routledge, 2011), p. 35.
10 Catherine Hall, *Civilising Subjects: Metropole and Colony in the English Imagination 1830–1867* (Chicago: University of Chicago Press; Cambridge: Polity, 2002), p. 16.
11 Sally Swartz, 'The regulation of British colonial lunatic asylums and the origins of colonial psychiatry, 1860–1864', *History of Psychology*, 13:2 (2010), p. 172.
12 Hall, *Civilising Subjects*, pp. 16–17.
13 Mark Finnane, 'The ruly and the unruly: Isolation and inclusion in the management of the insane', in Carolyn Strange and Alison Bashford (eds), *Isolation: Places and Practices of Exclusion*, Routledge Studies in Modern History (London and New York: Routledge, 2003), pp. 92–3; pp. 94–5.
14 See Waltraud Ernst, 'Madness and gender in nineteenth-century British India', *Social History of Medicine*, 9:3 (1996), pp. 364–7; Bronwyn Labrum, 'The boundaries of femininity: Madness and gender in New Zealand, 1870–1910', in Wendy Chan, Dorothy E. Chunn and Robert Menzies (eds), *Women, Madness and the Law:*

A Feminist Reader (London, Portland OR, and Coogee: GlassHouse Press, 2005); Catharine Coleborne, '"His brain was wrong, his mind astray": Families and the language of insanity in New South Wales, Queensland and New Zealand, 1880s–1910', *Journal of Family History*, 31:1 (2006), pp. 45–65.

15 Coleborne, 'Locating ethnicity in the hospitals for the insane', pp. 73–90.
16 Elspeth Knewstubb, '"Believes the devil has changed him": Religion and patient identity in Ashburn Hall, Dunedin, 1882–1910', *Health and History*, 14:1 (2012), pp. 56–76.
17 Table xiv, *Report of the Inspector of Lunatic Asylums on the Hospitals for the Insane* (1884), in *Victoria Parliamentary Papers* (hereafter VPP), 1885, v. 3 (John Ferres, Government Printer, Melbourne), p. 25; Table xiv, *Report of the Inspector of Lunatic Asylums on the Hospitals for the Insane* (1887), VPP, 1888, v. 2, part 1 (John Ferres, Government Printer, Melbourne), p. 29.
18 See Catharine Coleborne, 'Making "mad" populations in settler colonies: The work of law and medicine in the creation of the colonial asylum', in Diane Kirkby and Catharine Coleborne (eds), *Law, History, Colonialism: The Reach of Empire*, Studies in Imperialism (Manchester: Manchester University Press, 2001).
19 See for example Catharine Coleborne, 'Pursuing families for maintenance payments to hospitals for the insane in Australia and New Zealand, 1860s–1914', *Australian Historical Studies*, 40:3 (2009), pp. 308–22.
20 Emma Spooner, 'Digging for the Families of the "Mad": Locating the Family in the Auckland Asylum Archives, 1870–1911', unpublished Masters thesis in History, University of Waikato, 2006, p. 38.
21 Sally Swartz, 'Lost lives: Gender, history and mental illness in the Cape, 1891–1910', *Feminism and Psychology*, 9:2 (1999), pp. 152–8.
22 Jonathan Andrews, 'Case notes, case histories, and the patient's experience of insanity at Gartnavel Royal Asylum, Glasgow, in the nineteenth century', *Social History of Medicine*, 11:2 (1998), p. 280.
23 Coleborne, *Reading 'Madness'*, pp. 70–1.
24 Elsewhere, I compare the casebooks and case files of different colonial institutions including the Yarra Bend, Auckland, Gladesville and Goodna asylums, writing about the subtle differences between their styles, entries, conventions of doctors, the relative emphases placed on family information and committal papers, the role of patient correspondence, and ancillary sources; see Coleborne, *Madness in the Family: Insanity and Institutions in the Australasian Colonial World, 1860–1914* (Basingstoke and New York: Palgrave Macmillan, 2010), pp. 143–53; Coleborne, 'Reading insanity's archive: reflections from four archival sites', *Provenance*, 9 (2010), pp. 29–41.
25 The databases for the two institutions in this study were assembled separately using Microsoft Access. They have not been merged due to the establishment of slightly different data-entry practices over the period this research was conducted, making it more difficult to pool data and to represent data in visual formats. However, the chapter makes use of tables and other representations of the data contained in each case, sometimes also comparing institutions.
26 Lucy Chesser, 'A woman who married three wives': Management of disruptive knowledge in the 1879 Australian case of Edward De Lacy Evans', *Journal of Women's History*, 9:4 (1998), pp. 53–77; Ruth Ford, 'Sexuality and "madness": Regulating women's gender "deviance" through the asylum, the Orange Asylum in the 1930s', in Catharine Coleborne and Dolly MacKinnon (eds), *'Madness' in Australia: Histories, Heritage and the Asylum*, UQP Australian Studies (St Lucia: University of Queensland Press, 2003), pp. 109–19.
27 Henry Finlay, *To Have But Not to Hold: A History of Attitudes to Marriage and Divorce in Australia 1858–1975* (Annandale: Federation Press, 2005); Hayley Brown, 'Loosening the Marriage Bond: Divorce in New Zealand, c.1890s–c.1950s', unpublished Ph.D. thesis, Victoria University of Wellington, 2011; Roderick Phillips, *Divorce in New Zealand: A Social History* (Auckland: Oxford University Press, 1981).

28 Angela McCarthy, 'Ethnicity, migration and the lunatic asylum in early twentieth-century Auckland, New Zealand', *Social History of Medicine*, 21:1 (2008), pp. 47–65.
29 Coleborne, 'Locating ethnicity in the hospitals for the insane', pp. 73–90.
30 PROV, VPRS 7399/P1, unit 10, folio 145, 26 October 1894; VPRS 7399/P0, unit 15, folio 500, 17 September 1906.
31 Leonard D. Smith, 'Insanity and ethnicity: Jews in the mid-Victorian lunatic asylum', *Jewish Culture and History*, 1:1 (1988), pp. 28–9.
32 Ann Goldberg, 'The limits of medicalization: Jewish lunatics and nineteenth-century Germany', *History of Psychiatry*, 7 (1996), pp. 265–85.
33 Goldberg, 'The limits of medicalization', p. 266.
34 Goldberg, 'The limits of medicalization', p. 270.
35 Goldberg, 'The limits of medicalization', p. 275.
36 See '1881 Victorian Census', Revisiting Kew: Historic Explanations, 1 August 2012 http://rbkr.wordpress.com/2012/08/01/1881-victorian-census-11/, accessed 4 August 2014; see also Historical Census and Colonial Data Archive (HCCDA), Victorian Censuses 1865–1901, http://hccda.ada.edu.au/, accessed 4 August 2014. See letter by Mr C. P. Hodges at the end of the report, p. 183.
37 My sincere thanks to Dr Deborah Rechter for reminding me of the complex ethnic identities in colonial Victoria, and for pointing me to her own curatorial work about the Jewish peoples of colonial Melbourne. See materials in the permanent exhibition in the Zelman Cowen Gallery of Australian Jewish History, 'Calling Australia Home' at the Jewish Museum of Australia in Melbourne: www.jewishmuseum.com.au/exhibitions/permanent-exhibitions, accessed 18 November 2013.
38 See: www.teara.govt.nz/en/1966/hauhauism, accessed 20 June 2013.
39 For examples of the current scholarship in the field in the English context, see: www.geog.cam.ac.uk/research/centres/campop/occupations/, accessed 27 December 2013.
40 See for example the work outlined and summarised here: www.geog.cam.ac.uk/research/projects/occupations/britain19c/occupationsbritain/, accessed 27 December 2013.
41 *Annual Report on Lunatic Asylums of New Zealand*, AJHR, H-13 (1881), p. 16.
42 This is the language of the title of relevant tables in the official reports.
43 Akihito Suzuki, 'Lunacy and labouring men: Narratives of male vulnerability in mid-Victorian London', in Roberta Bivins and John V. Pickstone (eds), *Medicine, Madness and Social History: Essays in Honour of Roy Porter* (Basingstoke: Palgrave Macmillan, 2007), p. 119.
44 Suzuki, 'Lunacy and labouring men', p. 126.
45 Joseph Melling, 'Sex and sensibility in cultural history: The English governess and the lunatic asylum, 1845–1914', in Jonathan Andrews and Anne Digby (eds), *Sex and Seclusion, Class and Custody: Perspectives on Gender and Class in the History of British and Irish Psychiatry*, Clio Medica 73: The Wellcome Series in the History of Medicine (Amsterdam and New York: Rodopi, 2004), pp. 177–221.
46 Margaret Tennant, 'Elderly indigents and old men's homes 1880–1920', *New Zealand Journal of History*, 17:1 (1983), pp. 3–20; see Table 1 on p. 6.
47 *Report on the Lunatic Asylums of New Zealand*, AJHR, 1881, H-13, p. 11.
48 Angela Hawk, 'Going "mad" in gold country: Migrant populations and the problem of containment in Pacific mining boom regions', *Pacific Historical Review*, 80:1 (2011), pp. 74–5.
49 See Catharine Coleborne, 'Law's mobility: Vagrancy and imperial legality in the trans-Tasman colonial world', in Katie Pickles and Catharine Coleborne (eds), *New Zealand's Empire*, Studies in Imperialism (Manchester University Press, in press).
50 Gerard Curry, 'A bundle of vague diverse offences: The Vagrancy Laws with special reference to the New Zealand experience', *Anglo-American Law Review*, 1 (1972), pp. 523–36; Julie Kimber, 'Poor Laws: A historiography of vagrancy in Australia', *History Compass*, 11:8 (2013), pp. 537–50.
51 Dean Wilson, 'Community Violence in Auckland, 1850–1875', unpublished Masters thesis in History, University of Auckland, 1993, p. 27.

52 David Goodman, *Gold Seeking: Victoria and California in the 1850s* (Sydney: Allen & Unwin, 1994), pp. 76–7.
53 Norman Megahey argues this in 'More than a minor nuisance: Insanity in colonial Western Australia', in Charlie Fox (ed.), *Historical Refractions*, Studies in Western Australian History 14 (Crawley: University of Western Australia, 1993), p. 59.
54 Tim Cresswell, 'Embodiment, power and the politics of mobility: The case of female tramps and hobos', *Transactions of the Institute of British Geographers*, 24:2 (1999), p. 184.
55 James H. Mills, *Madness, Cannabis and Colonialism: The 'Native-Only' Lunatic Asylums of British India, 1857–1900* (London and New York: Macmillan and St Martin's, 2000); Lynette A. Jackson, *Surfacing Up: Psychiatry and Social Order in Colonial Zimbabwe, 1908–1968*, Cornell Studies in the History of Psychiatry (Ithaca: Cornell University Press, 2005).
56 Penelope Edmonds, 'The intimate, urbanising frontier: Native camps and settler colonialism's violent array of spaces around early Melbourne', in Tracey Banivanua Mar and Penelope Edmonds (eds), *Making Settler Colonial Space: Perspectives on Race, Place and Identity* (Basingstoke: Palgrave Macmillan, 2010), pp. 129–54.
57 See also Lorelle Barry and Catharine Coleborne, 'Insanity and ethnicity in New Zealand: Māori encounters with the Auckland Mental Hospital, 1860–1900', *History of Psychiatry*, 22:3 (2011), pp. 285–301; Bain Attwood, 'Tarra Bobby, a Brataualung man', *Aboriginal History*, 11:1–2 (1987), pp. 41–57.
58 PROV, VPRS 7400/P1, unit 5, folio 213, 24 September 1873.
59 PROV, VPRS 7400/P1, unit 12, folio 346, 11 August 1900.
60 PROV, VPRS 7399/P1, unit 10, folio 183, 19 December, 1894.
61 National Archives of New Zealand, Auckland (hereafter NANZ), Auckland Mental Hospital (hereafter YCAA), 1048/5 341, patient 1521, 22 December 1888.
62 Immigrants' Aid Society Minute Books, 1869–1871 (1870), p. 118.
63 Kirsten McKenzie, 'Opportunists and imposters in the British imperial world: The tale of John Dow, convict, and Edward, Viscount Lascelles', in Desley Deacon, Penny Russell and Angela Woollacott (eds), *Transnational Lives: Biographies of Global Modernity, 1700-Present*, Palgrave Macmillan Transnational History Series (Basingstoke and New York: Palgrave Macmillan, 2010), p. 77.
64 Radhika Mohanram, *Imperial White: Race, Diaspora, and the British Empire* (Minneapolis: University of Minnesota Press, 2007), pp. 169–70.
65 See for example work by McKenzie, 'Opportunists and imposters', pp. 69–81.
66 Goodman, *Gold Seeking*, p. 75.
67 See Catharine Coleborne, 'Passage to the asylum: The role of the police in committals of the insane in Victoria, Australia, 1848–1900', in Roy Porter and David Wright (eds), *The Confinement of the Insane: International Perspectives, 1800–1965* (Cambridge and New York: Cambridge University Press, 2003).
68 NANZ, Factsheet on Police Gazettes, http://archives.govt.nz/sites/default/files/Police_Gazettes.pdf, accessed 18 June 2013.
69 David Wright, 'Delusions of gender?: Lay identification and clinical diagnosis of insanity in Victorian England', in Andrews and Digby (eds), *Sex and Seclusion*, pp. 160–1. John Starrett Hughes agrees; see 'The madness of separate spheres: Insanity and masculinity in Victorian Alabama', in Mark C. Carnes and Clyde Griffen (eds), *Meanings for Manhood: Constructions of Masculinity in Victorian America* (Chicago and London: University of Chicago Press, 1990), pp. 53–66.
70 In addition, causes were recorded separately, meaning that a 'hidden' diagnosis, for example, suspected GPI, might lurk elsewhere in the patient record. In collating this data I have been careful to include and cross-check where possible such information.
71 James H. Mills and Satadru Sen (eds), *Confronting the Body: The Politics of Physicality in Colonial and Post-Colonial India*, Anthem South Asian Studies (London: Anthem Press, 2003).
72 See Mills, *Madness, Cannabis and Colonialism*.

73 Ngahuia Te Awekotuku, with Linda Waimarie Nikora, *Mau Moko: The World of Māori Tattoo* (North Shore NZ: Penguin Viking, 2007).
74 NANZ, YCAA 1048/6 237, patient 1954, 8 March 1894.
75 NANZ, YCAA 1048/10 2, patient 2895, 16 October 1903.
76 Brookes, 'Pictures of people, pictures of places', p. 32.
77 Brookes, 'Pictures of people, pictures of places', p. 30.
78 See PROV, VPRS 7399/P1, unit 6, folio 137, 7 May 1885.
79 Brookes, 'Pictures of people, pictures of places', p. 32. See also Stanley B. Burns, *Seeing Insanity: Photography and the Depiction of Mental Illness* (Burns Archive Press, 2007).
80 Brookes, 'Pictures of people, pictures of places', p. 36.
81 PROV, VPRS 7400/P1, unit 15, folio 5, 27 November 1906.
82 Rosemarie Garland Thomson, *Extraordinary Bodies: Figuring Physical Disability in American Culture and Literature* (New York: Columbia University Press, 1997), p. 5.
83 See for instance Maree Dawson's arguments about historically constructed forms of fear about racial degeneracy at the Auckland Mental Hospital from the 1850s to 1899: 'Halting the "sad degenerationist parade": Medical concerns about heredity and racial degeneracy in New Zealand psychiatry, 1853–1899', *Health and History*, 14:1 (2012), pp. 38–55.
84 Lorelle Barry and Catharine Coleborne, 'Insanity and ethnicity in New Zealand: Māori encounters with the Auckland Mental Hospital, 1860–1900', *History of Psychiatry*, 22:3 (2011), pp. 285–301; G. Eric Jarvis, 'Changing psychiatric perception of African Americans with psychosis', *European Journal of American Culture*, 27:3 (2008), pp. 227–52; Robert Menzies and Ted Palys, 'Turbulent spirits: Aboriginal patients in the British Columbia psychiatric system, 1879–1950', in James E. Moran and David Wright (eds), *Mental Health and Canadian Society: Historical Perspectives*, Studies in the History of Medicine, Health and Society (Montreal: McGill-Queen's University Press, 2008), pp. 149–75.
85 Coleborne, *Reading 'Madness'*, p. 67, pp. 52–3.
86 Desley Deacon, Penny Russell and Angela Woollacott, 'Introduction', in Deacon, Russell and Woollacott (eds), *Transnational Lives*, p. 2.
87 See, for instance, Coleborne, *Madness in the Family*.
88 Coleborne, *Reading 'Madness'*, pp. 57–79.
89 See my discussion about the production of 'otherness' in Coleborne, *Reading 'Madness'*, pp. 136–40.

CHAPTER FOUR

White men and weak masculinity: men in the public asylums, 1860s–1900s

In 1900, German man Ludwig Hesse was arrested in central Melbourne by police and taken to the Yarra bend. His behaviour included people witnessing him 'running around Little Bourke St' in only his night shirt in the early hours of the morning, calling out 'Shoot him, shoot him.' Hesse, aged fifty-one, was 'enfeebled by delusions of persecution'. At the Yarra Bend, he was taken out to work with the bricklayers and reportedly worked well, but he tried to escape a year later by picking a lock.[1] Like other white European men housed inside the institutions for the insane, Hesse was physically able, and was set to work as a form of rehabilitation. Forms of labour were important to the institutions, and were designed to determine 'wellness' among the institutional population. This practice would help to ameliorate anxieties about colonial masculinity and its failures.

Publishing more than twenty years apart about newcomers to the colony of Victoria, contemporary writers N. W. Pollard and W. J. Woods both suggested what other commentators had also come to suspect about the dangers inherent in migrant populations: that the weak, ill, dissolute, or lazy would find their way into the ranks of the colonial insane and needy. In his *Homes in Victoria* (1861) Pollard suggested that 'the lazy, the dissolute, and abandoned may and do find difficulty here, but they would and ought, to find difficulty anywhere, and Victoria is the last place in the world to which they should have come'.[2] Meanwhile, Woods wrote in his *A Visit to Victoria* (1886) that:

> Of men who fail in this country there are two classes – those whose failure is due to causes in themselves, and those who are too heavily handicapped by the overcrowding of our professions, trades, and crafts. The former would come to grief anywhere. The idler, the drunkard, the man without capacity, or without stability, or without energy, is less likely to prosper than in England. When a young fellow becomes reprobate at home, he should not be sent to Australia, for with fewer restraints upon him, and

far from his old friends, he is likely to rush with accelerated speed along the downward path.[3]

Their words hint at the supposed classes of men: there were men who would work hard but whose luck might turn on the local economy and their specific occupation or skill; and there were men who would fail because they were 'reprobate'. The 'ne'er do well' men depicted in the satirical images published in 1890 (see Figure 2.4 in Chapter 2) represented the form of masculinity despised by the hard-working, law-abiding Christian men who wanted their values to shape the new colonies.

Echoing the medical, scientific postulations of the period, both writers managed to hint at forms of masculinity which presented risks in the colonial environment. Writing about nineteenth-century Britain, John Tosh asserts that there were 'dominant' and 'subordinate' forms of masculinity, and that masculinity itself has been described as a form of 'social identity': as 'an aspect of the structure of social relations'.[4] Tosh goes on to examine forms of psychic identity for men, a theme also pursued in this chapter. Crucially, masculinity in the late nineteenth century was also an imperial identity.[5] In the imperial world, masculine weakness in the working classes was recognised as a failing of masculinity. British imperial masculinity 'was predicated on the possession of the idealised body – invulnerable, non-orific, youthful, white'.[6] White masculinity, then, can be situated at the intersection of class. The idealisation of masculinity took a variety of forms and was 'under siege' during periods of conflict and violence, with different nineteenth-century wars of empire destabilising the imperial myth of white masculine prowess and strength. The major problem was the oxymoronic white body: the poor and weak white man of empire.[7] Colonial forms of masculinity existed where the British had made themselves imperial outposts in a world that was based on racial difference, particularly where the white population was a minority.[8]

Yet in the white settler colonies of Victoria and New Zealand, how much did these ideas reverberate and take new forms? Edmonds suggests that Melbourne and the colony of Victoria came to exemplify the work of the British Empire, and that it followed that the colonial masculinities formed there were potent and symbolic.[9] Looking carefully at the ways that masculinity appears in the institutional record, the various forms it took, and how it became the subject of commentary, this chapter plots ways of understanding masculinity among the insane, and the model of masculinity proscribed for white colonial society.

New forms of masculinity in the period, observable in a variety of imperial social settings, in the different expectations for working men during the industrialising period, as well as being articulated through changing gender relations, all played into these ideas about the right kind of immigrant for the white settler colony.[10] Whiteness, a more or less 'invisible' ethnicity in the patient casebooks, found expression through the use of gender as a category in the patient case records. This chapter uses the tool of gender to explore the function and representation of whiteness as ethnicity, while at the same time it seeks to find out more about constructions and expectations of masculinity for nineteenth-century male inmates and their doctors. It is through the exploration of these two categories – 'male' and 'white' – in relation to each other that we might begin to understand the central preoccupations of contemporaries in their context. By using case materials in a qualitative analysis, the chapter examines the different ways in which we might begin to understand white European male patients against the backdrop of discursive formations of colonialism and masculinity. There were socially defined pressures on, and gendered expectations of men in the nineteenth century. Men who 'violated the norms of masculinity' were possibly more vulnerable to institutional confinement.[11] There are other ways of reading the evidence, too, which highlight differences between men and their sensitivity to the modes of masculinity of the day. Using both existing scholarship and new archival data, this chapter offers deeper interpretations of these historically specific and geographically located meanings of white masculinity.

The chapter takes a detailed look at who these men were: their occupations and social status, and then at their medical diagnoses, including sunstroke, mania and delirium tremens and alcoholism and also at GPI. It aims to show how the dominant (and some lesser but significant) medical diagnoses for colonial men, evinced through the data, tell us something about constructions of colonial masculinity and gender relations. In particular, the ways in which symptoms of mental illness were gender-specific, or aligned with gendered expectations of men and women, also helps to define the material here, with questions of masculine identity forming the focus of the chapter. Expressions of sexuality, and some of its manifestations outside and inside the institution, such as sexual vice in the form of masturbation, are highlighted against readings of masculinity in the period, and also linked to questions of medical diagnosis. Mental illness and behaviours can also tell us something about the gendered worlds of colonialism across the period. Male delusions, for instance, and specific allusions made to the world of machinery and mechanics, are read against the backdrop of urbanisation and industrialisation in the colonial setting.

Masculinity, insanity and colonialism

Two images of 'madmen' were both published in 1862 in the *Illustrated Melbourne Post* and suggest something of the meaning of white, institutionalised masculinity in the Australasian colonies in the nineteenth century. The first depicts a strong male inmate restrained by wrist and ankle cuffs on a bed; the other shows a feeble-looking male patient 'in the bag', another restraining device for the whole body in use during the period. Arguably, they present two kinds of men institutionalised as insane: those seen as physically strong, but manic and deranged, capable of violence; and those worn down, suffering from debility and disease, and protected against their own body's jerky, involuntary movements.[12] There were more than two 'types' of 'mad men' in the institutional populations of the insane of the period. Yet gender difference, and especially nuanced accounts of masculinity and illness in their social and cultural contexts, was not a topic privileged or made explicit by contemporary writers.

Although contemporaries had 'important insights' into the causes of male insanity, they did not, in their own recording of patient data, analyse the wider meanings of masculinity in colonial society.[13] These insights include the situations of single men, working in remote places and lonely; or married men whose illnesses related to the strains of relationships and families. Authorities also noted the appearance of syphilis among the insane men, and the higher incidence of 'sexual vice' among men when compared to women in the asylum.[14]

White male patients worked in the gendered occupations of the hospitals for the insane: in the garden or on the farm, and they were described as physically capable.[15] These men and similar examples derived from this present study across two colonial sites strike me as being what we might term the 'muscular insane'. The central tenets of the imperial practice of 'muscular Christianity' – a vigorous physical masculinity, with an emphasis on piety – could be said to have also permeated the discourses of the hospitals for the insane which, from the second half of the nineteenth century, were focused on the moral improvement of the insane through both religious practice and work therapies.[16] However, there were ambiguities around masculinity in the setting of the hospital for the insane. There were physically able male patients who could work in the outdoors, on the farm, and achieve considerable self-improvement through work therapies. This marked their bodies out as more successful, more curable, than some non-white bodies, including the few Chinese patients observed in my earlier study for colonial Victoria. And yet many white male patients also suffered extreme physical debility, either produced through poverty and ill health, or through the ravages of mental disease. These men lacked physical strength, thereby challenging expectations of colonial masculinity.

The ability to work hard and to exhibit the potential to be physically and mentally 'sound', as well as morally decent, were highly valued qualities for men in nineteenth-century imperial and colonial society in both Australia and New Zealand. However, as historians point out, not all men in the colonies were in continual employment; many found themselves down on their luck, and sought welfare assistance.[17] Indeed, weak masculinity arguably posed more of a threat to social order than weak femininity as colonists viewed it, especially given the emphasis on the success of white masculinity in the system of colonialism. Male migrant workers, mostly miners, were vulnerable to institutional controls around the Pacific region in the form of mental hospital records because of their tendencies to transience, border-crossing and highly masculine lives inside the complex and unstable social world of the gold-rush era.[18] Middle-class notions of respectability became increasingly important in the urban setting, and marked a growing 'intolerance' for unproductive behaviour, especially among men.[19] These ambiguities provide us with a way into the study of insanity and ethnicity by suggesting that the problems facing medical administrators were shot through with anxieties about colonial life, and concerns about the future health of the white colonial population.

Sunstroke was a phenomenon affecting men that was supposed to be a bodily vulnerability, but had external causes.[20] White male bodies occupied the discursive spaces of the colonies through a discussion of their physicality. During the 1870s, for instance, white male patients at the Yarra Bend admitted suffering from sunstroke reached as high as 16 per cent of the total male asylum population.[21] Asylum stories and family commentaries about those people who were institutionalised reveals a level of popular insight into the conditions of mental health and its causes, including understandings of the effects of sunstroke in the colonies.[22] Given colonial debates about white men and their unsuitability for physical labour in the tropics, at least until the late nineteenth century, the medical beliefs about sunstroke underline the general belief that climate and the physical environment affected the functioning of colonial masculinity. January heat, wrote one contemporary, was 'something dreadful, the sun scorches everything and burns it up and woe betide the man with big ears ... There has been known as many as nine men killed in Sydney in one week with sunstroke'.[23] In their medical arguments about the effects of the harsh climate in Australia, some colonists feared that Australia represented a real risk to the white male body, already out of place in the 'logic' of settler colonialism.²⁴ Cases of sunstroke at the Yarra Bend (thirty-eight men) show that sunstroke was more common among the men described as outdoor labourers or workers, and they were admitted from the 1870s onwards; one man, a German harbouring political delusions, was afflicted in India, while others were said to have been affected by the strong sun as boys. All the men, where a country of birth was listed, were born outside of Australia. At Auckland, men with sunstroke were all admitted in the 1890s or early 1900s: these five cases in the collated data reveal little about the way that sunstroke was regarded as either a 'cause' of insanity or as a diagnosis, but one of these men was pronounced 'sane'. These various cases of sunstroke do not amount to much in terms of knowledge about the condition or diagnosis, but they do suggest a level of thinking about exposure to the colonial sun. One example of 'colonial fever' in a man first admitted in 1859, and whose case continued at the Yarra Bend in 1885, reminds us of earlier notions of colonial madness, and the idea that the colonies might induce mental breakdown.²⁵

Many of the institutionalised men in the sample from the Yarra Bend asylum were described as feeble and weak. Debility and physical weakness among men obviously signified a loss of virility and masculinity. Many of these men were immigrants and were transferred from the Immigrants' Homes. These men were characterised in patient case notes as elderly, depleted of body and mind, and without family contacts in Australia; very little information about their previous histories accompanied the notes. To medical and colonial authorities they were most likely a sad reminder of the strains of migration to the new colony. They were also symbolic of other stresses present in colonial society, and especially ideas about the importance of white masculinity. Concerns over heredity, and the collection of family medical histories, posed the greatest problem for medical superintendents in these cases.²⁶

Perhaps the very 'masculinity' of the colonial man presented some problems for middle-class medical men. As William Howitt put it, writing about emigrants to Victoria in the 1850s, the men were a 'rough, rude, work-a-day set of fellows, very independent, and very unceremonious'.²⁷ Other contemporary writers to comment on masculinity included Thomas Dobeson, 'a refugee from industrial England', who observed and feared hyper-masculinity, its simmering violence and competitive swagger.²⁸ Another problem was the very mobility of white men and their inability to settle while the labour force was in transition, and while the needs for labour in the settler colony were, paradoxically, constantly changing and unsettled, in a state of 'excitement'. This contrasted with the vision for a formal, rational and highly controlled masculinity as performed by the constabulary and other official agencies of the colonial law and order machine.[29] In the 1850s, the Reverend Isaac Newton made an argument about masculinity in his discussion of the oak tree versus the hot-house flower: 'the oak had the fixity and dependability which the transitory men of Victoria so conspicuously lacked'.[30]

White masculinity took different forms, and was characterised by ethnicity and ethnic identifications. Contemporaries, for instance, sometimes referred to the Irish as dark-skinned. Writing about his adventures in the South Island of New Zealand, in the Canterbury district, Samuel Butler depicted the character of the superstitious 'old Irishman' at the hut where they camped, a man who saw ghosts, who was 'black and charred' and difficult to see in the half light.[31] This trope was repeated in other writing about colonial types; Irish men and women tended to be associated with dark skin, poverty, heavy drinking and sickness.

Manhood was displayed through heavy drinking, hard labour and rough speech.[32] The colonies were awash with alcohol.[33] Howitt and Dobeson both reported that drunkenness led to grave mistakes and hopelessness; Dobeson abhorred the results of a gang of men drinking 'a cargo of colonial beer' all night.[34] The abuse of alcohol was another aspect of colonial masculinity which contributed to institutionalisation. At the Yarra Bend, 186 cases of the total number of male cases were linked to the abuse of alcohol, while only fifty-one women were said to have problems with 'drink'. At Auckland, abuse of alcohol, alcoholism, drink and similar 'causes' of insanity were explicitly attributed to sixty-nine cases of men (compared to just fourteen of the women). Yet alcohol features in many more of the formal diagnoses for patients at both institutions, often combined with other diagnostic categories. Family violence, discussed later in this chapter, was often the result of excessive drinking bouts and binges, drinking episodes which also took their toll on men's mental health and brain function.

Alfred Newman, the self-appointed expert on medical theories in nineteenth-century New Zealand, whose ideas sometimes made their way into learned journals and earned an audience, articulated some ways of understanding masculinity in the colonies in a series of unintentionally humorous and flawed arguments about colonial men and drinking. For Newman, climate, propensity to drinking and the inherited characteristics of colonial men were bound up together: young colonial men in Victoria, New South Wales, Queensland and New Zealand, he argued, were simply 'unfit for drunkenness', their 'spareness of frame and general lack of vigour' revealing them as 'sober'.[35]

Other forms of addiction could take their toll on men. In a handful of cases, addictions such as excessive tobacco smoking, and the use of addictive substances including opium, combined with a poor diet and poverty, often produced delirious and malnourished specimens of men whose visible bodily decay marked on their sallow skins and sickly frames sent out to their institutional keepers anxious signals about men wasting away. Excessive alcohol consumption, especially of spirits, coupled with a poor diet, led to malnutrition. External causes, too, remind us of the dangers men faced in their work – such as exposure to copper fumes, lead, zinc and other toxic materials used in industry, some of which were reported in cases of sick men inside the institutions.[36] In 1909 Tom Billet, a painter, was brought to the Yarra Bend suffering from suspected lead poisoning, and craved open air and exercise; earlier at the same institution, in 1888, coppersmith James Drummond was brought by police believing he was being poisoned, and the cause of his illness was noted as copper poisoning, a fair deduction by the asylum doctors.[37] In a separate case in 1894, another man, George Lett, claimed to have been poisoned by tea tasting, which was his occupation.[38] Occupational categories can tell us other things, too, about patterns of colonial life and masculinity, as the chapter goes on to discuss below.

Occupations: masculinity and work

Occupational category is used here as a way to understand class identity in the institutional setting. Following from the previous chapter, this section teases out whether specific forms of institutional writing and categorising were common to specific groups. In addition, the theme of masculinity and work is potentially productive for the present study. The fact that labourers formed such a large population of the male insane suggests that working men were especially vulnerable to institutional committal.[39] Stephen Garton characterises the typical madman of the period as a 'maniacal labourer', with men roaming rural areas and remote stations likely to be arrested and policed for vagrancy among other 'offences', until, as Garton suggests, there was a population shift towards urban centres, making the new focus of male insanity the 'boarding-house, the city slum dwelling and the dock side pub'.[40] Both forms of the masculine insane can be found in the archival records examined for this study.

Victoria was built on the promise of plentiful labouring work. Described by contemporaries as a 'Paradise of Labour', Victoria's demand for labour from the 1850s was 'boundless' according to William Howitt, not surprising given his time in the colonies, as it seemed that every man had abandoned other forms of work for the diggings. Significantly, read in the light of the idea that Victoria was an imperial colony above others, the sort of conditions under which men would labour there, were, for Howitt, an 'Eden' when compared to the various colonial sites the English tended to seek out: the 'torrid desert', the 'pestilent swamp' and the 'frozen' regions all seemed uncivilised when held up against the colony's various disagreeable climatic aspects.[41]

Immigrant men in Victoria in the 1850s goldrush era who ended up in the Yarra Bend provide us with evidence for a discussion about the relationships between industrialising Britain, immigration, social change and masculinity. Colonial men valued independence; it became, briefly, the cornerstone of colonial masculinity.[42] Because it signalled the loss of this independence, the failure to find or to secure steady employment during periods of economic crisis was a trigger for male institutional committal. There was a new narrative about working men's fears of unemployment in Britain: labouring men expressed intense fears about their economic futures in the mid-1840s and early 1850s, in the midst of a new discourse of 'working-class manhood' that was undoubtedly imported to the colonies.[43] Labour in Victoria and New Zealand was highly seasonal, and thus demanded mobility and a willingness to be mobile, and it could interrupt family, friendship and domestic arrangements, and thereby induce loneliness and feelings of desolation. This was a pattern from the 1850s in Victoria, and also witnessed in Auckland and the North Island and across parts of New Zealand, as scholars have shown.[44] Single men, moving around for work, had limited access to a balanced diet of fresh foods and sources of nutrition, as a later section of this chapter shows.

Inside the hospitals for the insane, there were some opportunities for men to perform their masculinity in the colonial institutional setting through asylum labour. This was another way for the social differences among patients, particularly those based on class difference, to be used to force working patients to support the institutional economy.[45] Work was also gendered. Work was a dominant trope in the gendered discourses of insanity, and it was also a trope framed by expectations of ethnicity. In other colonial jurisdictions the non-white bodies of immigrant labourers were a contested domain, and became sites for debate about the suitability of bodies for specific forms of work in different spaces.[46]

Many of the men in both of these institutions resided in urban areas at the time of their committal. In Victoria, the gold mining regions and small towns north, west and east of Melbourne also generated small populations of the insane who ended up at the Yarra Bend, a situation that changed to some extent following the erection of new asylums that were built in regional areas from the 1860s and 1870s. At Auckland, the institutional population was drawn from a potentially wide catchment area north and south of Auckland, taking in remote areas and coastal parts of the North Island. But as with the Yarra Bend, the majority of inmates were also urban men and women.

The case notes of the Auckland asylum took details about the literacy of those admitted. At the Yarra Bend, it seems that no similar details about whether patients could read and write were routinely collated. Men at Auckland were recorded in the patient casebooks as literate – able to read and write – in fifty-four of the cases in the sample, which does not necessarily mean that other men without this annotation were illiterate. The detail does allow some insight into occupational categories of the period, with the literate men working at a range of often professional jobs. These include chemist, clerk, journalist, telegraph messenger, photographer, priest, Chief Justice (in just one case), solicitor, engineer, school master, school teacher and school student, book keeper, book binder, druggist, medical practitioner, commercial traveller and storekeeper. Labourers and gum diggers were also among those noted as literate. Of the fifty-four literate men, thirty-nine had registered birthplaces, and of those, most were born outside New Zealand, mostly in parts of Britain or in Europe. Although the Yarra Bend omits this type of information about literacy, from the cases of the men at Auckland who were described as literate, we might infer that men in similar occupations in Victoria were also literate. Whether levels of literacy, and occupational categories, tell us much more about the formation of identities inside the institution is open to debate: of the fifty-four cases noted for Auckland, just twelve were discharged recovered or improved, with five transferred to other institutions, and nineteen of these men died in the institution; of those who died, thirteen were single or widowed. Being literate did not guard against alcoholism, nor against other forms of instability; all of these men suffered from the same forms of mental illnesses as others in the institution.

Although it is not necessarily the case that men occupying these 'professional' and skilled positions were more likely to be urban dwellers, there is some evidence that urban men fashioned specific forms of masculine identity. The neurasthenic identity had not yet taken hold in the colonial institutions; at the Yarra Bend, only two men were diagnosed with either nervousness or hysteria, the closest categories to neurasthenia available in those listed in the cases for this study, while a handful of other patients were listed as having 'nervous' family members. Nervousness was sometimes attributed to urban life and the busy world of the city; but the few cases describing nervousness among men offer little in the way of a specific identity being fashioned for urban colonial men of the middle classes.[47]

Medical diagnoses: categories of the male patient

One of the major difficulties for the researcher lies in the interpretation of the many diagnostic categories used in institutions.[48] The diseases set out in patient diagnoses were sometimes overlapping physical and mental illness conditions: for instance, at the Yarra Bend, Thomas C. suffered sunstroke and then his melancholia set in, but he was also ill with tubercular disease.[49] Other men in the same institution, such as William R., aged seventy-two and originally from Glasgow, had been involved in accidents; he had suffered an injury to his head.[50] Organic brain disease affected many other men: Joseph R., a 'feeble old man' aged seventy-four, suffered from dementia.[51]

Age was a compounding factor in the many cases of dementia and illnesses of old age for male patients. At Auckland, seventy-four men in the sampled data were aged over sixty years. 'Old age' was listed as a cause for their confinement in just two cases, while thirty of the men were diagnosed with senile dementia, dementia with complicating factors such as melancholia, and dementia caused by old age. The sampled data shows that the Yarra Bend housed 219 men aged over sixty. Of these, fourteen cases were linked directly to old age and the stymied life worlds of the colonial elderly: living alone, living longer than a spouse and poor conditions. More formal diagnoses of these men, too, labelled them as suffering from dementia. Senility and dementia were the most common of these formal diagnoses at the Yarra Bend. More detail exists which includes references to the poor bodily conditions of the older inmates: one man had gangrene due to a foot abscess; others were feeble, lonely, or had alienated their families with odd behaviour, threats of violence, or had been wandering and restless.[52]

Brain and other physical injuries were more commonly listed as causes of insanity in the institution than historians have suggested. Colonial life was accident prone, and especially for men, who worked at physical occupations and sometimes in extreme conditions.[53] Among those men presenting with injuries and accidents at Auckland in the 1890s and early 1900s were an engineer, a horse trainer from the Waikato region, two millers, and a bush contractor. Again the notes for these men are spartan; but head injuries resulted in severe depression for Robert Frulove in 1909, while horse trainer Charles Napper was laid low for a time with 'trauma'.[54]

Men's delusions might also tell us something about masculinity, and these are briefly discussed here as they pertain to the diagnosis of 'delusional insanity'. More men than women were diagnosed as having delusions at the Yarra Bend and at Auckland. This was most likely the result of overindulgence with alcohol, as well as more men presenting with forms of paranoia and suspicion.[55] Men harboured suspicions of persecution, and some of their fears related to their domestic situations, as described later in this chapter. But the world was changing, and a few men believed they were in possession of heightened abilities to imagine mechanical inventions in delusions reflecting their times: in 1885, John Serastoun believed that he had 'an electric heart which ha[d] been transformed by the working of an electric machine', while Crawford Ferguson thought he had 'inventive power about boats, dental instruments, painting machines etc etc'. In an extreme case in 1894, partly because of his delusions that he should kill other people, 35-year-old Robert Brooke had 'delusions that a "flying machine" ha[d] been fastened to his body'.[56] Other 'male' delusions related to electricity, and at Auckland in 1900, Thomas Starr thought he was a 'theatrophone', or a machine that allowed people to hear live music from a stage performance through a telephone listening device, often available in public places.[57]

The diagnosis of GPI was primarily linked to men, and arguably became a hallmark of the colonial male profile in the institution. Nineteenth-century asylum doctors held views about masculinity and weakness (both physical and moral) or debility. Men diagnosed with the disease were viewed as possessing an inherent weakness of character. Cases of GPI present some interesting issues when read alongside other cases of male patients in the institution because of the questions they raise about male sexuality, physical decline and weakness. General paresis or paralysis of the insane (GPI), or the tertiary stage of syphilis, was considered a psychiatric disorder with an organic cause, and was a condition which affected around 25 per cent of those who contracted syphilis. It officially struck men aged between twenty and forty. It typically presented as psychotic episodes in affected men, with the onset of early dementia. Dr Frederic Norton Manning published his medical observations of the effects of GPI in 1880. Reflecting on the causes of asylum deaths, Manning noted that two organic diseases, *phthisis pulmonalis* and GPI or *paresis*, had particularly awful consequences for sufferers. GPI was a relatively new disease label in the middle of the nineteenth century and had been difficult to diagnose until the 1880s; indeed, for much of the nineteenth century there was uncertainty about its cause, and it was often only diagnosed after autopsy.[58] Writing about men with GPI at Auckland Asylum, Maree Dawson shows that theories about 'vice' and the lifestyles of colonial men were more readily attributed to cases of the disease than syphilis in the latter part of the nineteenth century.⁵⁹ This finding is borne out by looking at contemporary medical arguments, such as the account of the 'Premonitory Symptoms of General Paralysis of the Insane' by Dr Edward E. Rosenblum, the Senior Medical Officer at the Yarra Bend in 1892. Rosenblum's discussion of these symptoms was presented to the Intercolonial Medical Congress, and he posited that it was difficult to notice some of the early symptoms, which included migraines, sleeplessness and tremor, but in one case he described, the patient's tendency towards 'self-abuse' and 'sexual excess' were later read as examples of 'symptoms' or indications of the likely trajectory of the disease.⁶⁰ In only two cases – the 1903 case of 4-year-old John William Clarke at the Yarra Bend, and that of Edward Woolls in 1873 – was insanity and the GPI diagnosis linked to syphilis, noted in both cases as the cause of the mental disorder.⁶¹

The official asylum inspectors reports for 1909 show that a very small percentage of patients with GPI – less than 1 per cent – were housed in all of Victoria's institutions in that year, but the sampled data adds to the gaps in the overall official record for the time period. Cases of GPI present some interesting issues when read alongside other cases of male patients in the institution because of the questions they raise about male sexuality, physical decline and weakness. Ethnicity, too, was perceived as a useful category of analysis here: as Dr Ross noted in his 1889 address, the 'Australasians' suffered least from GPI, with immigrant English and Irishmen affected in greater numbers. Syphilis had become endemic in the major urban districts of Britain where larger number of prostitutes circulated in city districts, and where venereal disease was rife; men's working conditions of life meant they could easily access prostitutes in these areas. As the majority of patient cases show, the typical experience for men diagnosed with GPI was asylum admission at the point of severe debility, rapid physical and mental decline, and an institutional death, though some men died at home. The case notes for these men tend to be sparse, and repetitive. In the cases I describe here below, and as noted above, very few set out the cause of the affliction as either sexual behaviour or syphilis itself. It was, as Manning reported, an 'insidious' disease, and featured a 'strange mixture of sanity with moral aberration'. Sufferers tended to conceal their erratic behaviour, making the observations of family and physicians alike somewhat fraught. The disease ended in a descent into a calm and gentle dementia or mental weakness.⁶² It is likely that wives of men with GPI were unaware of the diagnosis, with syphilis grossly under-reported in the colonies.⁶³

Using a simple counting method, there are 110 men in the Yarra Bend sample with a clear diagnosis of GPI, or just over 6 per cent of the total male institutional population. However, the data shows that 'GP' or 'GPI', or 'GPI?' was listed as a complicating cause for mania, dementia, melancholia and a range of other diagnoses for a large number of the men where a diagnosis was listed (1,526 cases). This means that GPI may have been a much more widespread cause for mental decay among colonial men, many of them immigrants, than scholars have previously estimated. Over half of these 110 cases had a country of birth, with the vast majority born in England, Scotland or Ireland, and only three born in Australia. Most of these men were married, and their cases mention them living with wives and families. A few hailed from the Immigrants' Home or from prisons and other institutions. At Auckland, twenty cases of men with a clear diagnosis of GPI among 558 men, with a similar pattern of GPI noted as a complicating cause of mental illness, shows a smaller but still significant percentage of colonial institutionalised men with the disease at 3 per cent; most of these men were English.

The case of Alfred Crigan, a hairdresser aged thirty-two, invokes some of the contemporary language around cases of men who were in stages of moral and physical decay, such as those 'revolting' cases noted in the Immigrants' Home in the 1870s: Crigan was a married Englishman living in Footscray, a Western suburb of Melbourne, with his wife and children, when he was brought by police to the asylum. His 'habits' were said to be 'dirty and gluttonous' and he had to 'be carried about'. He had trouble swallowing and he died shortly after his admission to the asylum.[64] Most of these men were in a parlous bodily state; some were demented, others excitable and delusional; many slurred their speech and had trouble speaking, eating or moving their muscles. Their collective presence, and the growing use of the diagnosis of GPI by asylum doctors, may have suggested that immigrant men brought a distinct set of disease characteristics with them to the colonies.

Sexuality

The diagnosis of GPI, which related sexual behaviour and disease, is a useful one to illustrate some of the concerns held by nineteenth-century asylum doctors themselves about masculinity and debility. The subject of men and family life, and how masculine identities were formed in and outside of marriage and family relationships, is linked to this question of the diagnosis of GPI.[65] Western, imperial notions of appropriate sexuality and sexual expression emphasised the controlled male heterosexuality of the white European.[66] Tosh suggests that 'the dominant code of manliness in the 1890s' was 'hostile to emotional expression' and intolerant of gender ambiguity and homosexuality.[67]

This form of masculine sexuality can be linked to imperial frontiers, with their emphasis on power and control. Such normative sexuality – increasingly private, taking place in specific relationships – could hide and disguise white male violence against those weaker than themselves. It also promoted forms of inappropriate behaviour among young men, whose transgressions, in the form of sexual vice, appeared to hasten suspicions of mental illness in some cases. Male homosexuality existed, but was often invisible because of the predominance of men, and it was also censured by courts and in other ways through social mores for a long period of time.[68] In other cases, sexual expression could indicate illness because of its extremity. At the Yarra Bend, sixty-three cases of male insanity (compared with only two women) were linked to 'sexual excess', masturbation or self-abuse. The term onanism was also used. The vast majority of these men were single, and most were aged under thirty years. At Auckland, there were sixty cases of men linked to masturbation. Masturbation was associated with people of the lower classes.[69] The vast majority of these men were single and aged in their twenties. Only two of the cases of women mentioned overt sexual behaviour, one of them labelling it 'nymphomania' in a married woman in 1876.[70] Two cases of male 'debauchery' were listed at Auckland in 1891: Arthur Winders and Frederick Bould, but few details were recorded about their behaviour.[71]

However, in the case of Auckland patient William Drummond, a single cabinet maker aged thirty-six, one imagines a sadly closeted man unable to freely express his sexual identity; he showed 'no inclination for females' in 1903 and was admitted as an alcoholic patient.[72] Male homosexuality was illegal under laws which specified forms of assault, coercion and sexual acts including sodomy, but other sexual practices were also prohibited.[73] But men did have sex with other men, and were sometimes more open about their same-sex desires. Chris Brickell has provided a deep reading of the story of Percy Ottywell, a man who was committed to the Seacliff Asylum in 1891. Then aged twenty-two, he had been in a relationship with a younger man who was just fifteen. His behaviour was watched closely by Seacliff superintendent, Dr Frederic Truby King, who took an interest in the emotional dimension of the case, and who investigated Ottywell for aspects of 'weakness' usually attributed to men with 'perversions', such as masturbation, excessive smoking and drinking, among others, but found none.[74] Brickell concludes that Ottywell was not made marginal in the institution because of his sexuality or romantic attachments to men, but King sought his rehabilitation.[75]

Likewise, Brickell's examination of the playful worlds of New Zealand colonial men and their experimentation with cross-dressing, theatrical performances of gender identity, and close male friendships suggests that before the 1920s, male friendship was more fluid and affectionate than it later became. The emotional possibilities Brickell notices in his close reading of the photographic images produced by one man allows him to speculate about men more generally.[76] It was understood that puberty and its onset could also trigger male insanity. 'McDade the younger', a 15-year-old boy confined at the Yarra Bend in 1897, was a newspaper seller who had had a fit three years before, smoked excessively, and was diagnosed with 'insanity of puberty'.[77] Adolescent insanity was a category of illness made visible in the case records, and for young men, it possibly hinted at sexuality which threatened the acceptable social order. Of the four young men at the Yarra Bend diagnosed with 'adolescent insanity' or 'insanity of puberty', three openly masturbated. Alexander Dunn, aged seventeen when taken to the institution in 1909, not only masturbated but also swore at his mother and declared himself an anarchist.[78]

While the idealised 'language of domesticity'[79] was invoked as a way of settling fears about the wild independence of masculinity in the 1850s, domestic lives for some men could involve drudgery, unhappiness and burdensome responsibilities, just as domesticity did for women on a larger scale. Marital status figured in the official discussions about male insanity to an extent. While single men and their loneliness and transient lives may have appeared to dominate the record, married life could also occasionally be the source of other conflicts for colonial men. Of the 661 men at the Yarra Bend who were married, widowed or divorced, only twelve cases directly cited domestic troubles, family problems or marital discord. At Auckland, only five cases of the 228 married or formerly married men listed family or marital problems as causes of mental breakdown, with one most certain that a 'nagging wife' had caused a bout of melancholia in 1885.[80] 'Jealousy' and suspicion of wives did feature; men experiencing delusional symptoms reported feeling that their wives had been unfaithful or somehow presented a challenge to their masculinity. Whether or not parenthood featured as one aspect of male worry and domestic troubles is hard to determine from the case records and the sampled materials. Contemporaries did not make much attempt to link fatherhood to illness, or the work of parenting to men with mental illness. The institution did not routinely gather information about inmates' children. One way to find out about male familial violence is to examine the records of institutionalised women, who sometimes came to the institution for periods of respite from family strife. Women reported ill treatment by husbands in several cases, and complained about 'family trouble'; one woman, Mrs Charlotte Marsden, was confined with mania aged thirty at the Yarra Bend in 1885, and her two children were sent to an Industrial School, following the conviction of her husband who was jailed for bigamy.[81] Contemporary novels depicted this social narrative, too, drawing attention to the causes of insanity among women: one proto-feminist writer, Ellen E. Ellis, described her protagonist's visit to the Auckland asylum in her book published in 1882. The asylum matron told 'Mrs H' that there 'were more women in the house, deranged through the ill-treatment of their drunken husbands, than from all other causes put together'.[82] However fanciful or misguided about the causes of women's mental breakdown, the scene shows some awareness of the social impact of men's familial violence. Alcoholism among men contributed to female family misery.[83]

Men also suffered from grief, loneliness and fear. Wives, children and siblings died, creating a sense of extreme sadness in some colonial subjects, and this grief was possibly compounded by existing mental conditions like depression. The overwhelming impression gained from a scan of the large sample of data collated for this study is one of a population of people in need, of men in search of respite from the toils of colonial labour, family distress, and worry about work and income, especially for men of the working classes whose fortunes were challenged by this new economic world as the nineteenth century moved into the twentieth, with its accompanying mechanised labour and new forms of work and organisation.

Although historians have argued that masculinity was in transition in this period – from a 'rugged' form to one shaped by new ideas about domesticity and the role of men in domestic life – Angus McLaren finds that this was not the case in British Columbia in the early twentieth century.[84] Colonial societies still required strong masculine subjects: to perform labour, to tame colonial frontiers and wilderness. The oddly silent case of one man named Frances Hainler at Auckland in November 1909, who was described as having delusional insanity caused by 'physical inferiority', reminds us of the deeply inaccessible nature of these records, and of the currents of feeling about physical gendered identities in the period.[85] It therefore makes sense that men who were too weak to perform such work, or who shirked it somehow, were more vulnerable to surveillance and possible institutional confinement, as cases of wandering, mobile men show. Very rare cases of masculine insanity manifesting itself as hysteria, as the case reported in the *Intercolonial Medical Journal of Australasia* in 1897 suggests, also point to an emerging fixity of diagnostic categories in the period.[86]

WHITE MEN, WEAK MASCULINITY: PUBLIC ASYLUMS

Mobilised men: the male vagrant

Vagrancy was the most reviled form of mobility in this period in the colonies. The vagrant suggested predatory behaviour, a threat of criminality, and was prosecuted on those grounds, as my own and other scholarly work about male vagrancy shows.[87] James Cox, whose diary (1888–1925) of life in New Zealand presents an often bleak view of the lot of the working man in the colony, describes the life of vagrancy in detail. Written between 1892 and 1893, this part of his diary is rich with references to looking for shelter, sources of food and companionship, among other themes. The institutional case records provide much less detail about the life of vagrant men. Presumably because they were alone and without family, and because they had often been inside other social institutions, these men were admitted with few details about their lives, work or other descriptors. Very few of these records contain references to family in the colonies.

The admissions of men to the Immigrants' Home in Melbourne, discussed in Chapter 2, were a source of concern to colonists. It was this group of men, who had both not fulfilled the ambitions of settler colonial identity as strong and accomplished adventurers and workers, or settled family men, who presented a challenge to colonial society's sense of itself. In the Special Report based on an inquiry into the condition of the inmates resident in the Immigrants' Aid Society's Home in 1872, many older men were found to be suffering from poor health: 'Reckless living and exposure ... have caused many to become helpless for life', it lamented.[88] Peter Stewart and Thomas Witticombe found their way to the Yarra Bend from the Immigrants' Home on the same July day in 1891. Stewart was single, aged sixty, and had an 'accident to his head', and was referred to the asylum by the IAS and diagnosed with dementia. Witticombe was seventy-six, from Manchester, and a former labourer, who by the time he arrived at the Yarra Bend was 'demented, old and feeble', in the words of the case notes, and was later transferred to Sunbury Asylum in 1893. Nothing in their notes suggested reckless lives or abuse of alcohol, though many other men did fit the IAS description, as the casenotes for the Yarra Bend also make plain.[89]

At Auckland, one Irishman who called himself a protestant became a 'deserter' from a militia regiment and found himself labelled as a vagrant in May of 1903; he was one of only four men labelled as 'vagrant' at Te Whau.[90] There is some speculation that Irish Catholics pretended to be protestant so that they could be employed by the New Zealand militia, and earn social privileges including access to land, but many became deserters. At the Yarra Bend, while fifteen men were recorded as 'vagrant', a further four men were listed as 'tramps' or 'travellers'. The collective portrait of their experiences is one of a rough and dangerous life: many of these men had previously been imprisoned, or in benevolent and immigrants' homes, in other institutions for the insane or sleeping rough 'in empty houses', and they were uniformly brought to the institution by police or gaol warders. There were also wandering men who were characterised as escape artists, such as John Wilson who was a known 'wandering mendicant' with little moral 'sense', and described as 'mentally deficient' in 1891.[91] The rising number of homeless men in the late 1880s in Victoria, because of economic depression, was well known and vigorously debated by ministers, doctors and others with a social conscience.[92] Although not all those men who were homeless were labelled as 'vagrants' it is possible to find many other cases of men without fixed places to live: those listed as no fixed abode, or who were without any addresses (and recorded as having 'none') numbered twenty-four at the Yarra Bend. These men, too, were mostly brought by police (nineteen men of the twenty-four, with no other admitters listed for the remaining five men). George Weir had become a 'career inmate' by 1906 at the Yarra Bend: an alcoholic who did not know the 'day, month or year', he was described as 'frequently admitted into various asylums where he makes a quick recovery'.[93] Some vagrant men drew attention to themselves, such as Charles Jenour, an Englishman who 'went to the governor's residence to demand the rights and privileges of a titled person' and instead was arrested and confined in the Yarra Bend in 1891.[94]

Conclusions

This chapter has signalled the relative importance of arguments about whiteness in settler colonial institutions for the insane, given the focus in most studies of colonial insanity and psychiatry. It draws out some of the important historical debates of recent times in Australian and New Zealand national histories, too, by examining how institutional populations tell us more about the evolution of white identities for settler colonies, which were formed historically during the second half of the nineteenth century and which came to have deep meaning by the early twentieth century in various facets of colonial and later national life. 'Whiteness' was formed in the context of the mid-century belief in the racial identities of the 'Anglo-Saxon', which, as Edmonds suggests, came to be mobilised in British settler-colonial cities of the same period.[95] Marilyn Lake argues that historians must be attentive to the historical specificity around the formation of whiteness, also showing that white men were themselves constituting their own identities in relation to, and inside, the work of colonialism.[96] Immigration restriction legislation in the latter part of the nineteenth century, when white labourers sought to exclude non-white labour, are well known, and became a central tenet of the debate about immigration restriction by the end of the century.[97]

White masculinity, in the colonies of Victoria and New Zealand, was potentially flawed. The colonial conditions for men, with various pressures on their physical and mental worlds, could become appallingly stressful. The cases collected here and cited in this chapter reveal a population of broken men, rather than men who were always facing 'breakdown'. I argue that their stories offer us some insights into the gendering and 'racing' of the colonial society from which they come.

Medical constructions of gender and ethnicity have much to reveal about colonial identity making. This chapter reveals a set of formulations of identity through the fragments of casebook evidence available, and it has shown that some patterns emerge, as well as highlighting the relevance of single stories and 'cases' in the quest to fully understand how masculine identities were fashioned. Studies of ethnicity have most recently been situated at the nexus between the nation, the empire and discourses of racial hierarchy. This discussion has centred on the ways that settler colonialism developed notional meanings of whiteness as an ethnicity and characterised these through gendered identities: identities for men at work, in families and in bodily terms.

What emerges most strongly here is that institutional sites for those deemed most marginal to the workings of colonialism – such as the men deemed too weak or mad to work or to stay in their own homes and communities – perhaps paradoxically demonstrate the very flawed self-conception of colonial settler identity, its antithesis. As Warwick Anderson, writing about white male breakdown in tropical colonies, so effectively argues, the colonial setting provided a 'special resource for white male self-fashioning and its testing ground', as medical theories of 'instability' among men converged with ideas about the cultivation of white, civilising masculinity.[98]

By narrowing the focus of this chapter to white European men, this chapter does not mean to overlook other forms of masculinity; in Chapter 6, the intersections between gender, 'race'/ethnicity and class are examined in more depth through a discussion of non-white institutionalised peoples. These intersections also appear in the following chapter which focuses on white women and femininity, where ideas about whiteness are once more closely examined against the patient data in ways which show that scholars have not fully appreciated the implications of the question of sick, white colonial women in the context of settler colonial identity.

Notes

1. PROV, VPRS 7399/P1, unit 12, folio 330, 27 September 1900.
2. N. W. Pollard, *Homes in Victoria, or, The British Emigrant's Guide to Victoria, to Accompany Passage Warrants*, Vol. 1: *Victorian Institutions and Establishments* (Melbourne: Walker, May & Co., 1861), p. 10.
3. W. J. Woods, *A Visit to Victoria* (London: Wyman & Sons, 1886), pp. 54–5.
4. John Tosh, 'What should historians do with masculinity? Reflections on nineteenth-century Britain', *History Workshop*, 38 (1994), p. 194.
5. Tosh, 'What should historians do with masculinity?', p. 196.
6. Radhika Mohanram, *Imperial White: Race, Diaspora, and the British Empire* (Minneapolis: University of Minnesota Press, 2007), p. 166.
7. Mohanram, *Imperial White*, pp. 166–8.
8. Mrinalini Sinha, *Colonial Masculinity: The 'Manly Englishman' and the 'Effeminate Bengali' in the Late Nineteenth Century*, Studies in Imperialism (Manchester: Manchester University Press, 1995).
9. Penelope Edmonds, *Urbanizing Frontiers: Indigenous Peoples and Settlers in Nineteenth-Century Pacific Rim Cities* (Vancouver and Toronto: University of British Columbia Press, 2010), p. 182.
10. On definitions of 'manliness' in the period, including imperial and 'Anglo-Saxon' forms of manliness, see, for instance Michael Roper and John Tosh (eds), *Manful Assertions: Masculinities in Britain since 1800* (London and New York: Routledge, 1991), pp. 2–3; J. A. Mangan and James Walvin (eds), *Manliness and Morality: Middle-Class Masculinity in Britain and America, 1800–1940* (Manchester: Manchester University Press, 1987), pp. 2–3; and Mark C. Carnes and Clyde Griffen (eds), *Meanings for Manhood: Constructions of Masculinity in Victorian America* (Chicago and London: University of Chicago Press, 1990).
11. Barbara Brookes, 'Men and madness in New Zealand, 1890–1916', in Linda Bryder and Derek Dow (eds), *New Countries and Old Medicine: Proceedings of An International Conference on the History of Medicine and Health* (Auckland: Auckland Medical History Society, Pyramid Press, 1995), p. 209.
12. 'Yarra Bend Patient, in the bag', wood engraving by Charles Frederick Somerton *Illustrated Melbourne Post*, 26 June 1862; 'Hospital patient under restraint' wood engraving by Charles Edward Somerton *Illustrated Melbourne Post*, 26 June 1862. Both images feature as figures in Catharine Coleborne, *Reading 'Madness': Gender and Difference in the Colonial Asylum in Victoria, Australia, 1848–1888* (Perth: Network Books, Australian Public Intellectual Network, 2007), pp. 28–9.
13. Brookes, 'Men and madness in New Zealand', pp. 204–10.
14. Brookes, 'Men and madness in New Zealand', pp. 205–7.
15. Catharine Coleborne, 'Making "mad" populations in settler colonies: The work of law and medicine in the creation of the colonial asylum', in Diane Kirkby and Catharine Coleborne (eds), *Law, History, Colonialism: The Reach of Empire*, Studies in Imperialism (Manchester: Manchester University Press, 2009 [2001]), pp. 115–18.
16. On Christianity and masculinity, see Pamela J. Walker, '"I live but not yet I, for Christ liveth in me": Men and masculinity in the Salvation Army, 1865–90', in Roper and Tosh (eds), *Manful Assertions*, pp. 92–112; John Springhall, 'Building character in the British boy: The attempt to extend Christian manliness to working-class adolescents, 1880–1914', in Mangan and Walvin (eds), *Manliness and Morality*, pp. 52–74. Catherine Hall also locates the Christian Evangelical theorising of gender in her work *White, Male and Middle Class: Explorations in Feminism and History* (Cambridge: Polity, 1992), p. 86.
17. Miles Fairburn, *Nearly Out of Heart and Hope: The Puzzle of a Colonial Labourer's Diary* (Auckland: Auckland University Press, 1995); Annabel Cooper, 'Poor men in the land of promises: Settler masculinity and the male breadwinner economy in late nineteenth-century New Zealand', *Australian Historical Studies*, 39:2 (2008), pp. 245–61.

18 Angela Hawk, 'Going "mad" in gold country: Migrant populations and the problem of containment in Pacific mining boom regions', *Pacific Historical Review*, 80:1 (2011), pp. 64–96.
19 Bronwyn Labrum, 'The boundaries of femininity: Madness and gender in New Zealand, 1870–1910', in Wendy Chan, Dorothy E. Chunn and Robert Menzies (eds), *Women, Madness and the Law: A Feminist Reader* (London, Portland, OR, and Coogee: GlassHouse Press, 2005), p. 77.
20 This idea was prevalent from the 1850s; see David Goodman, *Gold Seeking: Victoria and California in the 1850s* (Sydney: Allen & Unwin, 1994), pp. 198–9.
21 Leigh Boucher, 'Masculinity gone mad: Settler colonialism, medical discourse and the white body in late nineteenth-century Victoria', *Lilith*, 13 (2004), pp. 56–7.
22 See Catharine Coleborne, *Madness in the Family: Insanity and Institutions in the Australasian Colonial World, 1860–1914* (Basingstoke and New York: Palgrave Macmillan, 2010), p. 38; p. 84; Queensland State Archives (QSA), Runcorn, Queensland, Wolston Park Hospital [formerly Goodna], A/45606, folio 126, Letter, 2 October 1885.
23 Graeme Davison and Shirley Constantine (eds), *Out of Work Again: The Autobiographical Narrative of Thomas Dobeson, 1885–1891*, Monash Publications in History 6 (Melbourne: Monash University, 1990), p. 25.
24 Patrick Wolfe, *Settler Colonialism and the Transformation of Anthropology: The Politics and Poetics of an Ethnographic Event*, Writing Past Colonialism (London and New York: Cassell, 1999), pp. 2–3; Lorenzo Veracini, *Settler Colonialism: A Theoretical Overview* (Basingstoke and New York: Palgrave Macmillan, 2010), pp. 26–7.
25 PROV, VPRS 7399/P1, unit 6, folio 159, July 1885. Stories of 'colonial fever' exist in other records, including a relatively detailed account of the deterioration and death of one man, H. Harvey, by several letter writers on a voyage to the Australian colonies in the 1860s; see National Library of Australia, Canberra (NLA), MS 4009, Eliza Kennison, Letters 1867–1868.
26 F. Norton Manning, 'A contribution to the study of heredity', *The Australasian Medical Gazette*, 17 July (1885), p. 266. See Coleborne, *Madness in the Family*, p. 59.
27 William Howitt, *Land, Labour, and Gold, or, Two Years in Victoria with Visits to Sydney and Van Diemen's Land* (Sydney: Sydney University Press, 1972 [1855]), p. 288.
28 See, for example, Davison and Constantine (eds), *Out of Work Again*, pp. 2, 24.
29 Dean Wilson, 'Well-set-up men': Respectable masculinity and police organizational culture in Melbourne 1853–c.1920', in David G. Barrie and Susan Broomhall (eds), *A History of Police and Masculinities, 1700–2010* (Abingdon and New York: Routledge, 2012), pp. 163–80.
30 Goodman, *Gold Seeking*, pp. 194–5.
31 Samuel Butler, *A First Year in Canterbury Settlement, With Other Early Essays*, edited by R. A. Streatfeild (London: A. C. Fifield, 1914 [1863]), pp. 78–9.
32 Frank Bongiorno, *The Sex Lives of Australians: A History* (Collingwood: Black Inc., 2012), p. 33.
33 Goodman, *Gold Seeking*, pp. 19–27.
34 Dobeson, *Out of Work Again*, p. 91.
35 A. K. Newman, 'Speculations on the physiological change obtaining in the English race when transplanted to New Zealand', *Transactions and Proceedings of the Royal Society of New Zealand* (30 September 1876), p. 41.
36 Michael Cannon, *Australia in the Victorian Age*, Vol. 3: *Life in the Cities* (Melbourne: Thomas Nelson, 1975), p. 269.
37 PROV, VPRS 7399/P0, unit 18, folio 458, March 1909; VPRS 7399/P1, unit 7, folio 190, 16 January 1888.
38 PROV, VPRS 7399/P1, unit 10, folio 112, 22 August 1894.
39 Stephen Garton, 'The dimensions of dementia', in Verity Burgmann and Jenny Lee (eds), *Constructing a Culture: A People's History of Australia Since 1788* (Ringwood: McPhee Gribble/Penguin, 1988), pp. 106–10.

40   Garton, 'The dimensions of dementia', pp. 67, 69.
41   Howitt, *Land, Labour and Gold*, pp. 284–5.
42   Goodman, *Gold Seeking*, pp. 149–50.
43   Akihito Suzuki, 'Lunacy and labouring men: Narratives of male vulnerability in mid-Victorian London', in Roberta Bivins and John V. Pickstone (eds), *Medicine, Madness and Social History: Essays in Honour of Roy Porter* (Basingstoke: Palgrave Macmillan, 2007), p. 127.
44   For his extended argument about the way 'domesticity' was both challenged and evoked as a stabilising force, see Chapter 5 of Goodman, *Gold Seeking*, pp. 149–87. For New Zealand, see Cooper, 'Poor men in the land of promises'; Miles Fairburn, 'Vagrants, "folk devils" and nineteenth-century New Zealand as a bondless society', *Australian Historical Studies*, 21:85 (1985), pp. 495–514; Miles Fairburn, *The Ideal Society and Its Enemies: The Foundations of Modern New Zealand Society, 1850–1900* (Auckland: Auckland University Press, 1989).
45   Geoffrey Reaume, *Remembrance of Patients Past: Patient Life at the Toronto Hospital for the Insane, 1870–1940* (Don Mills: Oxford University Press Canada, 2000), pp. 143–6.
46   James S. Duncan, *In the Shadows of the Tropics: Climate, Race and Biopower in Nineteenth Century Ceylon, Re-Materialising Cultural Geography* (Aldershot and Burlington: Ashgate, 2007), pp. 101–2.
47   Eighteenth-century texts attributed nervousness to the loss of masculinity or masculine characteristics, including physical labour; see Roland Pietsch, 'Hearts of oak and jolly tars? Heroism and insanity in the Georgian Navy', *Journal for Maritime Research*, 15:1 (2013), p. 76; Roy Porter, 'Nervousness, eighteenth and nineteenth century style: From luxury to labour', in Marijke Gijswijt-Hofstra and Roy Porter (eds), *Cultures of Neurasthenia: From Beard to the First World War*, Clio Medica 63: The Wellcome Series in the History of Medicine (Amsterdam and New York: Rodopi, 2001), pp. 31–49; Mathew Thomson, 'Neurasthenia in Britain: An overview', in Gijswijt-Hofstra and Porter (eds), *Cultures of Neurasthenia*, pp. 77–95; Katie Wright, 'The arrival of therapeutic culture in Australia: Modern life, masculinity and the problem of "nerves"', TASA Conference 2006 (The Australian Sociological Association), University of Western Australia and Murdoch University, 4–7 December 2006.
48   As David Wright argues, the more valuable route into understanding gendered diagnoses is by thinking about how the symptoms of those experiencing mental breakdown are ordered and described using gendered language. Such an approach also indicates the deep involvement of some family members, friends and even employers in the work of 'lay diagnosis'. See David Wright, 'Delusions of gender?: Lay identification and clinical diagnosis of insanity in Victorian England', in Jonathan Andrews and Anne Digby (eds), *Sex and Seclusion, Class and Custody: Perspectives on Gender and Class in the History of British and Irish Psychiatry*, Clio Medica 73: The Wellcome Series in the History of Medicine (Amsterdam and New York: Rodopi, 2004); and Coleborne, *Madness in the Family*.
49   PROV, VPRS 7399/P1, unit 2, folio 198, 1873.
50   PROV, VPRS 7399/P1, unit 10, folio 26, 1984.
51   PROV, VPRS 7399/P1, unit 10, folio 91, 1894.
52   PROV, VPRS 7399/P1, unit 6, folio 121, 27 March 1885; VPRS 7399/P1, unit 9, folio 54, 9 July 1891; VPRS 7399/P0, unit 18, folio 642, 29 January 1909.
53   John C. Weaver, *A Sadly Troubled History: The Meanings of Suicide in the Modern Age*, McGill-Queen's/Associated Medical Services Studies in the History of Medicine, Health, and Society (Montreal and Kingston: McGill-Queen's University Press, 2009).
54   NANZ, YCAA, 1048/11 184, patient 3878, 25 August 1909; YCAA 1048/11 149, patient 3843, 25 May 1909.
55   Labrum, 'The boundaries of femininity', p. 68.
56   PROV, VPRS 7399/P1, unit 6, folio 155, 26 June 1885; VPRS 7399/P1, unit 6, folio 147, 01 June 1885; VPRS 7399/P1, unit 10, folio 50, 17 March 1894.

57 NANZ, YCAA 1048/9 3, patient 2496, 12 May 1900.
58 Joel Braslow, *Mental Ills and Bodily Cures: Psychiatric Treatment in the First Half of the Twentieth Century* (Berkeley, Los Angeles and London: University of California Press, 1997), p. 73.
59 See Maree Dawson, 'National Fitness or Failure? Heredity, Vice and Racial Decline in New Zealand Psychiatry: A Case Study of the Auckland Mental Hospital, 1868–99', unpublished Ph.D. thesis, University of Waikato, 2013, Chapter 4, pp. 130–62. See also Maree O'Connor (née Dawson), 'Mobilizing Clouston in the colonies? General paralysis of the insane at the Auckland Mental Hospital and beyond, 1868–1899' (forthcoming).
60 Edward E. Rosenblum, 'Premonitory symptoms of general paralysis of the insane', *Intercolonial Medical Congress of Australasia*, Third Session (Sydney: W. M. Maclardy, Printer, 1892), pp. 670–1.
61 PROV, VPRS 7399/P1, unit 13, folio 22, 11 April 1903; and VPRS 7399/P1, unit 2, folio 196, 12 September 1873. Only one woman at the Yarra Bend, 26-year-old Lily Ivory, was also said to have syphilis; venereal disease was also mentioned in her record, which described her as nymphomaniac; VPRS 7400/P1, unit 11, folio 333, 26 March 1897.
62 F. Norton Manning, *Ten Years at Gladesville* (Sydney: Thomas Richards, Government Printer, 1880), pp. 4, 8, 10–12.
63 See Coleborne, *Madness in the Family*, pp. 83–4.
64 PROV, VPRS 7399/P1, unit 12, folio 320, 8 September 1900.
65 Jock Phillips, *A Man's Country? The Image of the Pakeha Male: A History*, Revised edn (Auckland: Penguin, 1996 [1987]).
66 Philippa Levine, 'Sexuality, gender and empire', in Philippa Levine (ed.), *Gender and Empire*, Oxford History of the British Empire (Oxford: Oxford University Press, 2004), p. 137.
67 Tosh, 'What should historians do with masculinity?', p. 196.
68 Bongiorno, *The Sex Lives of Australians*, p. 33.
69 Bongiorno, *The Sex Lives of Australians*, p. 43.
70 NANZ, YCAA 1048/5 89, patient 573, 21 October 1876.
71 NANZ, YCAA 1048/5 569, patient 1689, 15 April 1891; YCAA 1048/5 631, patient 1721, 14 September 1891.
72 NANZ, YCAA 1048/9 331, patient 2827, 9 April 1903.
73 Chris Brickell, 'Court records and the history of male homosexuality', *Archifacts* (October 25, 2008), p. 28.
74 Chris Brickell, 'Same-sex desire and the asylum: A colonial experience', *New Zealand Journal of History*, 39:2 (2005), pp. 158–78.
75 Brickell, 'Same-sex desire and the asylum', p. 173.
76 Chris Brickell, *Manly Affections: The Photographs of Robert Gant, 1885–1915* (Dunedin: Genre Books, 2012), pp. 154–5.
77 PROV, VPRS 7399/P1, unit 11, folio 185, 15 March 1897.
78 PROV, VPRS 7399/P0, unit 18, folio 30, 21 October 1909.
79 Goodman, *Gold Seeking*, p. 158.
80 NANZ, YCAA 1048/4 93, patient 1257, 22 July 1885.
81 PROV, VPRS 7400/P1, unit 8, folio 44, 23 January 1885.
82 Ellen E. Ellis, *Everything is Possible to Will* (London, 1882), p. 148. My thanks to Kirstine Moffat for this and other useful references to novels of the period.
83 Howard Le Couteur, 'Of intemperance, class and gender in colonial Queensland: A working-class woman's account of alcohol abuse', *History Australia*, 8:3 (2011), pp. 139–57.
84 Angus McLaren, 'Males, migrants and murder in British Columbia, 1900–1923', in Franca Iacovetta and Wendy Mitchinson (eds), *On the Case: Explorations in Social History* (Toronto, Buffalo and London: University of Toronto Press, 1998), pp. 175–6.
85 NANZ, YCAA 1048/11 217, patient 3911, 8 November 1909.
86 *Intercolonial Medical Journal of Australasia*, Vol. 2 (1897), p. 660.

87 See Fairburn, 'Vagrants, "folk devils"', pp. 495–514; Lionel Rose, *'Rogues and Vagabonds': Vagrant Underworld in Britain 1815–1985* (London and New York: Routledge, 1988); A. L. Beier, *Masterless Men: The Vagrancy Problem in England 1560–1640* (London and New York: Methuen, 1985); Catharine Coleborne, 'Law's mobility: Vagrancy and imperial legality in the trans-Tasman colonial world', in Katie Pickles and Catharine Coleborne (eds), *New Zealand's Empire*, Studies in Imperialism (Manchester University Press, forthcoming).
88 *Report of Sub-Committee of the IAS, Appointed on the 6th of June, 1873, to Examine into the Condition and Prospects of the Inmates – Male and Female – at Present Resident in the Immigrants' Home, Princes Bridge* (Flinders Lane West: Mason, Firth, & McCutcheon, General Printers, 1873), p. 4.
89 PROV, VPRS 7399/P1, unit 9, folio 55, 9 July 1891; VPRS 7399/P1, unit 9, folio 54, 9 July 1891.
90 NANZ, YCAA 1048/9 343, patient 2839, 23 May 1903.
91 PROV, VPRS7399/P1, unit 9, folio 39, 29 May 1891.
92 Roslyn Otzen, *Dr John Singleton, 1808–1891: Christian, Doctor, Philanthropist* (Melbourne: Melbourne Citymission, 2008), p. 46.
93 PROV, VPRS 7399/P0, unit 15, folio 460, 31 July 1906.
94 PROV, VPRS 7399/P1, unit 9, folio 36, 22 May 1891.
95 Edmonds, *Urbanizing Frontiers*, p. 181.
96 Marilyn Lake, 'On being a white man, Australia, circa 1900', in Hsu-Ming Teo and Richard White (eds), *Cultural History in Australia* (Sydney: University of New South Wales Press, 2003), pp. 110, 101.
97 Marilyn Lake and Henry Reynolds, *Drawing the Global Colour Line: White Men's Countries and the International Challenge of Racial Equality*, Critical Perspectives on Empire (Cambridge and New York: Cambridge University Press, 2008).
98 Warwick Anderson, 'The trespass speaks: White masculinity and colonial breakdown', *American Historical Review*, 102:5 (1997), p. 1346.

CHAPTER FIVE

Insanity and white femininity: women in the public asylums, 1860s–1900s

Miss Susan Cumming, aged twenty-two, was taken by her brother to the Yarra Bend Asylum in 1885. Although her occupation was noted as 'governess', her brother described her as a 'lady's companion' and said that she had met many men, but had few female associates; he thought it likely that she had been 'violated'. Her manic episode was brought on by hysteria, and had continued for more than two weeks before she was admitted to the institution.[1] Young women in service or working in homes as governesses in the colonies were thought by others to be vulnerable; their stories often do affirm this fear, but also show the circumscribed lives led by women in the period. Emma Thornton was aged thirty-three when she arrived at the same institution in 1906, and was living on the streets as a vagrant. The case notes remarked that she was 'defective': 'says she is 27, her mother 33, that her baby is her little brother ... hid knife in her breast ... when rescued she had a bunch of coloured rag which she said was very valuable'.[2] Several phrases here stand out in both cases: Cumming had been in the company of men, according to her brother, placing her at risk. Thornton was thought to be mentally 'defective', a central preoccupation of contemporaries when commenting on dependent women inside institutions. The institutional notes describe her as having been 'rescued', a significant comment given the prevalent view of women inmates in institutions, many of whom were seen as recipients of welfare and care which was not provided to them by colonial families.

The preceding chapter's discussion about masculinity signalled a range of themes through which we might examine the meanings of a gendered 'white identity' for the majority of the institutional inmates of the two institutions in the colonies examined here. White men who became welfare dependants, or who were unable to fulfil the ambitions for a strong and physical masculinity because they were weakened by mental disease, disappointed the gendered expectations of them, and seemed to undermine the ambitions of the white settler project to create a new society. Similarly, women had to be physically and mentally strong to help create a future population base; fears about the decline of the white birthrate in Australia and New Zealand in the late nineteenth century highlighted concerns about the fitness of white Europeans in the colonies and emergent nations of the Australasian world.

The fragility of gender roles in the colonies, in the wake of a 'project' of domesticity being fashioned for colonial women and men, possibly contributed to the stresses and strains of colonial life for both sexes.[3] Like the previous chapter, this chapter argues that whiteness found expression through gender in the patient case records. It uses gender as a category of analysis to explore the function and representation of ethnicity, at the same time finding out more about constructions and expectations of femininity for nineteenth-century women inmates and those around them, through both quantitative and qualitative evidence. Read together, these two chapters show gender in relationship and tease out some of the dominant strands of historiographical inquiry about gender and asylum confinement.

Specifically, this chapter examines the institutional identity of the white female patient through representations of the physical bodies of women, including asking questions about the emphasis on women's occupations, and on women's physical and reproductive health. It also plots the various diagnoses women received, also taking the stated causes of mental illness into account as a way of understanding the gendered dimensions of these diagnoses. How did women's mania and melancholia manifest as symptoms, and who noticed these? The diagnoses of puerperal insanity, and the problem of female imbecility, are addressed here to show that concerns over women's sexuality took different forms in the institution. Finally, the chapter examines the women who were labelled as vagrants and prostitutes and uses these themes to understand and gauge how aspects of 'white femininity' were causing alarm for colonial commentators. By thinking about the ways that women were characterised once they slipped into the world of the institutionally 'hidden', I suggest we might find out more about imperial gender relations in colonial situations.[4] This chapter also deals with the ways in which women were classified and grouped, as the previous chapter also suggested for men, but with a different set of inflections and emphases.

Femininity was used as a measure of sanity; how 'manageable' a woman was once inside an institution for the insane could determine the outcome of her hospitalisation.[5] Gendered prescriptions for women's behaviours and lives are located in occupational categories, bodily descriptions, ideas about female sexuality and sex roles, and in the interpretations of women's mental illness, all of which have received significant scholarly attention in many works of international history. This chapter places some emphasis on each of these themes in turn. There is much evidence, too, to show that most of these women were sick, and often very unwell with mental illness, and had been neglected or abused in some cases. Interpreting the way language was used about them is not offered here as evidence that they were wrongfully confined or imprisoned.

Femininity and colonialism

Colonialism brought new attention and focus on gendered roles for women which were formed in relation to economic status. While 'genteel' women worked hard to maintain their class status in the new colonies, fashioning homes, clothing and relationships based on class status and the performance of gentility, poor and working-class women simply had to survive and continue to feed themselves and their families. Many women worked in domestic situations; others were deserted by husbands, or thrown into ignominy by pregnancy out of wedlock. Still other women pursued freedom from marriage and, once widowed, carved out lives as publicans, boarding-house keepers or brothel keepers; the goldrush era provided some women with lucrative forms of work. Therefore women were afforded some new potential, and possibly even new freedoms, in the colonial world.

Yet much of this activity among women of all classes was still controlled by imperial and colonial notions of respectability. The Immigrants' Home in Melbourne in the 1870s reported with frequency on the conditions of the 'classes' of women it housed: the deserted wives, the widows, the young women with babies and the pregnant unmarried women. This tendency to imagine women in classes continued into the asylum and other institutional sites. The powerful work of the 'classing gaze' was and is a way to separate 'respectable' from 'unrespectable' women and to categorise them, with the effect of penalising some women.[6] Respectability was a powerful marker of social divisions in the period; the 'ideal of respectability was amongst the most important cultural baggage brought to Australia by immigrants hoping for dignity and prosperity in a new land'.[7] Respectability was heavily gendered. As Bronwyn Labrum put it, in her study of gender at the Auckland Asylum, 'another set of factors, specifically linked to their having crossed the boundaries of acceptable feminine behaviour, ran through many of the cases involving women'.[8] Femininity was 'enforced' inside the institution.

We could argue, then, that femininity was given new and specific expression in the colonies. But inside the institutions, specific forms of gendered behaviour mattered and were expected or used as a measure of inmates' identities. The mixing of women from all walks of life inside the public institutions for the insane perhaps gave some members of society pause for thought, given the emphasis on keeping different classes of women separate.[9] The identity of the white woman inmate was not static: an overview of her 'profile' in the institutions discussed here shows variations in age, class, marital status, ethnicity and experiences of family life and work.

The white woman inmate

Contemporary writers often focused on the negative effects of colonial life on the health of white women, such as Dr Mingay Syder's commentary about the bodies of women exhausted by 'ovarian excitement, frequent miscarriages ... of worn out constitutions and of prostitutes, accidents of childbearing'.[10] It was the female body, then, which signalled the potential for crisis, given its role in contributing to mental disease and mental breakdown. Colonial medical discourse seemed preoccupied by 'difference'.[11] This preoccupation with forms of difference – most notably gender, class and 'race' or ethnicity' – arguably became more pronounced as the nineteenth century continued.[12] Medical writing presented gendered and embodied forms of madness.[13] Ethnicity, sexuality and class were all embodied in the records of the institutional women, and represented in patient cases. The female body in particular became the site of much fashioning of notions of pathology across Britain, Europe and elsewhere, as feminist historians show.[14] The 'primacy' of biological, sex difference was consolidated and intensified through medical writings, as well as in social theory, in the nineteenth century.[15] Bodily differences, too, such as size, deformity or disfigurement, or bodily markings, are important as we consider the way that the body was a central trope of colonial discourse and used in aspects of social organisation and institutional classification.[16]

Ethnicity, on the other hand, has been used less frequently to shed light on gender proscriptions in the imperial world. Previous chapters show that immigration to the colonies shaped the institutional populations. One of the striking features of the data collated for this study is the low number of women who were non-white when compared with the male institutional population. Women whose racial identities were blurred or ill-defined, or who were Māori, are described in the final chapter of this book, but the vast majority of the women in this study's sample were white, Anglo-European. But the differences among this dominant group are important, as the book has also argued. Within the studies of unassisted immigration, some scholars suggest, English women have been less visible than other migrants, partly because they played roles as wives or helpmeets to husbands and other men. Information about women's lives as migrants was recorded less often than information about men.[17]

Imperial ideas about 'race' and difference circulated and possibly shaped colonial institutional treatments and record-keeping.[18] Some historians argue that the Irish were a colonised people, with the language around their identities particularly racialised.[19] Irish women inside English institutions for the insane in this period, argues Elizabeth Malcolm, were already disadvantaged by virtue of their class and cultural differences and the gulf between them and their male, middle-class doctors was stark.[20] It was Irish women, too, who generated the most anxiety around 'moral character' in various international debates about immigrants.[21] In addition, Irish people, together with some other ethnic groups such as Jewish people in Britain, were regarded as more susceptible to mental breakdown and characterised as violent, dirty and resistive to asylum regimes.[22] Some of these negative ideas about 'Irishness', as one form of difference, were continued in the new colony. The criticisms of single women Irish immigrants to Victoria show how ideas about ethnicity shaped and distorted notions of gender.[23] In his study of Port Phillip, *Garryowen's Melbourne*, for instance, 'Garryowen', a pseudonym for Irishman Edmund Finn, reports on Irish orphan girls brought as immigrants to the colony in the late 1840s to balance the sex ratio and to provide labour, and he shows how colonial newspapers had unfairly treated these girls and alleged they were harlots, immoral and dishonest.[24] The 'English' constitution of the new colony meant that ingrained attitudes towards Irish remained, and resurfaced at different moments, and took on special meanings in relation to Irish women.

There were more Irish women at the Yarra Bend than at Auckland, but both groups tended to attract attention for their ethnicity: for instance, direct references to ethnicity exist in more than half of the thirty-three women noted as Irish at Auckland. In the colonial institutions, some Irish women were described as provoking comment about being 'troublesome' and too talkative.[25] This meant they could be treated harshly, often right from the time they were young girls and women: brought to the Yarra Bend aged twenty-five from a nearby 'children's home', Ellen Dwyer's body showed various marks and bruising upon admission; these were said to be marks from 'being strapped by a leather strap'.[26] Other Irish women were described in ways which suggested a heightened awareness of them as 'Irish', including the ready use of the 'Irish' category in the records indicating ethnicity, or in references to their experiences: at Auckland, one 67-year-old Irish Catholic woman, Mrs Susan Quick, 'spoke of English treatment of Irish Catholics' in 1903, showing her own awareness of the social, political and cultural inequities between the two peoples.[27] The shared characteristic of many female inmates in general was their poverty and failing bodily health. However, Irish women earned comments which drew attention to their bodies in very direct ways: in 1879, an Irish woman admitted to the Yarra Bend, aged forty-three, but without a name, came with her 'clothes so full of vermin that they had to be destroyed'. Moreover, her body was 'covered in a rash' assumed to be 'the result of sexualizing'.[28] Other Irish women came with histories of 'vagrancy and intemperance', or living 'in a filthy condition', or were said to be heavy drinkers.[29] The narrative of Rebecca Aitken, brought to the Yarra Bend in April of 1900 aged thirty-one, shows how the lives of single Irish women working as domestic servants were shaped by misfortune and poor circumstance. Annie's notes mention that 'she left Ireland a little over 12 years ago' and that she had just given birth to a male child. She had also lost a female child six months before, and was imprisoned at Christmas suspected of poisoning herself. After just a few months at the Yarra Bend, she was transferred to Ballarat Asylum in September of 1900.[30]

Still other women had come to the colony from Germany, Italy, Spain, Denmark and other places: several German women at the Yarra Bend were married, suggesting they had accompanied men to Victoria. Their notes suggest a dislocation in place, with melancholia a defining feature of their cases. Annie Peers continually called out in German in 1891; other women in this group suffered from religious delusions.[31] Among the German women at both institutions were Lutheran and Catholic women, and while the practices of chapel and 'moral therapy' revolved around generally Christian precepts, the provision of Lutheran services was not common.

If the 'dominant' ethnicity was 'British', who were the white women in the majority? 'Locating' ethnicity involves looking at the various signs and signals of ethnic difference before 'ethnicity' was a popular concept or term. Accent, language, appearance, names, as well as behaviours, religious faith, the content of delusions and so on, are all clues to embodied and lived 'identities' shaped by place and notions of belonging. But the primary way that institutions thought about national identity concepts was through birthplace, and the details gathered about places of birth, sometimes including county, town or city, tell us much about the collective identities of the majority of inmates, at least among those where information was recorded.

'British' women included, then, the 121 English women at the Yarra Bend, many of them born in London, Birmingham or Manchester (32) with the vast majority from London. These were women from cities, not farming areas. Their occupations ranged from domestic servant, housewife and shopkeeper to laundress, factory hand and teacher. While one woman believed her marriage certificate showed she was related to the Queen, another woman feared the 'Fenians' were attacking. Several women had delusions about time and place, thinking they had come directly from parts of England, or believed themselves to still be living there. In 1885, the 'worry of home' continued to affect one woman, Elizabeth Hornby, who was 'in a very restless condition, the worry of home has upset her'. As the patient's husband appeared to be supportive (she was released on probation to him at least twice), it seems likely that 'home' refers to England.[32] The distance of these women from extended family appears frequently in the notes kept by the asylum recorders, reminding us of the relevance of these points about dislocated families, migration and mental health. Now that these women were institutionalised, they were no longer able to be effective envoys of their white identity; they were reduced, perhaps, to seeing their lives in the colonies as a form of imprisonment exacerbated by their actual confinement.

Occupations

The complexities involved in analysing female occupations in historical context have been outlined by historians interested in occupational structures over long periods of time. Given that, as historians show, women have often been assumed to be in part-time employment, or defined through their marital status, the challenge to fully understood women's work outside the home in the past has been immense.[33] Here, I have selected some categories of female occupations which received attention in the colonial world, including the dominant and more marginal careers of women, to explore the meanings of colonial women's identities as evinced through the institutional record. The evidence, however imprecise, is nonetheless suggestive, and tells us new things about colonial women inside institutions.[34]

Domestic service

Domestic service was critical to the maintenance of the English class structure in the nineteenth century. In the middle of the century, domestic servants 'formed the biggest category of employed persons' in Britain.[35] During the nineteenth century and particularly in the period under investigation, from the 1870s onwards, huge numbers of women took their place among the mobile journeyers crossing the ocean in search of new opportunities, and many of them were looking for work as domestic servants.[36] Many of these women were unmarried: as single women of empire, they became 'free agents' in their search for new lives.[37] They were sought after in Australia as servants, being well-trained and superior, at least in the eyes of colonists and settlers who wished to employ good domestic help.[38] However, this was changing over the period 1870 to 1910; by 1911, as the colonial Census data shows, more women in the younger age group of fifteen to nineteen years were choosing factory work, while older women continued to work in domestic service.[39] Nonetheless, the number of women inside the institutions whose occupation was listed as domestic servant is evidence of their continued presence in the labour force, if not their relatively vulnerable status inside homes and households, where younger women might be victims of male predators, and also, conflicts with other women.[40] This type of vulnerability and conflict could leave them more prone to mental distress. They also lived outside their own family situations, another constant concern of asylum doctors and administrators.[41]

The majority of domestic servants admitted to the Yarra Bend in the period were single women. Of the 269 women designated as domestic servants (or similar explicit label of paid domestic work outside the home) 170 were single, and 141 of these were aged between fifteen and forty-five. In their childbearing years, these women were likely to have experienced sexual contact with men outside marriage. The euphemistic 'trouble', listed as a cause of insanity for 40-year-old Catholic Mary Farrell, hid what appeared to be an unmentionable experience; Augusta Hugg was noted by police as having two children 'though unmarried'.[42] Among the thirty-six women at the Auckland Asylum who had been domestic servants before their institutional committal were twenty-two single women.[43] Although pregnancy was not recorded in any of their cases, these women had suffered disappointment in love, and one had experienced puerperal insanity, suggesting she had been pregnant.

Governess employment

The Female Middle Class Emigration Society was formed in London in 1862. Women emigrated between the early 1860s and the mid-1880s under the auspices of this scheme, and found their way to most Australian colonies and capital cities, and to New Zealand. Patricia Clarke's research into these women through their letters and some additional surviving documentation shows that some women had a poor start in the colonies looking for governess work, their situations already precarious because of problems with governess employment in

Britain. Some women were, for example, already stymied by a relative lack of experience, or by problems with colonial climates.[44]

The governess 'crisis' in 1850s Britain, discussed by Joseph Melling, identifies some useful points for understanding the presence of teachers and governesses in the institutions of the later period. An evolving class structure in Britain in the middle of the nineteenth century meant that some educated women were poised between domestic work or teaching work inside the home, which meant their domestic roles as single women were blurred and ambiguous.[45] In the opening example for this chapter, for instance, Susan Cumming's brother does not describe her as a 'governess', but instead as a 'lady's companion'. There may not have been a 'distinctive' colonial narrative of 'the governess', as had happened in England, but there were women who possibly also occupied a peculiar status inside the domestic spaces of colonial homes before they appeared inside institutions. Sybylla, the central character in Miles Franklin's novel *My Brilliant Career*, exemplifies this particular colonial identity for educated but lower- to middle-class women who were caught between needing to earn a living once they were of age and unmarried, and who keenly felt the unpleasant and risky situations they encountered as single women in colonial homes.[46]

Accounts of living in the colonies by governesses who came from Britain in the period underscore this point, with women encountering difficult and lonely situations in the bush, or finding colonial towns and cities unpalatable. Most well known is the account of Louisa Geoghegan, who arrived in the colony of Victoria to find work for the wealthy Irish squatter family, the Hines, in the western districts of Victoria's wheat fields in the 1860s. Geoghegan disliked Australia, calling it an 'out-of-the-world place', but she persevered with her employment and relationship with the Female Immigration Society. Other women railed against the culture of the colonies and campaigned at length to return to England. 'I cannot like the Colony or the people. More and more I dislike both', complained Rosa Phayne in 1871.[47] From the point of view of the 'genteel ladies in training', who were educated by governesses in the colonies, the role of the governess was but one of several ways in which gentility was learned and proscribed for young women in the homes of the wealthy.[48]

The Yarra Bend and Auckland asylums both took in governesses, teachers, music teachers and women involved in religious orders. Their educational achievements could become, at times, a source of difficulty: the idea of 'over work' or 'over study' was sometimes cited as a cause of mental breakdown among both women and men. At the Yarra Bend, 'mental labour' was mentioned in a few cases of women, among them, one governess, two teachers and two domestic servants.

Anna Fraser, a servant, was believed to be affected by 'novel reading' in 1894. The governess, Annie Luibher, had an 'overtaxed' brain due to 'spiritism' in 1885. Housemaid Millicent Pearce, aged thirty in 1909, came to the Yarra Bend with an anxious family in the background. Her sister wrote a letter asking that she not see anyone who might upset her, if the Medical Superintendent believed them to be distressing to her sister 'in any way'; she also requested information about her sister's well-being. Millicent was still in the asylum in 1922.[49] Female literacy was mentioned in just thirteen cases at Auckland, and these women were almost all known to be teachers. 'Overstudy' was mentioned in just one of these cases: Miss Edith Mary Hawkeswood, aged nineteen, who was living in Auckland and admitted to the institution in 1891, but no formal diagnosis was ever recorded in her case.[50]

Barmaids and hotel keepers

By contrast, the barmaid, like the factory girl, was at risk of danger by virtue of her employment situation. Aligned with the prostitute, the working barmaid in Victoria in the 1880s became one subject for scrutiny during the Royal Commission on Employees in Factories and Shops which ran between 1882 and 1884, when the final report was released.[51] Medical evidence about the working conditions in pubs argued that the long hours and social consequences for women working both on their feet, in the constant company of men, and surrounded by temptation to drink, was bound to have deleterious effects on young women.[52] Yet it was difficult to 'police the boundaries' of women's work in the period, as women moved into a variety of employment situations both inside and outside, in public worlds traversed by men, and were experiencing more freedoms with increasing urbanisation in the latter part of the nineteenth century.[53] Women working and living in hotel environments experienced other forms of conflict and tension.[54]

'Barmaid' was listed as an occupation in just a few cases at the Yarra Bend, along with 'Hotel keeper', 'publican' and 'publican's wife'. Of the total of eight hotel workers listed, two barmaids were diagnosed as alcoholics: Ada Jane Handley had a 'careless and irresponsible' manner, and was 'violent when in a temper'; before her admission, she 'had been drinking heavily and [been] out all night'.[55] Such a description supported the fears about hotel work for women: that it led women to poor lifestyles, alcohol abuse and made them more likely to 'go off the rails'. Married German hotel keeper, Henrietta Fulder, had developed signs of GPI a year after her admission to the Yarra Bend, suggesting that she had also been in contact with men with syphilis.[56] Yet the fact that so few women were admitted as hotel workers (with only four at Auckland) shows that this profession was not, in itself, destined to drive women mad. The preponderance of married women with insanity caused by the conditions of married life, childbirth and related domestic worries was far more striking in social terms than the 'diseased barmaid'.

Other occupations listed for women at both institutions, such as milliner (sometimes listed as hat maker), seamstress, factory hand or worker, tailoress, needlewoman, bootmaker, shirtmaker and grocer or fruiterer, remind us of the growing diversity of women's work in the period, especially from the late 1870s and 1880s in the colonies. However, the urban identities of women pursuing independent, waged work outside the home are very difficult to examine using just the scant descriptions of these women in the institutional record. Additional analysis of their presence in the social and economic worlds of the colony in relation to existing studies of gender and labour might tell us more about their colonial identities.[57]

Dependants

Women also came to the institution as the wives or daughters of men whose professions were noted in the record. As the previous chapter suggested, these women were dependants on men, and their identities were formed in relation to their status as wives or daughters; in relation therefore to men. Such identities also need further teasing out to be fully understood as aspects of identity formation. For example, the category of 'settler's daughter' was one defined in relation to respectability. Although the number of cases where a woman's profession was listed explicitly as a 'wife' – or 'married woman', or a wife of a man of a certain profession – was relatively small, many more 'wives' existed in the institution.

A number of women were described as 'wives' under the heading 'occupation'. In 1903, Louisa Rankin spent time at the Yarra Bend Asylum. The wife of a farmer at Morwell, in Gippsland, Rankin had spent long periods of time alone 'in the bush'. Gippsland was settled in the 1860s but was still remote from urban areas; east of Melbourne by coach or train, it took several hours to make the journey to the city. Most of the farming districts surrounding the small town of Morwell were also at a distance. Rankin's sister commented that 'she has a child three weeks old' and that Louisa herself was said to be 'stranger in her manner' as she had 'lived in the bush almost alone for long periods' (due to her husband's occupation). In her story, then, being the wife of a farmer was less than 'respectable': it had involved her losing social contacts and going mad with loneliness.[58] The designation of 'wife' could also indicate that others were available to intercede on behalf of these women, as in the case of 21-year-old Elizabeth Hagley, taken to the Yarra Bend in 1906 following childbirth, whose brother wrote to ask that she be allowed out on trial. He suggested that he and his 'sister would do everything that will please her'.[59] It also possibly signalled to institutional authorities the fact that these women were of lesser or greater status: the wife of a clergyman or missionary, for example, might be seen as more educated than the wife of a small farmer; conversely, wives of small farmers were known to contribute much to their family incomes through their own labour, and were sometimes admitted suffering from exhaustion.

The designation 'settler's wife' seems to connote a different meaning about status, especially when used in New Zealand. Three 'settler's wives' admitted to Auckland stand apart from the wives of farmers or labourers, and suggest elevated class identities in the context of the period. Though the three committals of Emma Watson, admitted in 1870, Jane Clarke, admitted in 1873, and Rose Lowe, admitted in 1903, were separated by thirty years, the meaning of the term settler's wife had not diminished over time.[60] Daughters, those women described as 'living at home', contributed to the domestic work of the household in unpaid capacities.

One final label attributed to some women was 'lady'. Elizabeth Chambers Wallace, thirty-seven, was admitted to Auckland with melancholia due to a 'fright' in 1897.[61] Other 'ladies' included three at the Yarra Bend, at least one of whom appeared to have lived in and around the British Empire and become idle and depressed. Miss Frances Brady, a New Zealand-born lady, was single, aged thirty-six, when taken with acute mania to the Yarra Bend. She seems to have suffered an attack onboard a ship in 1879 (the *S.S. Rotorua*) and by the time she went to the Yarra Bend, she was 'in a delicate state of health'. She was removed on probation in 1880, but died ten days later. The very melancholic widowed Elizabeth Tonsmore, aged fifty-three, imagined 'her brain [was] permanently injured from drinking gin every morning (which she does not do)'. Finally, Miss Rose Stanley, whose residence was listed as 'India' for the previous sixteen years, and who had 'never done any work', went to the Yarra Bend in 1903. Her sister stated that Rose's state was 'a relapse of similar troubles in India (believes she has been bayonetted and that bits of iron are lodged in her body)'. She was later transferred to Ballarat Asylum in August of the same year.[62]

Medical diagnoses: categories of the female patient

The previous chapter suggested that there were specific diagnoses that more often pertained to men to show how institutional and medical 'identities' were formed through medical diagnoses. Again, this chapter seeks to simply locate women's most common mental illness diagnoses inside a discussion about the ways in which these categories could be used and interpreted, without aiming to provide an exhaustive discussion of medical diagnoses or meanings of specific illnesses. The rise of a discussion about the 'mental defective' was beginning in the late nineteenth century, and it took hold in the first two decades of the twentieth. The effective 'care and control' of women inmates began to take place in separate institutions, built in the first decades of the twentieth century.[63] Mentally defective women were among those who posed the greatest concerns for the well-being of families, the future colony, and who represented a drain on the welfare economy. Allied to concerns about mental defect, open displays of inappropriate sexuality were reviled. The majority of women inside institutions had experienced forms of mental breakdown that sprang from their lives as wives and mothers, and were both social and biological in origin. Their stories form an important part of this discussion about the ways that ordinary life presented mental illness challenges to women from all walks of life.

Mental defects among women

The special report of the Immigrants' Aid Society committee appointed in August 1872 to examine the Immigrants' Home, as noted in Chapter 2, mentioned women 'sick and incompetent from mental defect', which was an often-repeated phrase in the annual reports of the IAS.[64] The incompetence of women to care for infants or for older children, should they become mothers, was certainly frightening. Mental defects were often inherited, and contemporaries noted, too, the hereditary nature of mental illness in general, concerned to avoid its repetition.[65]

Diagnoses such as 'imbecile', 'feeble-minded', 'idiot' or 'idiocy' were more straightforward than other diagnoses, insofar as the records show a specific clarity about the labels used, rather than listing various possibilities. These diagnostic categories could also be complicated by other conditions such as epilepsy. At the Yarra Bend, fifty women were confined as imbeciles, idiots or feeble-minded. Where ages were known, the majority were aged in their teens or twenties (twenty-seven women), with a few older (nine), and the oldest inmate was aged fifty-eight. Fourteen of the women were under fifteen years of age. The children were at risk in their homes, and at the Yarra Bend, of unscrupulous adults; one girl reported 'sexual tampering'.[66] Several were later transferred to Kew Asylum's Idiot Ward. The older girls and women worked in domestic situations, but were reportedly physically weak, small, or 'abnormal', or were mentally slow and unable to process simple tasks, and had finally drawn the attention of someone in their world who had thought it better to admit them to an institution.

Many of the notes about the women with mental defects suggest overtones of protection, although some of these women were capable of working. Dinah Foodes, eighteen, had reputedly been disordered 'since birth', and although she was 'strong and robust in person', she had 'a strong sexual development' and it was 'difficult to prevent her mixing with low company'.[67] Jane Gibney, who was twenty-three, was described as 'abnormally small', and was 'apparently a girl who has always been weak-minded'.[68] Phrases drew attention to the concerns about intellect: 'power of mind imperfect'; 'always as dull as a child'; 'mental development much below the average'.[69] At Auckland, twenty cases of women with similar diagnoses show a trail of inquiry about heredity and some clues as to family patterns of imbecility in a few cases.[70] In Victoria, some of the younger inmates had spent time in Industrial Schools. Attention to their needs as potentially 'unproductive' citizens shaped their lives inside institutions after committal. The bodily shapes and sizes of women played into their diagnoses in some cases. Said to be 'somewhat small and malformed', Blanche Delman was twenty when she was taken to the Yarra Bend in 1897. Diagnosed with 'acute mania', nothing more is known about Blanche or her social situation.[71]

Sexuality and disease

Open displays of sexuality were guaranteed to increase the likelihood of asylum committal for women. The close association with such displays, and the fear of the contamination of sexually transmitted disease by prostitutes, was rife in the contemporary imagination. Sexual vice was perceived as a non-western trait, so when white women exhibited such transgressive behaviours, they were immediately censured. But drawing on the lengthy history of medical beliefs about women's bodies, an excess of sexuality was seen to be harmful, and was also linked to their delinquency.

In New Zealand, female immigrants incited debates about 'loose women' in the nineteenth century. The enticement to single women to emigrate to the colonies came because of the need for men and women to procreate to sustain the white British Empire.[72] Single women arriving as immigrants in the South Island, where many lone men outnumbered women on goldfields, as elsewhere, in the 1860s, were monitored for 'character' and moral behaviour. The suggestion was that their single status made them more susceptible or even likely to become prostitutes.[73] This colonial belief had a longer history: in the 1840s, Caroline Chisholm, campaigner for women in the colonies, intervened to improve conditions for female immigrants after speaking with women in the Sydney Immigrants' Home. Her descriptions of the pressures on young women coming to the colonies was an evocative account of poor living conditions, young women vulnerable to the world of the growing city, and the prevalence of the belief that single women immigrants were women of 'bad character'.[74] Chisholm campaigned for the 'protection' of girls who came to the colonies, because her impression was that without parental influences, they were likely to 'lose character and become burdensome to the public'.[75]

How shocking it must have seemed in 1885 that Mrs Nellie Armstrong would indulge in 'indolent behaviours and often [go] about almost in a state of nudity'.[76] Taken to the Yarra Bend from her home in Faraday Street in Carlton by a friend, Nellie was diagnosed as 'manic'. Women's sexual excitement was linked to hysteria and mania, and played a role as both a cause of mental breakdown and also an outcome of it. At Auckland Asylum, three women were admitted whose sexuality was expressed through masturbation, rumoured 'nymphomania' or caused by 'adolescence'. Many women came with bodies displaying marks of violence, injuries, open sores or rashes, including Emily Voss who had bruises on her body when she was admitted; she had 'lost all sense of modesty and decency'.[77] There were eighteen women admitted to the Yarra Bend with GPI. Most were married, and aged over thirty-five, and they came from a variety of social and occupational backgrounds, including a teacher and one brothel keeper. Presenting with similar symptoms to the male population with GPI, these women had difficulty in swallowing, were frail, scarred and delusional, and most (thirteen) died inside the asylum.

Family and domestic worries

White women had become agents of colonisation. With white men, they were to form a new society of families and landowners, people who would produce and reproduce themselves as the new governing group.[78] But for the women who experienced severe anxieties about their domestic situation, or who suffered ill-treatment at the hands of husbands or other men, the erosion of confidence and physical and mental health took its toll. Married women whose mental breakdown had been caused by a form of domestic strife were likely to be middle-aged and working in the home as housewives. Their melancholia about desertion, the deaths of children, illnesses of husbands, among other worries, conveyed a pattern among institutionalised women. Jessie Wright, aged thirty, had come to the Yarra Bend in 1900, 'despondent in appearance; negligent in dress'. She was said to have neglected her household duties, and 'wander away from home'.[79] The notes suggested the cause of her illness to be 'ill treatment by husband'. Previously hospitalised at both Kew Asylum and the Yarra Bend, and taken by police, it is possible that Wright was seeking asylum in the institution; however, there was also uncertainty as she was said to have 'delusional melancholia'. Similar cases show how difficult it is to know how far women's confinement was shaped by male controls of the domestic situation. However, like men, women could find marriage stifling and disappointing; they were more vulnerable to sexual and physical violence and to social disapproval when they did not conform as wives.

Younger women's identities could be affected by lack of opportunity to marry, or by the breakdown of romantic and social relationships which resulted in their loss of status in the eyes of others. Several women were found to be 'disappointed in love', and most of them – but not all – were single women aged under thirty. Very little detail was recorded about their cases at Auckland, but at the Yarra Bend, these women were variously reported as mentally ill following 'love affairs', 'disappointment in love' and 'love matters'. One woman, Rose McEvoy, who lived at a hotel in East Melbourne, was taken to the Yarra Bend by her brother-in-law suffering from mania at the age of seventeen, in 1906. Sexuality was on her mind: she accused her sister of being 'unpure'. She felt she has been accused of 'being a fallen woman' and appeared to be frightened of her relatives, and thought that she was watched by 'several men'.[80] Like her, 24-year-old Mary Northorpe, a domestic servant in St Kilda, had possibly suffered abuse or been let down by a man: she called on God to 'save' her in 1888.[81]

Women faced biological changes in their lives: of these, the stages of pregnancy and childbirth, and later, menopause, could bring about the most profound mental disturbances. A variety of terms was used to describe such changes, including: for childbirth, 'parturition', 'confinement' and lactation; menopause was expressed as 'change of life', 'ovarian trouble' and 'climacteric'. At the Yarra Bend, the many cases of women for whom these life changes had created severe mental distress remind us of the stresses of women's biological lives.

Puerperal fever inside asylums, or in relation to mental health, has received more specific historical attention than the menopause.[82] Puerperal insanity was also a formal diagnosis, whereas the menopausal 'change of life' was more often viewed as a cause of mental breakdown. Among those diagnosed with puerperal insanity, most, though not all, were married women. Following childbirth, these women were sometimes very unwell with sepsis and fever, showed signs of mental distress, threatened their infants, or were simply physically unable to care for them. There were forty such women at the Yarra Bend, among them women very weak, emaciated, feverish and some who were violent. 'Confinement' in pregnancy and birth was listed as the direct cause in fewer than half of these cases, though no cause was listed for the others. Cases of puerperal insanity at Auckland more routinely accounted for the illness by listing childbirth or the associated biological events of childbirth, such as lactation, as the cause of the illness for the twenty-one women in the data sampled. In both institutions, some women with puerperal insanity had been ill with some form of insanity prior to childbirth, suggesting a link between forms of insanity.

Debates about women in childbirth in British medical journals of the period tended to test ideas about women's femininity and propriety, as well as the biological basis for the 'disease' of puerperal fever.[83] Whether or not women were seen to be 'respectable', or affected by 'vice' and poor lifestyle, were factors that became part of a larger discussion about women's biological vulnerability to insanity.[84] Heredity was also examined, and signalled a family weakness. Of the Yarra Bend women diagnosed with puerperal insanity, a number were noted to have insane relatives, such as Georgina Barker, whose family 'admitted' that her father was also insane.[85] Read in the context of the early twentieth-century movement to ensure that white rates of childbirth would grow, concerns about women becoming insane after childbirth were perhaps provoked by the increasing emphasis on the meanings of inherited mental illness for population health.

Fifteen women experiencing the 'change of life' were taken to the Yarra Bend aged in their late thirties, forties and fifties with mania and melancholia, having lost interest in husbands, families or with deluded ideas about their identities; likewise, at Auckland, fifteen women in the same situation were hospitalised in mid-life and later, and that institution used the term 'climacteric' and 'menopause', neither of which was used in the sampled data for the Yarra Bend. The menopause affected women socially as well as in biological terms; their lives as potential mothers had ended, and they faced growing older, sometimes with fear.

Older women were also at risk in colonial society because of social ideas about their status, and the very real likelihood of their being alone and surviving a spouse by some time. The case of the 72-year-old widowed Annie Owen, who had a 'poor idea of time and place', sums up the experience of many older women inside the institutions for the insane.[86] At the Yarra Bend, 151 of the women in the sampled data were aged over sixty. Of those women, sixty-nine were widowed. Widows were often forced to turn to charity in colonial cities and towns, particularly during the years of economic depression in the 1890s in both colonies.[87] Interestingly, a number of these women were transferred to the institution from other social, medical or religious institutional sites in Victoria, including the Immigrants' Home, the Benevolent Asylum and the Melbourne Hospital. All considered to have dementia or diagnosed as senile, the women in this smaller group were among the most vulnerable in colonial society. Among the group of older women more generally were women whose mental conditions had made them distant or suspicious of family, or who feared for their own safety through their delusions about – or the realities of – their situations. No longer able to work, in many cases, they presented the colonial state with a population to manage.

Vagrant women and prostitution: gendered mobility

Feminist historians assert that the meanings produced around formations of sexuality can be traced along imperial routes.[88] The very politics of colonisation – the imperial project – were deeply implicated in the creation of meanings around sexuality. For example, prostitutes became, as Philippa Levine asserts, a category of woman watched and regulated in Contagious Diseases legislation across colonial sites.[89] Therefore it is useful to scrutinise the various ways in which colonial institutional records ascribed meanings to particular sexualities and bodily health. Just as Irish women were identified with notions of immorality, so too were the working-class women of empire. Terms such as 'prostitute', 'vagrant' and 'dissolute' possessed productive power inside a gendered institutional language.[90]

Women occupied public spaces on different terms to men.[91] Women moving around urban areas or in parks at night might be unfairly tagged as 'harlots', but Australian colonial society tended to see prostitution as both inevitable and also, sometimes, necessary.[92] The colonial mental hospitals used the explicit label of 'prostitute' relatively rarely, although other women in the pages of the institutional records, as noted above, raised questions of female propriety, transgressive sexuality and morality in a general sense. Where the label was used, it highlighted not only colonial worlds of female dependency and need, but also concerns over the identities of women in social spaces.

Prostitutes came with life stories marked on their bodies. Elizabeth Smith, aged thirty-four and married, arrived at the Yarra Bend Hospital for the Insane from the inner city suburb of Fitzroy in 1909 and was described as a prostitute, though a question mark raised issues about her status. Notes about her in the case book include her tendency to almost continually talk using 'obscene language'. She had 'tattoo marks on both arms', looked 'to be suffering from effects of drink', and called out for her sister. On her person, she carried a letter to her father with a message for her husband and sister.[93] Another, 'M. J.', aged seventeen, was pregnant, and 'suffering from secondary syphilis with [a] sore throat', while other women came in various states of pregnancy or

[156]

with infants: Annie O'Brien, who was 'very unsteady on her feet', gave birth in the institution in 1894.[94]

Vagrant women evoked still other institutional responses. Over the course of the nineteenth century middle-class meanings of 'respectability' increasingly became benchmarks for the poor and socially disenfranchised, issues which impacted upon the institutionalisation of some poor, homeless, drunk or similarly 'unproductive' citizens in the colonial context.[95] The vagrancy laws in Victoria and New Zealand were used to police both prostitutes, and also lower-class women who moved in and out of *de facto* relationships.[96] 'Respectability' meant, for some women of the middle and upper classes, keeping themselves away and separate from women of the lesser ranks, a practice of social distinction pilloried in the satirical press of the era.[97] The 'persistent mobility' of these less respectable women challenged expectations of settlement and white settler culture.[98] Among the vagrant women at the Yarra Bend was German woman Auguste Shase, whose case notes were virtually empty, suggesting she was somewhat inaccessible to observers.[99] One Irish woman admitted to the Yarra Bend Lunatic Asylum in March 1897 earned the unique label of 'Dissolute Vagrant' as her occupation.[100] Vagrant women, and those described as prostitutes, were often brought to the Yarra Bend from other social institutions, including Salvation Army Homes or Benevolent Asylums, again suggesting the strength of this network of welfare provision which included the hospitals for the insane. The criminal justice system, too, was part of this provision. At Auckland, among the very few women described as vagrants, one example echoed the cases of women whose lives were spent in contact with police or the law: 63-year-old Kate Hinch, admitted in July 1900, was released in November. Her notes read that within a week of discharge, she was at the Police Court, charged as 'drunk and disorderly', and that she had spent most of her life in prison.[101]

Conclusions

Understanding these different aspects of the identities of white women inmates in the colonial hospitals for the insane presents a particular challenge of interpretation to historians. Women were the future: their childbearing capacity was ultimately the most important of their productive abilities. Yet their roles as wives, mothers and small farmers, as workers and as respectable citizens, were significant in the new colonies. These women were also being held up against an 'idealised Victorian femininity'.[102] To see these women become weakened by mental illness and its associated physical impacts, as well as unable to support the white men of the colonies, was to witness a display of the failure of settler colonial ideals. Although there are emerging understandings embedded in these materials about mental illness and its causes, I suggest that the information about these women is relatively limited, and needs to be read against and inside the colonial discourses of welfare and poverty, and its prevention.

The theme of 'rescue' should now be revisited. When Dr John Singleton told the story of the suicidal woman he met in inner-city Melbourne, in the Collingwood Watch-house, a woman who was brought to him as a possible 'lunatic' to be certified, he told a story of redemption and the rescue of a woman from institutional confinement.[103] An image accompanied the story: titled 'Saved from Suicide', it depicted a woman facing away from the doctor, touching her forehead with closed eyes, downcast; the doctor stood behind her proffering a 'jug of hot tea'.[104] There were other stories, too, of rescuing women from drunken husbands; and children from unkind fathers. Singleton's work was on the streets, mediating between families and institutional spaces. Rescue could happen through missions, through homes for fallen women, through the efforts of the benevolent asylums, and it could take place inside the hospitals for the insane. In New Zealand, too, women who became dependent upon charity and the kindness of others were understood through their 'female sex'.[105]

This theme of 'rescue' emerges throughout the cases of women who had fallen on hard times, with the institution for the insane just one of the agencies among the several that impoverished women might encounter during their lifetimes. This idea of women as a colonial population who needed to be rescued – from men, from poverty, or from themselves – distinguishes women inmates from men, and seems to suggest that women were more likely to be perceived as subjects of institutions, even though fewer women in fact occupied institutions than men across the period studied here, in part due to population imbalance, at least in the earlier part of the period. White women were perceived as among the most 'deserving' of the needy in the colonies. Whether this hand of charity was extended as naturally to non-white women is less clear in the institutional records examined for this study. The following chapter highlights the plight of Māori women, and those whose racial identities were blurry or indistinct.

Notes

1 PROV, VPRS 7400/P1, unit 8, folio 105, 22 September 1885.
2 PROV, VPRS 7400/P1, unit 14, folio 259, 14 March 1906.
3 David Goodman, *Gold Seeking: Victoria and California in the 1850s* (Sydney: Allen & Unwin, 1994), p. 167.

4 By 'hidden', I mean to examine the ways that individuals and groups were institutionalised and thus hidden from everyday view, but therefore also became part of the colonial archival record: see Catharine Coleborne, 'Reading insanity's archive: Reflections from four archival sites', *Provenance*, 9 (2010), pp. 29–42. I also allude here to the term used by historian Raymond Evans, in 'The hidden colonists: Deviance and social control in colonial Queensland', in Jill Roe (ed.), *Social Policy in Australia: Some Perspectives 1901–1975* (Melbourne: Cassell, 1976), pp. 74–100.
5 Catharine Coleborne, '"She does up her hair fantastically": The production of femininity in patient case-books of the lunatic asylum in 1860s Victoria', in Jane Long, Jan Gothard and Helen Brash (eds), *Forging Identities: Bodies, Gender and Feminist History* (Nedlands: University of Western Australia Press, 1997), pp. 57–9.
6 Lynette Finch, *The Classing Gaze: Sexuality, Class and Surveillance* (Sydney: Allen & Unwin, 1993), p. 47.
7 Janet McCalman, *Struggletown: Public and Private Life in Richmond, 1900–1965* (Carlton: Melbourne University Press: 1985), p. 20.
8 Bronwyn Labrum, 'The boundaries of femininity: Madness and gender in New Zealand, 1870–1910', in Wendy Chan, Dorothy E. Chunn and Robert Menzies (eds), *Women, Madness and the Law: A Feminist Reader* (London, Portland, OR, and Coogee: GlassHouse Press, 2005), p. 69.
9 Penny Russell, *A Wish of Distinction: Colonial Gentility and Femininity* (Melbourne: Melbourne University Press, 1994), p. 167.
10 C. Mingay Syder, *The Voice of Truth in Defence of Nature: And Opinions Antagonistic to Those of Dr Kilgour, Upon the Effect of the Climate of Australia Upon the European Constitution in Health and Disease* (Geelong: Heath and Cordell, 1855), p. 24. Syder also remarked that Europeans had made the Indigenous women 'barren', p. 29.
11 Megan Vaughan, *Curing Their Ills: Colonial Power and African Illness* (Stanford: Stanford University Press, 1991), pp. 3–4.
12 As argued in Coleborne, *Reading 'Madness'*.
13 Jacqueline Leckie, 'The embodiment of gender and madness in colonial Fiji', *Fijian Studies*, 3:2 (2005), pp. 311–36. See also Leckie, 'Unsettled minds: Gender and settling madness in Fiji', in Sloan Mahone and Megan Vaughan (eds), *Psychiatry and Empire*, Cambridge Imperial and Post-Colonial Studies (Basingstoke and New York: Palgrave Macmillan, 2007).
14 Leckie, 'The embodiment of gender', p. 99.
15 Ann-Louise Shapiro, *Breaking the Codes: Female Criminality in Fin-de-Siècle Paris* (Stanford: Stanford University Press, 1996), pp. 96–7.
16 James H. Mills and Satadru Sen (eds), *Confronting the Body: The Politics of Physicality in Colonial and Post-Colonial India*, Anthem South Asian Studies (London: Anthem Press, 2003), p. 1.
17 Nicole McLennan, 'Glimpses of unassisted English women arriving in Victoria, 1860–1900', in Eric Richards (ed.), *Visible Women: Female Immigrants in Colonial Australia*. Visible Immigrants: Four (Canberra: Division of Historical Studies and Centre for Immigration and Multicultural Studies, Australian National University, 1995), p. 62.
18 Laura Tabili, 'A homogeneous society? Britian's internal "others", 1800–present', in Catherine Hall and Sonya O. Rose (eds), *At Home with the Empire: Metropolitan Culture and the Imperial World* (Cambridge: Cambridge University Press, 2006), p. 69.
19 Christine Kinealy, 'At home with the Empire: The example of Ireland', in Hall and Rose (eds), *At Home with the Empire*, p. 92. See also Anne McClintock, *Imperial Leather: Race, Gender and Sexuality in the Colonial Contest* (New York and London: Routledge, 1995), pp. 52–3.
20 Elizabeth Malcolm, '"A most miserable looking object" – the Irish in English asylums, 1851–1901: Migration, poverty and prejudice', in John Belchem and Klaus Tenfelde (eds), *Irish and Polish Migration in Comparative Perspective* (Essen: Klartext Verlag, 2003), p. 130.

21 A. James Hammerton, 'Gender and migration', in Philippa Levine (ed.), *Gender and Empire*, Oxford History of the British Empire (Oxford: Oxford University Press, 2004), p. 161. Laura Tabili also writes about the use of language to describe the Irish in Britain; see Tabili, 'A homogeneous society?', p. 63.
22 Malcolm, '"A most miserable looking object', pp. 130–1. See also Carol Anne Reeves, 'Insanity and Nervous Diseases Amongst Jewish Immigrants to the East End of London, 1880–1920', unpublished Ph.D. thesis, University of London, 2001, p. 29.
23 Hammerton, 'Gender and migration', p. 161.
24 Edmund Finn, 'How Port Phillip was peopled', in Maggie Weidenhofer (ed.), *Garryowen's Melbourne: A Selection from* The Chronicles of Early Melbourne, 1835 to 1852 (Melbourne: Thomas Nelson, 1967), pp. 171–3.
25 PROV, VPRS 7400/P1, unit 6, folio 37, 12 July 1879.
26 PROV, VPRS 7400/P1, unit 13, folio 338, 15 July 1903.
27 NANZ, YCAA 1048/9 361, patient 2857, 28 June 1903.
28 PROV, VPRS 7400/P1, unit 6, folio 61, 13 September 1879.
29 PROV, VPRS 7400/P1, unit 17, folio 4, 14 August 1909; VPRS 7400/P1, unit 17, folio 502, 15 July 1909.
30 PROV, VPRS 7400/P1, unit 12, folio 315, 4 April 1900.
31 PROV, VPRS 7400/P1, unit 10, folio 94, 11 September 1891.
32 PROV, VPRS 7400/P1, unit 8, folio 62, 4 April 1885.
33 Jacob Field and Amy Erickson, 'Prospects and preliminary work on female occupational structure in England from 1500 to the national census', Occupations Project Paper (2009), The Cambridge Group for the History of Population and Social Structure, Department of Geography, University of Cambridge, www.geog.cam.ac.uk/research/projects/ occupations/categorisation/, accessed 1 August 2014.
34 I use the term 'imprecise' because my work here is not to exhaustively classify and group occupations but to show how some of these women's lives tell us about their institutional identities.
35 Liza Picard, *Victorian London: The Life of a City 1840–1870* (New York: St Martin's Press, 2005), p. 120.
36 Emma Robinson-Tomsett, *Women, Travel and Identity: Journeys by Rail and Sea, 1870–1940*, Gender in History (Manchester and New York: Manchester University Press, 2013), pp. 18–19.
37 Jan Gothard, *Blue China: Single Female Migration to Colonial Australia* (Melbourne: Melbourne University Press, 2001).
38 Beverley Kingston, *My Wife, My Daughter, and Poor Mary Ann: Women and Work in Australia* (Melbourne: Thomas Nelson, 1975), p. 30.
39 Kingston, *My Wife, My Daughter*, pp. 48–9.
40 See Russell, *A Wish of Distinction*, pp. 170–1. On domestic servants with stories of fear and abuse by men, see Catharine Coleborne, *Madness in the Family: Insanity and Institutions in the Australasian Colonial World, 1860–1914* (Basingstoke and New York: Palgrave Macmillan, 2010), p. 90.
41 See Coleborne, *Madness in the Family*, p.52.
42 PROV, VPRS 7400/P1, unit 8, folio 78, 5 May 1885; VPRS 7400/P1, unit 13, folio 302, 17 February 1903.
43 A larger number of women were listed as working in the home, home duties, household work and related terms, but this commentary is confined to those designated as servants.
44 See Patricia Clarke, *The Governesses: Letters from the Colonies 1862–1882* (Sydney, Wellington, London and Boston: Allen & Unwin, 1985), pp. 14–15.
45 Joseph Melling, 'Sex and sensibility in cultural history: The English governess and the lunatic asylum, 1845–1914', in Jonathan Andrews and Anne Digby (eds), *Sex and Seclusion, Class and Custody: Perspectives on Gender and Class in the History of British and Irish Psychiatry*, Clio Medica 73: The Wellcome Series in the History of Medicine (Amsterdam and New York: Rodopi, 2004), p. 181.

46 Miles Franklin, *My Brilliant Career* (Melbourne: William Blackwood & Sons, 1901).
47 See Clarke, *The Governesses*, pp. 103–8; p. 105; pp. 114–15.
48 Russell, *A Wish of Distinction*, p. 145.
49 PROV, VPRS 7400/P1, unit 11, folio 3, 8 July 1894; VPRS 7400/P1, unit 8, folio 67, 18 April 1885; VPRS 7400/P1, unit 17, folio 410, 5 Mary 1909.
50 NANZ, YCAA 1048/5 669, patient 1747, 26 November 1891.
51 Diane Kirkby, *Barmaids: A History of Women's Work in Pubs* (Cambridge, New York and Melbourne: Cambridge University Press, 1997), p. 71.
52 Kirkby, *Barmaids*, pp. 72–3.
53 Kirkby, *Barmaids*, p. 75.
54 Di Hall, 'Irishness, gender and household space in "An up-country township"', in Lindsay J. Proudfoot and Michael M. Roch (eds) *(Dis)Placing Empire: Renegotiating British Colonial Geographies*, Heritage, Culture and Identity (Aldershot and Burlington: Ashgate, 2005), pp. 81–97.
55 PROV, VPRS 7400/P1, unit 14, folio 287, 2 June 1906.
56 PROV, VPRS 7400/P1, unit 11, folio 336, 3 April 1897.
57 See for instance Raelene Frances, *The Politics of Work: Gender and Labour in Victoria, 1880–1939* (Cambridge, New York and Melbourne: Cambridge University Press, 1993).
58 PROV, VPRS 7400/P1, unit 13, folio 355, 7 September 1903.
59 PROV, VPRS 7400/P1, unit 14, folio 297, 21 June 1906.
60 NANZ, YCAA 1048/1 225, patient 170, 21 November 1870; YCAA 1048/2 177, patient 308, 7 January 1873; YCAA 1048/9 335, patient 2831, 29 April 1903.
61 NANZ, YCAA 1048/7 99, patient 2196, 13 February 1897.
62 PROV, VPRS 7400/P1, unit 6, folio 103, 25 December 1879; VPRS 7400/P1, unit 10, folio 41, 3 April 1891; VPRS 7400/P1, unit 13, folio 346, 3 May 1903.
63 These included Tokanui Hospital, which, while it was not specifically designated for 'imbecile' patients, did take a large percentage of persons in the category from 1912; see Adrienne Hoult, 'Institutional Responses to Mental Deficiency in New Zealand, 1911–1935: Tokanui Mental Hospital', unpublished Masters thesis, University of Waikato, 2007.
64 *Report of Sub-Committee of the IAS, Appointed on the 6th of June, 1873, to Examine into the Condition and Prospects of the Inmates – Male and Female – at Present Resident in the Immigrants' Home, Princes Bridge* (Flinders Lane West: Mason, Firth, & McCutcheon, General Printers, 1873), p. 2.
65 See Coleborne, *Madness in the Family*, pp. 54–9.
66 PROV, VPRS 7400/P1, unit 13, folio 347, 11 August 1903.
67 PROV, VPRS 7400/P1, unit 7, folio 38, 3 July 1882.
68 PROV, VPRS 7400/P1, unit 12, folio 11, 10 June 1897.
69 PROV, VPRS 7400/P1, unit 13, folio 332, 29 June 1903; VPRS 7400/P1, unit 7, folio 37, 3 July 1882.
70 The formal patient casebook pro forma at Auckland made more strenuous attempts to record the family history; see Coleborne, *Madness in the Family*, p. 147. Mental defects later became associated with sexual vice and degeneracy, and with racial fitness. Maree Dawson shows how congenital idiocy was constructed at the Auckland Asylum, pointing to the development of colonial discourses around national health. See Dawson, 'National Fitness or Failure? Heredity, Vice and Racial Decline in New Zealand Psychiatry: A Case Study of the Auckland Mental Hospital, 1868–99', unpublished Ph.D. thesis, University of Waikato, 2013, pp. 163–92.
71 PROV, VPRS 7400/P1, unit 12, folio 39, 24 August 1897.
72 Philippa Levine, 'Sexuality, gender and empire', in Levine (ed.), *Gender and Empire*, p. 137.
73 Charlotte Macdonald, 'The "social evil": Prostitution and the passage of the Contagious Diseases Act (1869)', in Barbara Brookes, Charlotte Macdonald and Margaret Tennant (eds), *Women in History: Essays on European Women in New*

Zealand (Sydney: George Allen & Unwin, 1986); see also Judith A. Allen, *Sex and Secrets: Crimes Involving Australian Women Since 1880* (Melbourne and Oxford: Oxford University Press, 1990). These arguments have also been made by feminist historians in Australia writing about convict women in a strong strand of historiography about female convicts, sexuality and gender; see for example Joy Damousi, *Depraved and Disorderly: Female Convicts, Sexuality and Gender in Colonial Australia* (Cambridge and Melbourne: Cambridge University Press, 1997), pp. 9–33.

74 Caroline Chisholm, *Female Immigration Considered: In a Brief Account of the Sydney Immigrants' Home* (Sydney: James Tegg, 1842).
75 Chisholm, *Female Immigration Considered*, Preface.
76 PROV, VPRS 7400/P1, unit 8, folio 48, 18 February 1884.
77 PROV, VPRS 7400/P1, unit 13, folio 43, 21 November 1900.
78 Catherine Hall, 'Of gender and empire: Reflections on the nineteenth century', in Levine (ed.), *Gender and Empire*, p. 67.
79 PROV, VPRS 7400/P1, unit 13, folio 51, 26 December 1900.
80 PROV, VPRS 7400/P1, unit 14, folio 262, 19 March 1906.
81 PROV, VPRS 7400/P1, unit 9, folio 142, 30 August 1888.
82 Hilary Marland, *Dangerous Motherhood: Insanity and Childbirth in Victorian Britain* (Basingstoke and New York: Palgrave Macmillan, 2004); elsewhere I touch on the history of puerperal insanity at the Yarra Bend, see Coleborne, *Reading 'Madness'* pp. 52–3.
83 Commentaries about puerperal fever also appeared in the *Intercolonial Medical Journal of Australasia*, and were focused on sepsis and treatment: see Vol. 1 (1896), p. 87; Vol. 2 (1897), p. 184; Vol. 7 (1902), p. 191.
84 Maree Dawson, 'National Fitness or Failure? Heredity, Vice and Racial Decline in New Zealand Psychiatry: A Case Study of the Auckland Mental Hospital, 1868–99', unpublished Ph.D. thesis, University of Waikato, 2013, pp. 193–222.
85 PROV, VPRS7400/P1, unit 7, folio 47, 27 July 1882.
86 PROV, VPRS 7400/P1, unit 14, folio 252, 6 March 1906.
87 Shurlee Swain, 'The poor people of Melbourne', in Graeme Davison, David Dunstan and Chris McConville (eds), *The Outcasts of Melbourne: Essays in Social History* (Sydney, London and Boston: Allen & Unwin, 1985), p. 96.
88 See Philippa Levine, 'Sexuality and empire', in Hall and Rose (eds), *At Home with the Empire*, p. 122; Levine, 'Sexuality, gender, and Empire', in Levine (ed.), *Gender and Empire*. See also Ann Laura Stoler, *Race and the Education of Desire: Foucault's History of Sexuality and the Colonial Order of Things* (Durham, NC, and London: Duke University Press, 1995); Philippa Levine, *Prostitution, Race and Politics: Policing Venereal Disease in the British Empire* (New York and London: Routledge, 2003).
89 Levine, *Prostitution, Race and Politics*, Chapter 7.
90 Levine's work *Prostitution, Race and Politics* argues for the possibilities inherent in comparing colonial sites, and usefully signals the importance of colonial and imperial constructions of social categories such as 'the prostitute' in both medicine and law; see Levine, pp. 4, 17.
91 Bettina Bradbury and Tamara Myers (eds), *Negotiating Identities in 19th and 20th Century Montreal* (Vancouver and Toronto: University of British Columbia Press, 2005), p. 1.
92 Frank Bongiorno, *The Sex Lives of Australians: A History* (Collingwood: Black Inc., 2012), pp. 44–5.
93 PROV, VPRS 7400/P1, unit 17, folio 278, 13 January 1909.
94 PROV, VPRS 7400/P1, unit 7, folio 79, 6 November 1882; VPRS 7400/P1, unit 10, folio 333, 12 March 1894.
95 Labrum, 'The boundaries of femininity', p. 77.
96 Bongiorno, *The Sex Lives of Australians*, p. 45.
97 Russell, *A Wish of Distinction*, pp. 167–8; p. 175.
98 Antoinette Burton, 'Introduction: The unfinished business of colonial modernities', in Antoinette Burton (ed.), *Gender, Sexuality and Colonial Modernities*,

Routledge Research in Gender and History (London and New York: Routledge, 1999), p. 2. Both Lynette A. Jackson and James H. Mills are intrigued by the 'women interrupted' or travelling women in the different colonial societies they examine; Jackson examines mobile women who were arrested 'out of place' in Southern Rhodesia (now Zimbabwe), while Mills studies the 'wanderers' in the context of colonial India who were taken into asylum care; see Lynette A. Jackson, *Surfacing Up: Psychiatry and Social Order in Colonial Zimbabwe, 1908–1968*, Cornell Studies in the History of Psychiatry (Ithaca: Cornell University Press, 2005), p. 17; pp. 99–128, p. 189; James H. Mills, *Madness, Cannabis and Colonialism: The 'Native-Only' Lunatic Asylums of British India, 1857–1900* (London and New York: Macmillan and St Martin's, 2000), pp. 68–9.

99   PROV, VPRS 7400/P1, unit 5, folio 134, 7 May 1873.
100 PROV, VPRS 7400/P1, unit 11, folio 327, 9 March 1897.
101 NANZ, YCAA 1048/9 29, patient 2521, 14 July 1900.
102 Waltraud Ernst, 'European madness and gender in nineteenth-century British India', *Social History of Medicine*, 9:3 (1996), p. 365.
103 On Singleton's role in female rescue, see also Roslyn Otzen, *Dr John Singleton, 1808–1891: Christian, Doctor, Philanthropist* (Melbourne: Melbourne Citymission, 2008), pp. 34–6.
104 John Singleton, *A Narrative of Incidents in the Eventful Life of a Physician* (Melbourne: M. L. Hutchinson, 1891), pp. 222–3.
105 See Margaret Tennant, *Paupers and Providers: Charitable Aid in New Zealand* (Wellington: Allen & Unwin/Historical Branch, 1990), pp. 103–26.

CHAPTER SIX

The 'Others': inscribing difference in colonial institutional settings

Born in New Zealand in 1875, Mrs Alice Sainsbury was taken by her husband to the Auckland Mental Hospital in 1903 suffering from puerperal insanity. Her mother's relatives were said to be consumptives, indicating, at least to contemporaries, some weakness of body. More worryingly, her mother had also experience puerperal insanity, and had become 'permanently insane', and Alice's own father had committed suicide.[1] Alice herself appears to have 'recovered' in the same year as her committal. Perhaps her future story would be brighter than that of her parents. Her doctors may well have speculated and hoped for this outcome, given the contemporary preoccupation with racial fitness, degeneration of the white 'race' and the health of populations. 'The time will soon come', wrote Anthony Trollope of his journeying through the colonies of Australia and New Zealand, 'in which the colonial will be stronger than the home flavour. It is of interest to inquire whether the race will deteriorate or become stronger by the change'.[2]

These words provide evidence of what Catherine Hall and others have described as an emerging 'grammar of difference' around empire, one that had to be constantly uttered to help maintain white identities in power.[3] It was the presence of the white insane that the colonies feared, worried about, and found at times detestable; the feeble, the mentally deranged, and the demented alike. The white men and women whose worlds had become small and confined by institutional walls were a signal of the decay of the 'race' for some commentators. As the two previous chapters have shown, healthy whiteness was formed in relation to its ideal, but it was also defined through what it was not, as this chapter now explains. 'Whiteness' therefore needs to be understood relationally, and as being in the process of articulation in this period.[4] White ethnicity was rarely explicitly described, something this book has also suggested in its account of colonial settler populations inside the institutions for the insane. Nor was whiteness, as Hall notes, uncomplicated or simply understood. Whiteness was the 'norm', and its instability, threatened by pollution, posed grave doubts about its future.[5] In general, too, there was a sense of the unpredictable about mental health; at a public meeting of the Auckland Institute in the 1890s, one speaker reminded listeners that public vigilance was important: 'the lot of the insane to-day might be any man's to-morrow, through fright, joy, grief, or a break-down in running the pace that kills in modern industrial life'.[6]

This chapter deals with the processes of discursive marginalisation of certain social, ethnic and cultural identities that occurred inside institutions. By using the term the 'Others', this chapter refers to the contemporary symbolic creation of an institutional 'opposite', and the forging of differences within the institutional populations studied here, to assert forms of authority and colonial identity. What processes of 'making foreign' some of those institutionalised people were at work, and how are these discernible?[7] Gender difference, as Mrinalini Sinha asserts, can become symbolic of cultural differences: Sinha's example was the 'effeminate Bengali' in the context of British imperial power in Bengal.[8] Whereas the previous two chapters largely dealt with gender, ethnicity and whiteness, given the vast majority of the institutional population was European, this chapter now examines the non-white population, as well as those who were in cultural minorities, and also again uses gender as a way of interpreting these groups. In particular, it examines two specific populations of the insane, unevenly represented across the two institutions in this timeframe: the Chinese as a subset of the asylum population, a larger number of whom were hospitalised at the Yarra Bend; and the Māori insane at Auckland, a group which highlights the comparative absence and silence about Indigenous inmates in the Victorian institutional context.

Thus far, this study has engaged with aspects of social identity expressed in medicine through and inside the institutional setting. Along the way, the study has also invoked aspects of the emerging discursive anxiety about the colonial-born and insanity, which in the early twentieth century led to mental hygiene movements in Australia and New Zealand. Therefore, the chapter also interrogates the ways that the medical establishment created both fixed and shifting categories of 'social identity'. Theories about colonial-born populations of the mad, specific migrant groups, and the intersections between these, produced a new composite identity for the institutional populations of the insane in the colonial context. The term 'hybrid' was used by contemporaries to explain the different inheritance of the colonial-born insane; they were not migrants themselves, and benefited from the positive circumstances of their birthplaces, but also took from their forebears the tendencies and characteristics of their kin, meaning that some were more susceptible to insanity than others.

This short chapter also touches on the rise of mental hygiene movements and their exponents, offering some insight into what were future glimpses of the treatment of the insane in emerging national contexts in the late nineteenth and early twentieth century in the separate colonial sites explored here. It ends on the note of very briefly prefiguring the form and content of Australian and New Zealand discourses of managing the insane which had emerged across the period of this study.

Existing studies of mobile peoples show that in different places, attempts to draw legal and medical distinctions between categories of person were bound up with concerns about population control and management.[9] For instance, historical studies of the Chinese as a diasporic people who not only moved through places, but also settled in them, show that the presence of Chinese triggered social unease among the European population, even while they intermarried and created settler families of their own.[10] Legislation controlling the immigration of Chinese was introduced relatively early in Victoria, in 1855, and in New Zealand, a similar law was also introduced in 1881.[11] Imperial legislation enforced for the purpose of controlling immigration to the colonies included the Passengers Act (1855), which aimed to ensure safe passage for migrants across the empire. In New Zealand, the Imbecile Passengers Act (1882) created specific provisions for controlling the entry to New Zealand of any person 'lunatic, idiotic, deaf, dumb, blind or infirm' who might later become a dependant upon charitable or government public institutions: it did this by requiring a bond from the person responsible for the ship discharging any such person.[12] In Australia, the Immigration (Restriction) Act of 1901 highlighted a new national attention to the restriction of a range of 'unwanted' immigrants, including those with mental illness.[13]

Whether the views expressed about immigrants in the 1870s demonstrate that colonial governments were moving towards concepts of mental hygiene, as Chapter 1 hinted, is debatable. There were far more pronounced concerns expressed surrounding immigration and insanity by the early twentieth century. Although the Imbecile Passengers Act in New Zealand was in force from 1882, in the Australian colonies the Immigration (Restriction) Act of 1901 introduced the concept of restricting immigration on mental health grounds, showing that it was in the final decades of the nineteenth century that such emphasis came to be placed on the way immigration was being viewed as contributing to the health concerns of national entities. Scholarship has highlighted the way that insanity became part of immigration restriction, and the ways in which 'insanity clauses' across places made certain forms of 'exclusion' from immigration 'lawful'.[14] This was a global issue by the 1920s. For example, different reports produced in North American jurisdictions shows a heightened awareness of the implications of mental illness among new immigrants. In Canada, a 1909 report by Peter Bryce, the Chief Medical Officer for the Department of the Interior, Ottawa, outlined the prevalence of insanity among immigrants.[15] A United States Treasury Department publication authored by surgeon Walter L. Treadway and published in 1925 showed that twenty-two years of data on aliens arriving in the country was gathered to examine patterns of mental health among new arrivals.[16] Both reports display interest in the rates of insanity among specific groups, but the Treadway report spends more time developing theories about psychopathology and race, and also examines the concept of mental hygiene in more depth.

By linking immigration and mental health, these reports, and others like them, indicated that worldwide interest in the mental health of migrants was one aspect of a new public health approach to insanity emerging over the later decades of the nineteenth century. Arguably, therefore, insanity was being viewed as evidence of the dangers of empire-wide population movement over the second half of the nineteenth century. The establishment of the colonial institutions for the insane was but one step in the direction of accumulating knowledge about the insane at close proximity, with the insane immigrants among their number.

The Chinese at the Yarra Bend

The Yarra Bend was the first asylum in the colony of Victoria, and operated from the 1850s, but by 1901 it was just one of several large public institutions for the insane in the colony. Others were established in the 1870s outside of urban Melbourne, as well as another metropolitan institution nearby at Kew, established in 1876. Therefore, other institutions came to house large numbers of inmates over time, including Chinese attracted to the goldfields of Victoria. While there was a group of Chinese inmates at the Yarra Bend, there was only one case of a Chinese inmate in the sampled data for Auckland Asylum, and therefore here, the discussion centres on Victoria and the Chinese in particular.[17] There were different forms of masculine identity in the institution, as I show elsewhere. White male patients were often able to work in the asylum, achieve 'recovery' and then attain their discharge from the asylum. By contrast, the Chinese were sometimes feminised and also characterised through their difference, both bodily difference and linguistic difference, and were also observed as a threat inside the institutional spaces of the Yarra Bend.[18] An official inquiry into Kew

Asylum in 1876 also reported that European patients disliked sharing the space with the Chinese patients. The fact that institutional authorities commented on this suggests that authorities considered separate spaces and classifications based on ethnicity as well as diagnosis.[19] Norman Megahey, writing about populations of the insane in Western Australia, finds a similar pattern of Chinese inmates being identified primarily through their racial difference.[20]

There were thirty-two Chinese-born inmates in the large sample of patient case data from the Yarra Bend, which is a small but statistically consistent number of 4 per cent when compared to the institutional population of Chinese as a whole in Victoria. Indeed, despite the worry over the number of Chinese patients exhibited in the official reporting by asylum inspectors in the 1870s and 1880s, the Chinese actually represented only a tiny percentage of the asylum population, and were not becoming a problem population in terms of their number. The overt worry about them as an institutional group came from the initial 'influx' of Chinese to the goldfields in the mid-1850s. Although most of these Chinese lived outside of the city in rural areas, over time, with the decline of alluvial mining from 1880, they came to reside in urban Melbourne, a shift which reminded the now dominant urban European population of their existence.[21] By 1901, then, the year of the Federal Immigration Restriction Act, over a third of all Victoria's Chinese lived in Melbourne. The sampled data shows that most Chinese admitted to the institution were confined in the 1870s, with thirteen coming from gold mining districts of rural Victoria, and all aged between their late twenties and mid-forties. Of the ten men admitted in the 1890s, most were on average much older (with the oldest man sixty-nine) suggesting they had come in the 1850s and stayed longer than other gold miners, and perhaps had fewer social connections to provide them with support, given the high masculinity of the Chinese population.[22]

As well as looking at when they came to the institution, we can find out who brought them there. Of these thirty-two men, twenty-one, or around 65 per cent, were admitted by police, with one of those admitted by a gaol warder; this matches the trend in the wider male institutional population, which is not surprising, since police admitted the majority of patients in the period. Almost 70 per cent of the male population at large, excluding Chinese, were admitted by police or a gaol warder. Police often assisted European families, too, with the admission and transportation of the insane.

Perhaps the institutional outcomes for Chinese inmates can tell us something more. Of these men, seven were discharged, and eleven of them died: of physical causes including pneumonia, dysentery, brain disease and GPI. A formal diagnosis was given to twenty-two of these men: most had dementia, others were diagnosed with mania, and few were diagnosed with melancholia, with only one formally diagnosed with GPI. Again, this matches the general population, suggesting that diagnostic categories were consistent here with the European population. In the general male population, almost 23 per cent were discharged, and 30 per cent died, again showing parallels with the Chinese male outcomes. However, more men in the general population – at least in the sample for this study – were formally diagnosed with GPI.

So far, then, the Chinese appear much the same as the general male population; nothing startling characterises these men statistically. What about who they were? Little information exists to tell us where these men came from but we know that most came from the Guangzhou province, and were Cantonese-speaking, and 'Canton' is inscribed in the case notes of a few patients. These Chinese inmates were all male, and their occupations also indicated a common pattern of Chinese sojourner lives: they were miners, and had come to work in the Victoria goldfields, but also (less often) worked as market gardeners, labourers, hawkers, cooks and in a couple of cases, farmers. Questions about their occupations help to amplify the readings of masculinity set out in Chapter 4 of this study, since the majority of white men in the institution were labourers, but clusters of occupational categories emerge for white men that show a much greater participation in the waged labour force than women, Chinese or other ethnic minority groups. Notably, inside the institution, none of these men were given work duties to perform, unlike many of their white male counterparts. Most of these men came from the areas designated as 'Chinese' in the colony: either (for the most part) the goldfield towns, the Chinese Camp at Bendigo, or the Little Bourke Street area of the city in Melbourne.

The numbers alone tell us little about the 'differences' ascribed to these men; for a deeper reading of their 'otherness' we need to look more closely at their notes, which are, in most cases, also sparse. Going further, and looking for specific ethnicity 'labels' applied to these inmates, we often find the recording of their identities as 'Chinese', where other inmates are given no ethnic identifier, but more often this is evident through the use of the designation of 'pagan' and occasionally 'heathen' for their chosen religion. Whether or not the Chinese believed in 'God' was worthy of a special entry in the *Census for Victoria* in 1881 in the form of a letter from C. P. Hodges, who was an official colonial Chinese interpreter.[23] Chinese men were also addressed as 'Ah', an Anglicised form of naming as prefix which was a familiar form of identifying a person as 'you', showing the homogenisation of Chinese that took place in the minds of the institutional scribes as details about them were recorded.

Two contrasting stories highlight small moments of difference. Ah Tan was a single man of twenty-two when he was admitted to the Yarra Bend in 1885 by police from Queenscliff, northwest of Melbourne on the coast. He was a French polisher, the only Chinese man in the sampled cases with that profession, and he was reportedly destructive, manic, and tore off his clothes; he also went through 'all sorts of antics with his hair down about his shoulders'. Interestingly, he was the only Chinese man in this group to be allowed out on trial, suggesting that someone outside the institution interceded on his behalf. There is no record of his release, but given the limitations of this data, it is possible that he was released following his trial leave and the selected case notes do not reflect this.[24] Descriptions of physical features suggest that bodily difference was one code for racial difference. For example, the length of Chinese men's hair was commented on more than once: in 1888, Ah Lou, who was a 41-year-old married hawker, was brought to the Yarra Bend from the urban area of Melbourne following a suicide attempt in gaol, where he had tried to hang himself using his pigtail.[25] He was later discharged recovered. Another man tried to strangle himself with his pigtailed hair when he arrived.[26] The sexuality of Chinese men was also questionable, with Chinese accused of luring white women into 'slavery' and prostitution, using drug addiction as their bait.[27] Thus perhaps one man's delusion that he 'had 12 wives' made the authorities wonder about him in 1894.[28]

Linguistic difference was always remarked upon. Interpreters were used on a few occasions. The use of interpreters inside social and medical institutions, and the Licensing Courts, was well established by the 1890s in Victoria, with interpreters used across these institutional spaces. Hawkers, most of whom were Chinese, Indian, Afghan and Syrian, had to apply for a licence and were required to answer questions in English in the space of the courtroom. Sadly, the institutions for the insane note the use of interpreters only in passing, but these traces also present what Nadia Rhook, drawing upon the work of socio-linguists, suggests as a form of 'linguistic markedness' inside an institutional 'node of empire'.[29] Among the cases of Chinese men in the institution, there are frequent mentions of the inability to speak English, difficulty in understanding, confusion about the institution, clarifying the content of delusions, among other barriers to effective communication. One man, 42-year-old William Ah Kew, did not 'understand what is being done to him'. Authorities complained that 'nothing can be elicited though he appears to be able to speak English fairly well'. Said to have a history of violence', there was also the possibility that William was 'promiscuous'.[30] That the mad were also linguistically 'other' in these cases, and in a smattering of cases of non-English speaking inmates in general, created more potential for marginalisation and distancing and ultimately, one imagines, a poverty of institutional care.

The composite picture of this group of Chinese men suggests a few interpretive possibilities. Following the framework of the 'hidden colonists', we can see that through their designation as 'pagan', these men were viewed as morally ambiguous. They were men without women but were also possibly sexually ambivalent, as signalled through mentions of their hair; they were difficult to understand and to know because of their linguistic difference. One of these men also swore profusely in other languages – at least, it seemed to his interpreters that he was being profane. A few of these men were frightened: they did not understand what was happening to them, and they did not understand local laws – several of these men had already been in gaol or police lockups. Their delusions also indicated fears of violence and conflict, possibly borne out of realities on the Victorian goldfields. They knew other Chinese men also inside the institution; references to other 'Chinamen' being their countrymen show up too. Their identities were puzzling because they were out of place: one man, known as 'George Thompson' carried a letter with him indicating his Chinese name, and that he had sought refuge in the Wesleyan church out of fear, and that he had a wife in China.[31] These fragments of identity, read inside the prism of the wider social world of the institution and its context, tell us much about the social dislocation of these men.

The Māori insane at Auckland

In contrast with the group of Chinese men at the Yarra Bend, there were very few Aboriginal inmates in the Victorian institution, and none at all in the data sampled for this study. However, while there were very few Chinese inmates at Auckland in the period, there was a sizeable group of Māori patients, a group which constituted a quarter of those patients known to be born in New Zealand in this sampled data. The different conditions and practices of colonialism across Victoria and the other colonies of Australia when compared with New Zealand go some way towards explaining this anomaly. Notably, for the Māori insane at Auckland, there was no hesitancy on the part of the medical authorities in attributing an ethnic label or category. There were forty-eight Māori brought to Auckland Asylum in the sample for this study, of a total of seventy-two Māori in the asylum by 1900.[32] This sample, then, includes a large number of the Māori known to be in the institution. Located in New Zealand's North Island, Auckland was a catchment area for most of the North Island population from the Waikato region and everywhere north, which meant that higher concentrations of

Māori people were part of the catchment area when compared to institutions elsewhere in the country, leaving aside Wellington's institution at Karori in the lower North Island. There were, though, very few Māori in New Zealand asylums overall. The population of Māori people was in decline between 1840 and 1860, due to disease and clashes with settlers, but by 1870 it had stabilised. Following the violence of the land wars, and cultural attack, the population of Māori was at its lowest point in 1896, at an estimated 42,000 people, compared with 703,000 Pākehā (Europeans).

The Māori inmates at Auckland's Te Whau asylum came from all over the North Island: from as far away as Gisborne on the East Coast; from west of Auckland, from the Waikato region in the south, and from Taupo, even further south, in one instance, in 1909. More Māori than European inmates were brought to the institution by police. Police brought twenty-three Māori, and one was taken in by 'friends and police'; two others were taken to the institution by other Māori. For the remaining Māori inmates, no detail was collected about their admission or those who admitted them. Overall, the data sample reveals that 53 per cent of Māori were admitted by police, compared with just under 20 per cent of non-Māori. Among the Māori patients brought by Māori to the institution was the single gum digger Hami Te Herenga whose family lived in Huntly in the Waikato region south of Auckland. Te Herenga was violent, and was brought to police by other 'natives' because he needed restraint.[33]

The rates of Māori institutional death and discharge also tell us something about this group. Where we have data, we know that around one-third of all patients died in the institution. Rates of death for Māori were about the same, but rates of phthisis or tuberculosis among Māori were higher than for other inmates when we look at recorded deaths and causes of death: seven of seventeen Māori died with phthisis or tubercular disease, or 41 per cent, compared with just five of the 130 non-Māori deaths, or 3 per cent. There is a parallel here with Canadian research about Aboriginal inmates by Bob Menzies and Ted Palys, reminding us of the plight of Indigenous institutionalised peoples.[34]

Gender is also a significant category when we examine the Māori inmate population. Most of these Māori inmates were men: thirty-five men and thirteen women. This means that more Māori men were slightly more vulnerable to committal than European men (72 per cent compared with 65 per cent). Looking at their occupations tells us that they were working in contact with Europeans: they worked as labourers and as gum diggers, digging Kauri tree gum, mostly in Northland, and on farms (with twenty-one cases of these two occupations). This contact with Europeans as employers perhaps explains their committal to a European institution. Some of these Māori men retained tribal status as 'chief', at least insofar as the casebook was concerned; one was described as 'semi-civilised', and a few others were classified with the occupation of 'Aboriginal'. Of the Māori women, where an occupation was noted, it was either 'domestic service' or 'Aboriginal native'. These women were mostly married, suffering from what was labelled 'depression' in several cases, or melancholia, and were aged between seventeen and seventy.

Again, there are just a few hints of their differences from the dominant group of European patients among this sampled population. Most Māori had converted to Christianity, but a few (three in this sampled data) followed the Hauhau faith led by Te Ua, a Māori prophet and political activist in the period. Hauhauism was practised by the followers of one of several Māori religious sects of the period and was the faith of the Paimārire Church.[35]

Just as happened with the Chinese inmates in Victoria, ethnic difference was signalled by the use of another language, and again, institutional interpreters were employed. Some Māori patients spoke both English and Māori, a language which was then discouraged, and later, actively denied in native schools from 1867. There was an occasional blurring of the lines when it came to racial identity: the case of 'Kanaka Jack' in 1900 shows that it was important for the institution to note where racial designation was uncertain. Hoani Kuni, a male patient aged thirty-eight who worked as a gum digger, was noted by police as 'not a pure Maori but a kanaka' and was known to them for more than ten years.[36] William Wilson was a 'congenital idiot' aged thirty-six, and described as a 'half caste' Māori but had 'typical Maori features', perhaps confusing to the institution given his own preoccupation with his parentage: 'he imagined one of his parents was English.'[37]

There are also hints of the separate meaning of madness for Māori: 'porangi' is a term used in one case in 1900 which highlights a tribal conception of heredity, explaining that the Māori woman Ruita was not the first in her family to exhibit the tendency to insanity.[38] In one final example, child sacrifice was noted in the case of male patient Hemi Ngarano in 1897, which most likely represented his insanity rather than an alien, culturally specific practice, but it was confirmed that he spoke good English, to reinforce the oddness of the moment.[39] In addition, Ngarano was said to have been affected by 'religion', but no religious faith was listed for him. Two of the oldest patients here, both aged seventy, were widowed, and although no diagnosis was offered in either case, it was possible they were both victims of old age and the loss of family connections. Interestingly, of the forty-eight Māori inmates, only forty-two were given a formal diagnosis, and in perhaps three cases, it was the opinion of the doctor that these inmates were not insane. Two men, Apera Taitu and Tea Peter, were said to have insanity triggered by 'tribal matters' or 'tohunga', showing the scant knowledge of Indigenous affairs and practices (though some curiosity) on the part of the asylum's doctors. Little more is said about either man's case.[40]

Writing about the Aboriginal insane in the colonial institutions in Australia, Caitlin Murray contends that doctors were more concerned about the category of whiteness than they were about the Indigenous peoples.[41] The decline of the Indigenous 'races' symbolised the coming of the whites and their eventual eclipse and survival in the new colonies, as the 'sad' but inevitable loss of the Native peoples took place. There is little in the patient case records of the Māori described above to suggest that the European doctors in this period were especially concerned about their illnesses, or puzzled as to why they were suffering from European diseases of the mind, including conditions such as 'melancholia', given their status as 'native' peoples. In other words, it is tempting to speculate that in this situation the mental health of the Māori peoples was not upmost in the minds of the European doctors who treated them. This is interesting when we look at the gendered identities of the Māori women inmates at Auckland. Although, as Chapter 5 argued, there are only fragmented and suggestive pieces of evidence in the records of confined white women inside institutions, historians show that it was the white birthrate which bothered contemporaries at the end of the nineteenth century.[42] There were few concerns about the women inside the Auckland Asylum whose identities as Māori mothers, separated from their whānau (families) in the event of puerperal insanity, were further confused by the impact of institutional confinement in a Pākehā space.

Hybrids: the colonial-born insane

By the end of the nineteenth century, the Report of the Inspector of Lunatic Asylums for the Hospitals for the Insane in Victoria sounded a gloomy note. 'The increasing number of certified lunatics in every civilized country', intoned J. V. McCreery, 'is a startling and dispiriting sequel to the hopes entertained in the middle of the century as to the results to be obtained from the scientific and humane treatment of the insane.'[43] However, McCreery agreed with all the other commentators on the subject when he explained that it was not so much an increase in mental disease as an 'accumulation' of cases over time; the fact was, institutions had become home to a vast number of incurable and chronically ill patients or those with life-long congenital conditions. They had also been for a long time a stopping place for some of those mobile colonial peoples whose fortunes did not include family support or for whom systems of leave and absence had not functioned well.

Postcolonial scholars remind us that identities 'in-between' or *hybrid* create important fissures in water-tight conceptions of racial identity. It was the hybrid identity of the person of indeterminate race which challenged notions of fixity, shattered artificial distinctions between self and other, and reminded colonial society of its own inability to retain and force segregation. Somewhat paradoxically, the visible and undeniable reminders of mixed-race children in the Australian colonies tended to force the issue in political terms, with Aboriginal Child Removal Policies of the twentieth century directly related to late nineteenth-century anxieties about miscegenation, which were also reinforced by the Immigration Restriction Act in newly federated Australia in 1901, and New Zealand's legislation restricting the entry of non-white immigrants in the same period.

Inside the institution, mixed-race identities threw into relief the finer distinctions being made between inmates. It was not always possible to carefully ascribe identities and to make sense of who people really were; indeed, a certain amount of identity blurring went on inside the asylums anyway, through practices such as forgery, disguise and the use of aliases, as I describe in Chapter 3. There are a handful of indeterminate cases of hybrid identities which illustrate these uncertainties. For example, in 1897, a woman named Jenny Ah Yen arrived at the Yarra Bend Lunatic Asylum from the Chinese camp on the goldfields of Castlemaine, northwest of Melbourne, where she had reputedly worked as a prostitute.[44] Her body was extensively scarred, and she was in a 'base' physical condition. She was aged thirty-six, and although she came with a Chinese surname, the question mark inscribed next to her 'single' marital status suggests some uncertainty around her marital status, and also therefore her ethnicity. Was she a Chinese woman, or a European woman who had taken a Chinese name, and then reverted to single status? With her religious background described as 'Church of England', the latter identity seems possible. Delusional for two months, apparently following her opium-smoking habit, Jenny was brought by police to the institution, where she died two months later, with her death attributed to brain and lung disease. Traces of incomplete identities abound in the records for the reasons I described earlier: white and non-white inmates alike were represented only through the details that were known about them. But in the reporting by colonial medical administrators and personnel, one possible answer to the question raised by mixed-race identities lay in highlighting the racial differences inside the institutions as a way of understanding mental disease for the dominant white population.

The contemporary medical preoccupation with the health of white subjects was reinforced in the nineteenth century by examining the colonial-born, or 'hybrid' populations of the insane, as Dr Chisholm Ross asserted in the late nineteenth century. In both Australia and New Zealand, the emergence of national discourses of mental hygiene by the early twentieth century shifted the focus from the immigrants of the nineteenth century to the colonial stock of the future national health. Just how these problems were played out in separate 'colonial' spaces, and whether the approaches to psychiatric institutional care and treatments changed as a result, is yet to be fully examined. Local practices of psychiatry took their place among the plethora of imperial ones, and insanity was now viewed as an inherent feature of all new societies. However, it is clear that the emerging interest in the colonial-born and insanity led to mental hygiene movements in Australia and in New Zealand. The medical establishment, then, created both fixed and shifting categories of 'social identity'. Theories about colonial-born populations of the mad, specific migrant groups, and the intersections between these, produced a new composite identity for the institutional populations of the insane in the colonial context. The term 'hybrid' was used by contemporaries to explain the different inheritance of the colonial-born insane; they were not migrants themselves, and benefited from the positive circumstances of their birthplaces, but also took from their forebears the tendencies and characteristics of their kin, meaning that some were more susceptible to insanity than others.

Elsewhere I have described the special interest shown in the question of the 'race' and ethnicity of the insane in the colonies at the Intercolonial Medical Congress of Australasia in 1889.[45] For example, Dr Chisholm Ross examined the patient registers at Gladesville for the ten years between 1878 and 1887 to determine whether any particular patient nationalities dominated the admissions. It was a preoccupation of a number of medical men of this era. In 1885, the *Australian Medical Journal* briefly noted an item under 'Local Subjects', commenting that the Chairman of the Lunacy Commission, Ephraim Zox, had obtained a return of inmates from four institutions: Sunbury, Yarra Bend, Ararat and Kew, with a view to looking closely at the 'nationalities and creeds' of those confined inside the colony's hospitals for the insane.[46] It was the identities of the colonial born which stood out for Ross. Although they were 'of no special race', with their 'marked hybridity' confusing to contemporaries who wanted to apportion the incidence of insanity to racial categories, it is this very 'hybridity' which had come to obsess institutional authorities over time.[47]

The structure of the population, with younger people born in the colonies, and asylum admissions dominated by older people, especially those immigrants described in the earlier chapters of this book, the desire of contemporaries to understand, capture and categorise insanity through the prism of 'race' was particularly complicated.[48] Ross tried to examine categories of patients including 'Irish' and 'Chinese', and he had suspicions that there were more Chinese mad than asylum admissions alone revealed, perhaps because they were 'harboured by their countrymen'.[49] His ultimate conclusion was that the hybridity of 'Australasians', meaning those colonial-born to immigrant parents, possibly protected them from insanity, along with their environment, their diets, their conditions of life and their lack of worry, all of which also shaped their responses to mental challenges. He listed 'self-reliance' and 'self-confidence' as two of the colonial attributes that held madness at bay.[50] The fears of those advising the 'weak' emigrants in the middle of the nineteenth century that colonial life would cause them hardship, cited in previous chapters here, seem to support this idea: the second generation of these immigrant families had learned to adapt, to survive and to harness their innate racial superiority but in new ways for colonial life.

These ideas had some support among other medical professionals, including those in New Zealand. In his report on the colony's populations of the insane for 1905, Dr Frank Hay considered the relatively low incidence of insanity in the New Zealand-born populace when compared with its frequency among new arrivals. Yet, as suggested earlier here, Hay was not talking about Māori. The gaze was firmly directed at white subjects, and the mental health of Māori attracted little attention at all in any of the official reports or inquiries into insanity statistics. In 1908, the detailed use of statistics to amplify and correct Hay's work by Segar similarly turned a completely blind eye to the issue of Indigenous peoples and insanity. He was concerned with whether or not Europeans born in the colonies were less susceptible to insanity. He also worried about European women's propensity to insanity in the colonies, and was keen to measure it against women of Britain, finding that the populations of women born in New Zealand and women born in Britain had roughly the same percentages of insanity.[51]

These ideas mattered when it came to developing policies of 'mental hygiene' from the late nineteenth century onwards, and into the early twentieth century. With the investigation of racial differences came the interrogation of bodily difference, the emergence of categories of disability and mental deficiency.[52] Mental deficiency was defined in the Australian and New Zealand institutions at around the same time through both legislative change, but also institutional practices. The accrual of meanings around 'idiocy', 'imbecility' and 'feeble-minded' by the early twentieth century signalled a shift in thinking about institutional populations and ideal groups for asylum or mental hospital care. Made visible through the Mental Defectives Act in New Zealand (1911), and later legislation in Victoria, Australia in the 1920s, as well as through an official inquiry into mental defectives and sexual offending in New Zealand in 1924, this shift was linked to a 'patchy' assemblage of eugenic ideas in Australia and New Zealand which failed to become truly influential as policy.[53] Unlike Britain, where the Mental Deficiency Act of 1913 led to discussions about segregation of the 'feebleminded' in separate institutions, as occurred in North America, such moves to segregate inmates in asylums in the colonies were less successful, although some separate institutional spaces for those inmates who were categorised as having congenital mental deficiency did exist in close proximity to larger institutions.[54]

A collection of terms used to define and classify these congenital conditions appeared in the patient casebooks in both of the public institutions discussed in this study. The list included 'idiocy' (idiot, idiotism), 'imbecility' (imbecile), weakness of intellect, mental enfeeblement and feebleminded. Cases of patients confined in mental hospitals who were diagnosed using these labels were often sparse, and suggestive of worries about heredity, poverty and family dysfunction, though not always. This language of the nineteenth-century institution symbolised a coming discourse of the body and its idealisation in the twentieth century. Defined as 'congenital idiocy', hereditary mental deficiency was emerging as a distinct concern for the medical authorities in institutions in Australia and New Zealand before the twentieth century. Mental deficiency was understood as a twin inheritance of biology and poor 'habits of life', and centred on the family as one cause of degeneration. Historians show that the case notes of the institutionalised came to reflect nascent medical theories of the period, in knowledge spanning the British Empire and its colonial institutional spaces and their physicians.[55] This preoccupation with family histories of mental illness, and in particular, congenital conditions, is evidenced through the patient casebook pro forma at both the Yarra Bend and at Auckland, as I note in other discussions about the form and content of the patient records, both in terms of familial observations of the person admitted to the institution, but also in terms of details collated about the likelihood of heredity.[56]

Conclusions

Non-white peoples, including Chinese and Indigenous peoples, were a minority of inmates in public institutions for the insane, not because they were excluded from them, but because they were already in a minority in the wider colonial population. What was the place, then, of non-whites in the discourses and practices of the institution? Although the evidence in the casebooks for any sustained discussion of their identities is relatively slight, this chapter has engaged with these texts to argue that the analysis of these populations using social and cultural history techniques can tell us about the formation of colonial identities: both for the insane, and for colonial society more broadly.

Social differences were inscribed in colonial patient records. In the Introduction to this book, I asked whether social distinctions, such as those applied to individuals in the official records, meant anything to their reporters and recorders. If social institutions in fact inadvertently 'produced' social identities, and we later, modern scholars have over-interpreted their significance, then what was the purpose of keeping fulsome records, even though they varied in their levels of detail, and were strangely uneven and haphazard? The vagaries of the colonial archive certainly reflect the chaos of admission, and the daily work of the institutions, which strived to maintain order yet failed, from time to time, to know as much as they wished to know about their inmates. Yet the continued production of these casebooks and reports also had a social impact. Practices of inscription reinforced power, as Chapter 3 showed; such textual productions were part of a larger apparatus, and formed the substance or 'stuff' of the assemblages of power which both infused and knitted colonial societies together. Social identities were, we know, mobilised by contemporaries in legislation and inside institutions, and were also often expressed through the outcomes of institutional confinement.

Understanding just how social identities have been formed and transformed over time has implications for the study of power.[57] If the 'empire' was also a 'cultural project', then its articulation of identities becomes vital to picking apart its exclusions, inclusions, separations and relations.[58] By interrogating the 'imperial turn' with closer attention to the institutional populations described this study, we can shed light on the formation of ideas about perfection and imperfection in colonial populations; populations which were striving to measure themselves against their old world models and with a view to replicating them at least in part.

Notes

1 NANZ, Auckland Mental Hospital (hereafter YCAA), 1048/9 356, patient 2852, 18 June 1903.
2 Anthony Trollope, *Australia and New Zealand*, Vol. 1 (London: Dawsons of Pall Mall, 1873), p. 479.

3   See Catherine Hall, *Civilising Subjects: Metropole and Colony in the English Imagination 1830–1867* (Chicago: University of Chicago Press; Cambridge: Polity, 2002), pp. 17–18. Hall is quoting from Frederick Cooper and Ann Laura Stoler (eds), *Tensions of Empire: Colonial Cultures in a Bourgeois World* (Berkeley and Los Angeles: University of California Press, 1997).
4   Anna Curthoys, 'White, British and European: Historicising identity in settler societies', in Jane Carey and Claire McLisky (eds), *Creating White Australia* (Sydney: Sydney University Press, 2009), p. 23.
5   Catherine Hall, 'Of gender and empire: Reflections on the nineteenth century', in Philippa Levine (ed.), *Gender and Empire*, Oxford History of the British Empire (Oxford: Oxford University Press, 2004), p. 49.
6   F. G. Ewington, 'The treatment of lunatics, historically considered', *Transactions and Proceedings of the Royal Society of New Zealand*, Vol. 27 (6 August 1894), p. 675.
7   Claudia Gronemann, 'A hybrid gaze from Delacroix to Djebar: Visual encounters and the construction of the female "other" in the colonial discourse of Maghreb', in Harald Fischer-Tiné and Susanne Gehrmann (eds), *Empires and Boundaries: Rethinking Race, Class, and Gender in Colonial Settings*, Routledge Studies in Colonial History (New York and London: Routledge, 2009), pp. 150–1.
8   Mrinalini Sinha, *Colonial Masculinity: The 'Manly Englishman' and the 'Effeminate Bengali' in the Late Nineteenth Century*, Studies in Imperialism (Manchester: Manchester University Press, 1995).
9   Catharine Coleborne, 'Legislating lunacy and the body of the female lunatic in 19th-century Victoria', in Diane Kirkby (ed.), *Sex, Power and Justice: Historical Perspectives on Law in Australia* (Melbourne: Oxford University Press, 1995), pp. 86–98; 'Making "mad" populations in settler colonies: The work of law and medicine in the creation of the colonial asylum', in Diane Kirkby and Catharine Coleborne (eds), *Law, History, Colonialism: The Reach of Empire*, Studies in Imperialism (Manchester: Manchester University Press, 2001), pp. 106–22; Angela Hawk, 'Going "mad" in gold country: Migrant populations and the problem of containment in Pacific mining boom regions', *Pacific Historical Review*, 80:1 (2011), pp. 64–96.
10 Kate Bagnall, 'Rewriting the history of Chinese families in nineteenth-century Australia', *Australian Historical Studies*, 42:1 (2011), pp. 63–4.
11 An Act to Make Provision for Certain Immigrants (No. 39 of 1855), known in Victoria as Chinese Immigration Act (1855); in New Zealand, the Chinese Immigrants Act (1881) was followed by the Immigration Restriction Act (1899).
12 Imbecile Passengers Act (1882); see also a brief reference to this legislation in Angela McCarthy, 'Ethnicity, migration and the lunatic asylum in early twentieth-century Auckland, New Zealand', *Social History of Medicine*, 21:1 (2008), p. 50. See also 'Immigration chronology: Selected events 1840–2008', New Zealand Parliamentary Research Library, www.parliament.nz/en-nz/parl-support/research-papers/00PLSocRP08011/immigration-chronology-selected-events-1840–2008, accessed 1 August 2014.
13 As described by Alison Bashford and Sarah Howard, 'Immigration and health: Law and regulation in Australia, 1901–1958', *Health and History*, 6:1 (2004), pp. 97–112. Bashford links this legislation to eugenic concerns in Australia.
14 Alison Bashford, 'Insanity and immigration restriction', in Catherine Cox and Hilary Marland (eds), *Migration, Health and Ethnicity in the Modern World*, Technology and Medicine in Modern History (Basingstoke and New York: Palgrave Macmillan, 2013), p. 19.
15 Peter H. Bryce, *Insanity in Immigrants* (Ottawa: Government Printing Bureau, 1910).
16 Walter L. Treadway, *Mental Hygiene with Special Reference to the Migration of People*, Public Health Bulletin (Washington: Government Printing Office, 1925).
17 Mr James Kay: see NANZ, YCAA 1048/5 326, patient 1496, 16 July 1888.

18 Catharine Coleborne, *Reading 'Madness': Gender and Difference in the Colonial Asylum in Victoria, Australia, 1848–1888* (Perth: Network Books, Australian Public Intellectual Network, 2007), pp. 138–9.
19 See Coleborne, 'Making "mad" populations in settler colonies', pp. 106–22.
20 Norman Megahey, 'More than a minor nuisance: Insanity in colonial Western Australia', in Charlie Fox (ed.), *Historical Refractions. Studies in Western Australian History* 14 (Crawley: University of Western Australia, 1993), p. 53.
21 *Census of Victoria* (1881), p. 18.
22 Chinese welfare and missionary organisations did exist, but a detailed discussion of these is outside the scope of the present study.
23 *Census of Victoria* (1881), p. 183.
24 PROV, VPRS 7399/P1, unit 6, folio 182, 14 October 1885.
25 PROV, VPRS 7399/P1, unit 8, folio 27, 30 November 1888.
26 PROV, VPRS 7399/P1, unit 11, folio 300, 7 December 1897.
27 Frank Bongiorno, *The Sex Lives of Australians: A History* (Collingwood: Black Inc., 2012), p. 103.
28 PROV, VPRS 7399/P1, unit 10, folio 37, 22 February 1894.
29 Nadia Rhook, 'Listen to nodes of empire: Speech and whiteness in Victorian hawker's license courts', *Journal of Colonialism and Colonial History*, 15:2 (2014). Project Muse, http://muse.jhu.edu.ezproxy.waikato.ac.nz/journals/journal_of_colonialism_and_colonial_history/v015/15.2.rhook.html, accessed 1 August 2014.
30 PROV, VPRS 7399/P0, unit 18, folio 130, 11 December 1909.
31 PROV, VPRS 7399/P1, unit 11, folio 175, 24 February 1897.
32 Lorelle Barry and Catharine Coleborne, 'Insanity and ethnicity in New Zealand: Māori encounters with the Auckland Mental Hospital, 1860–1900', *History of Psychiatry*, 22:3 (2011), pp. 285–301.
33 NANZ, YCAA 1048/9 1, patient 2494, 7 May 1900.
34 Robert Menzies and Ted Palys, 'Turbulent spirits: Aboriginal patients in the British Columbia psychiatric system, 1879–1950', in James E. Moran and David Wright (eds), *Mental Health and Canadian Society: Historical Perspectives*, Studies in the History of Medicine, Health and Society (Montreal: McGill-Queen's University Press, 2008).
35 See: www.teara.govt.nz/en/1966/hauhauism, accessed 20 June 2013.
36 NANZ, YCAA 1048/8 357, patient 2482, 27 March 1900.
37 NANZ, YCAA 1048/10, patient 2922, 8 December 1903. Emma Spooner, 'The mind is thoroughly unhinged': Reading the Auckland Asylum Archive, New Zealand, 1900–1910', unpublished Honours dissertation, University of Waikato, 2004, p. 21.
38 NANZ, YCAA 1048/8 321, patient 2465, 31 January 1900.
39 NANZ, YCAA 1048/7 130, patient 2228, 7 May 1897.
40 NANZ, YCAA 1048/9 391, patient 2885, 21 September 1903; YCAA 1048/7 145, patient 2246, 6 August 1897.
41 Caitlin Murray, 'Settling the Mind: Psychiatry and the Colonial Project in Australia', unpublished Ph.D. thesis, University of Melbourne, 2012, pp. 98–118.
42 Philippa Mein Smith, 'Blood, Birth, Babies, Bodies', *Australian Feminist Studies*, 17:39 (2002), pp. 305–23.
43 *Report of the Inspector of Lunatic Asylums, Hospitals for the Insane, Victoria* (1899) Victoria Parliamentary Papers (Robert S. Brain, Government Printer, Melbourne, 1900), p. 13.
44 The 'Chinese Camp' was well known and had persisted from the 1860s. For histories of rural Victoria and the Chinese, see *Dragon Tails: New Perspectives in Chinese Australian History*, a Special Issue of *Australian Historical Studies*, 42:1 (2011); PROV, VPRS 7400/P1, unit 12, folio 54, 27 September 1897.
45 Catharine Coleborne, *Madness in the Family: Insanity and Institutions in the Australasian Colonial World, 1860–1914* (Basingstoke and New York: Palgrave Macmillan, 2010), pp. 40–1.
46 'Local subjects', *Australian Medical Journal*, 7 (1885), p. 95.

47 Chisholm Ross, 'Race and insanity in New South Wales, 1878–1887', *Transactions of the Intercolonial Medical Congress of Australasia* (1889), p. 850.
48 For additional commentary about this idea see Elizabeth Malcolm, 'Mental health and migration: The case of the Irish, 1850s–1990s', in Angela McCarthy and Catharine Coleborne (eds), *Migration, Ethnicity and Mental Health: International Perspectives, 1840–2010* Routledge Studies in Cultural History (New York and Abingdon: Routledge, 2012), pp. 15–38.
49 Ross, 'Race and insanity', p. 852.
50 Ross, 'Race and insanity', pp. 852–3.
51 H. W. Segar, 'Insanity: Some comparative statistics', *Transactions*, 41 (Auckland: Auckland Institute 1908), pp. 221–30.
52 See Catharine Coleborne, 'Disability in colonial institutional records', in Michael A. Rembis, Catherine Kudlick and Kim E. Nielsen (eds), *Oxford Handbook of Disability History* (Oxford: Oxford University Press, forthcoming).
53 See Stephen Garton's summary of laws across the Australian colonies in 'Eugenics in Australia and New Zealand: Laboratories of racial science', in Alison Bashford and Philippa Levine (eds), *The Oxford Handbook of the History of Eugenics* (Oxford and New York: Oxford University Press, 2010), pp. 246–7. On New Zealand's mental deficiency law, see Adrienne Hoult, 'Intellectual disability: The patient population of Tokanui, 1912–1935', in Catharine Coleborne and the Waikato Mental Health History Group (eds), *Changing Times, Changing Places: From Tokanui Hospital to Mental Health Services in the Waikato, 1910–2012* (Hamilton: Half Court Press, 2012), p. 54.
54 Kew Cottages, for example, opened adjacent to the Kew Metropolitan Asylum to house children with intellectual impairment in 1887. See Corinne Manning, 'Imprisoned in State care? Life inside Kew Cottages 1925–2008', *Health and History*, 11:1 (2009), pp. 149–71.
55 Maree Dawson, 'Halting the "sad degenerationist parade": Medical concerns about heredity and racial degeneracy in New Zealand psychiatry, 1853–99', *Health and History*, 14:1 (2012), 38–55.
56 Coleborne, *Madness in the Family*, p. 147; pp. 54–9.
57 See the journal *Social Identity* and its self-description at www.tandf.co.uk/journals/carfax/13504630.html, accessed 27 May 2011.
58 Gavin Lucas, *An Archaeology of Colonial Identity: Power and Material Culture in the Dwars Valley, South Africa*, Contributions to Global Historical Archaeology (New York: Springer, 2006), p. 185.

CONCLUSION

In 1891, Charles Daniels, aged thirty-eight, was taken to the Yarra Bend Asylum by police from the Immigrants' Home. Believing he was 'on board a ship', he was partly paralysed on admission, and diagnosed with GPI. Born in England, he was a labourer, and without any family in the colonies.[1] Like the many other brief vignettes of institutional lives presented in this book, his story captures some of the aspects of the multiple narratives of insanity in the imperial world: those who travelled to the colonies came on ships with small cell-like berths. Other immigrants whose stories are told in this book came to worlds peopled by others who they found to be both strange and, at times, sympathetic. Their stories of identity formation are told in this volume through the careful accretion of details from institutional case records about them.

Victoria and New Zealand were two colonies of the British Empire in the process of social and cultural formation in the period under examination here. That process produced social institutions and their populations as part of a wider set of structures: the overlapping assemblages of institutions and their shared apparatus of care and control. This book has argued that by teasing out the role of the institutions for the insane – one inside a web of welfare institutions – in the formation of colonial identities, historians might ask new questions about the colonial and the national past.[2] Who were the insane of the British Empire? Their stories have the potential to shed new light on the literature of the 'imperial turn', and add to the many accounts now of 'transnational lives', 'moving subjects' and of medicine and gender in the imperial age. If there was, as Catherine Hall asserts, a 'complex web of gender relations across the [British] Empire', the evidence from the institutions for the insane might help to more fully explain how this web functioned inside colonial spaces, how it was articulated and contributed to the formation of colonial identities.[3]

Australia and New Zealand were remarkably diverse societies with complicated immigration histories, even while they aspired to visions of homogeneity and privileged a 'white' identity over time. Arguably, colonial social and medical institutions perpetuated and even refined social differences and distinctions in their efforts to make sense of the presence of need and illness in the population. This occurred in spite of the fact that the colonial asylums discussed here were public institutions, and took people from all walks of life, thus signalling the collapse of such distinctions between classes of person; they were also multi-racial sites of the institutional treatment of insanity. The brief stories about immigrant women and men, from all walks of life, as well as the mobile lives of prostitutes and vagrants provided here, underscore the notion that immigration processes created 'complex diasporas'.[4] The visible and invisible identities in these records, such as the taken-for-granted identities of white Europeans who were the focus of most anxiety in the official reports of institutions, further complicate these diasporic worlds of the colonists.

This book has returned to the rich scholarly exploration of ideas about patients and constructions of them through official case records to uncover new interpretations of this material in the Australian and New Zealand context, with the aim to examine the way that social differences were produced inside the colonial institutions for the insane. It has done so with an awareness of the work already produced around the gendered patient, but it also extends the analyses of institutional sources in the process. It argues that in their constructions of patients' bodies and behaviours, clinical case records produced new social identities and categories for those who were institutionalised. Cases, then, had a productive power. In their quest to identify colonial subjects through institutional medical confinement, forms of social difference were notable to contemporaries. Whether these social differences came to affect treatment and discharge rates for different inmates of institutions also needs to be assessed in future scholarship.[5]

Scholars have implicitly but consistently argued since the early 2000s that institutions effectively produced people in social categories, especially as they were (and are) obsessed with collecting details about individuals and arranging these into tables, using them to measure institutional populations. Power (and thus powerlessness) became 'intelligible' through the bodies of individuals, as Michel Foucault suggested.[6] My argument is that institutions operated with existing formulations of 'social identity' but produced these within the medical context as coexistent with pathology; that is, they equated some social categories with 'disease', mostly mental, but also physical.[7] Further and more detailed research and analysis of some of the many cases only

CONCLUSION

suggestively drawn upon for parts of this book will help to illustrate the ways that disease and colonial identity were produced alongside each other over time. However, despite historians' ability to weave together a reading of a patient case for the purpose of creating a short narrative, such as that of Jenny described above in Chapter 6, we might also say that individuals, in some senses, defied social categorisation. Just as individual cases remind us of this problem, so too did social groupings within the populations of the insane.

Narrating the stories of individuals, as opposed to featuring the stories and collective 'experiences' of groups as patterned by the data collated for this study, has involved negotiating a sometimes tense boundary between different forms of historical narrative. In writing about 'Europeans' I have also come to see the differences between groups of people as layered by notions of age, gender, occupation and marital status. Diagnostic categories, too, suggest groupings that might disguise the variations in and duration of a mental illness episode for individual sufferers. It has been, as reinforced by contemporary writing, difficult to distinguish some peoples from their collective identities: the 'Chinese', for instance, occupied a specific discursive space as Chinese inmates but their individuality is relatively muted. And perhaps the great number of the insane became the 'mad' and 'institutionalised', too, both at the time and in later historical accounts, in ways that extinguish their identities as individual people.

Additionally, this book has argued that by using 'mobility' as an interpretive framework, the relevance of the histories of insanity around empire can be understood in a new light. Traditionally applied to migration histories, but reimagined more recently as a new lens through which historians might view moving ideas, currents of intellectual change, and the transfer of institutional practices and discourses, the turn to 'mobility' has enabled historians to think again about the imperial world of migration with a different appreciation of the meanings of movement. The mobility of peoples made shifting and chimera-like identities out of imperial subjects, who passed through places on their way to becoming new colonial 'settlers', and whose movement was sometimes the cause of their discontent. This book has suggested that we might usefully think about its extension to the study of migrants in and out of place, and across sites and locations, to investigate how migration processes themselves produced complex and contradictory meanings around mobility and movement. Future work could productively examine the multi-layered nature of the concept of colonial mobility in ways which enhance and highlight our understandings of the 'multiplicity of relationships to place' in the past.[8] Without mobility, settlement had little to hit against, or to define the very importance of 'settling' and 'settlers'. It was in the impact of movement and mobility that settler colonies found and made their own meanings of settler culture.

The two urban and institutional sites studied in this book provide opportunities to examine categories of colonial identity. Both Penelope Edmonds and Philippa Levine, looking across colonial sites by using transcolonial modes of inquiry and analysis, find evidence for the closer attention being paid by contemporaries to the social categories of 'vagrant', 'prostitute' and to those of mixed race.[9] By adding 'lunatic' and 'insane' to this list of emerging marginal social categories, and reading these against the descriptors in the patient case records, the different chapters in this book show how colonial social identity was constantly being formed in relation to an institutional identity. In other words, we might find evidence of social identities for colonial populations being formed inside the social institutions, but we also find new categories of identity being formed through the process of institutionalisation and confinement.

The gendered and raced identities of the insane in Melbourne and Auckland have been the major focus of this book. The fact that gender relationships were fragile, in flux and changing in the transition not only from old worlds to the new colony, but in the shift towards modernity as the nineteenth-century world became increasingly mechanised and industrialised, meant that gender relations in particular were under scrutiny. While more opportunities for work emerged for both men and women, women's worlds, like the lives of the non-white subjects in this study, were still constrained and limited by expectations of them as more subservient. White women were to be rescued and rehabilitated into family life, a life framed by middle-class expectations of settler identity. Vagrant women, prostitutes or alcoholic women, whose lives had been violent and difficult, were on the very fringes of consciousness for institutional authorities. It was difficult to break out of the mould for many of the women whose stories are threaded throughout this book; Chinese men, too, had fewer opportunities to belong outside their 'group' and were classed as Chinese rather than viewed as colonial men in search of new futures. Among the Indigenous subjects of the institutions, Māori women and men led lives that were barely visible. Where these collided with those of Europeans they met across a linguistic and cultural divide that registered or reflected very little empathy in the institutional records and reports.

One of the critical contributions of New Zealand and Australian scholars to the debates around the institutionalisation of the insane has been to question the scholarly implications of the work of English historian Elaine Showalter, who argued that madness was increasingly

CONCLUSION

feminised in the Victorian era; this meant that historians tended to assume that women were in fact over-represented among institutionalised populations everywhere.[10] In particular, Bronwyn Labrum shows that men were committed more frequently than women to Auckland Mental Hospital in the second half of the nineteenth century, and Barbara Brookes finds similar patterns for institutions in the South Island of New Zealand. Stephen Garton also comments on the way that colonial populations of the insane in New South Wales were different to those in the British context. In New South Wales, young, single men were more likely to be committed than women in the colonial era.[11] Joanna Besley and Mark Finnane indicate that colonial Queensland's largest institution at Goodna was home to a substantial population of white men, with women inmates comprising 40 per cent of admissions until the 1930s.[12] So despite the existence of a powerful myth that women were highly vulnerable to asylum committal by 'cruel' husbands and fathers, the reality was that men numerically dominated colonial populations and found their way into the hospitals for the insane in greater numbers. Their vulnerability to institutional confinement was also shaped by their mobility outside the space of the home, as Brookes explains, a point also noted by contemporary medical observers who saw women's domestic role as protecting them from the harsher aspects of the peripatetic and rough life of the male labourer or miner.[13] Gender was an enduring and productive category in the shaping of patient identities through space, regulations, treatments and attitudes. Another argument previously made about the gendering of nineteenth-century insanity concerns the etiology of insanity and how it was tied to notions of the gendered body. The way that prescriptions for gender continued to define female insanity, for example, paid scant regard to the realities of asylum statistics as outlined by historians, with theories about the female bodily propensity towards insanity entrenched in asylum discourse. However, interestingly, there is evidence that male bodies were also caught up in discussions about 'the body', as arguments about labouring white men and sunstroke show.[14]

Finally, as the Introduction to this book argued, scholars have shown an appreciation for the formation of whiteness in colonial societies where white Europeans were in a minority but in power. In those worlds, whiteness was barely articulated while colonial governments spent time worrying over non-white populations, their health and their control. Yet this book has shown that in white settler colonies, the appearance of whiteness in the colonial record, in the archives of the social institutions set aside for Europeans and 'others' was both highly visible and yet also opaque. What *was* whiteness, to the administrators of the hospitals for the insane?

INSANITY, IDENTITY AND EMPIRE

Although whiteness can be shown to have been formed across the colonies through shared immigration restriction practices, few historians have examined the link between the institutional populations of the weak, needy and mentally ill and the discursive work of identity formation. The very 'instability' of whiteness around empire, as Catherine Hall suggests, means that it must also be read and understood in relation to the other categories of identity at work in the colonies; settler societies, Hall argues, depended on 'particular ideas ... of manliness and femininity'.[15] Gender categories were also forged through class divisions and 'played an important part', writes Hall, 'in unifying the middle class' in England in the nineteenth century.[16]

Colonial identities were not formed in isolation but were delineated inside the context of the imperial world, and were part of a larger fabric of identities which patterned the mobile world of this period. This book has set out to show that the intersections between 'white' identities and other forms of social identity, including gender, sexuality, class, ethnicity (and hybridity) and religion, helped to delineate and invent whiteness in these settings. These 'axes of differentiation' produced hierarchies and layers of power for colonial societies.[17] Such forms of identity would then have a much wider set of meanings for the emerging colonial nations of the twentieth century.

Notes

1 PROV, VPRS 7399/P1, unit 8, folio 316, 12 January 1891.
2 Leigh Boucher, Jane Carey and Katherine Ellinghaus suggest that by looking closely at 'whiteness', historians might ask new questions about colonial and national histories: see 'Historicising Whiteness: Towards a New Research Agenda', in Leigh Boucher, Jane Carey and Katherine Ellinghaus (eds), *Historicising Whiteness: Transnational Perspectives on the Construction of an Identity*, Melbourne University Conference and Seminar Series 16 (Melbourne: RMIT Publishing, in association with the School of Historical Studies, University of Melbourne, 2007), p. xii.
3 Catherine Hall, 'Of gender and empire: Reflections on the nineteenth century', in Philippa Levine (ed.), *Gender and Empire*, Oxford History of the British Empire (Oxford: Oxford University Press, 2004), p. 52.
4 A. James Hammerton, 'Gender and migration', in Levine (ed.), *Gender and Empire*, p. 179.
5 My thanks to Caitlin Murray for raising this question with me.
6 Jann Matlock, *Scenes of Seduction: Prostitution, Hysteria, and Reading Difference in Nineteenth-Century France* (New York: Columbia University Press, 1994), p. 3.
7 For my wider use of the term 'social identity', see Catharine Coleborne, 'Locating ethnicity in the hospitals for the insane: Revisiting case books as sites of knowledge production about colonial identities in Victoria, Australia, 1873–1910', in Angela McCarthy and Catharine Coleborne (eds), *Migration, Ethnicity, and Mental Health: International Perspectives, 1840–2010*, Routledge Studies in Cultural History (New York and Abingdon: Routledge, 2012), pp. 73–90.
8 Tony Ballantyne, 'On place, space and mobility in nineteenth-century New Zealand', *New Zealand Journal of History*, 45:1 (2011), p. 59.

CONCLUSION

9   Penelope Edmonds, *Urbanizing Frontiers: Indigenous Peoples and Settlers in Nineteenth-Century Pacific Rim Cities* (Vancouver and Toronto: University of British Columbia Press, 2010), p. 244; Philippa Levine, *Prostitution, Race and Politics: Policing Venereal Disease in the British Empire* (New York and London: Routledge, 2003).
10 Elaine Showalter, *The Female Malady: Women, Madness and English Culture, 1830–1980* (Michigan: Pantheon Books, 1985).
11 Bronwyn Labrum, 'The boundaries of femininity: Madness and gender in New Zealand, 1870–1910', in Wendy Chan, Dorothy E. Chunn, and Robert Menzies (eds), *Women, Madness and the Law: A Feminist Reader* (London, Portland, OR, and Coogee: GlassHouse Press, 2005); Barbara Brookes, 'Men and madness in New Zealand, 1890–1916', in Linda Bryder and Derek A. Dow (eds), *New Countries and Old Medicine: Proceedings of an International Conference on the History of Medicine and Health* (Auckland: Pyramid Press, 1995); Stephen Garton, *Medicine and Madness: A Social History of Insanity in New South Wales, 1880–1940* (Sydney: New South Wales University Press, 1988).
12 Joanna Besley and Mark Finnane, 'Remembering Goodna: Stories from a Queensland Mental Hospital', in Catharine Coleborne and Dolly MacKinnon (eds), *Exhibiting Madness in Museums: Remembering Psychiatry through Collections and Display*, Routledge Research in Museum Studies (New York and London: Routledge, 2011), pp. 116–36.
13 Brookes, 'Men and madness', p. 209.
14 Leigh Boucher, 'Masculinity gone mad: Settler colonialism, medical discourse and the white body in late nineteenth century Victoria', *Lilith*, 13 (2004), pp. 51–67.
15 Hall, 'Of gender and empire', in Levine (ed.), *Gender and Empire*, pp. 49, 52.
16 Catherine Hall, *White, Male and Middle Class: Explorations in Feminism and History* (Cambridge: Polity, 1992), p. 95.
17 Hall, 'Of gender and empire', p. 49.

BIBLIOGRAPHY

Primary material

Auckland War Memorial Museum, Auckland
Auckland Hospital and Charitable Aid Board, MS 287 91/40
Auckland Ladies' Benevolent Society, MS 92/52, Minute Book 1884–1985
Auckland Ladies' Benevolent Society, MS 877, Annual Reports

National Archives New Zealand, Auckland
YCAA 1048/1-17, Auckland Provincial Lunatic Asylum/Auckland Lunatic Asylum/Auckland Mental Hospital Casebooks 1853–1916

National Library of Australia, Canberra
MS 4009, Eliza Kennison, Letters 1867–1868

Public Record Office of Victoria (PROV), Melbourne
VA 2864, Lunacy Department (Chief Secretary), 1905–1934
VA 2863, Hospitals for the Insane Branch, 1867–1905
VA 2839, Yarra Bend (Asylum 1848–1905; Hospital for the Insane 1905–1925)
VPRS 7399, Case Books of Female Patients, 1862–1912
VPRS 7400, Case Books of Male Patients, 1872–1912
VPRS 7446, Alphabetical list of patients in asylums, 1849–1885
VPRS 7556, Admission warrants: Male, 1848–1925; Female, 1848–1855; 1896–1904
VPRS 7562, Admission warrants: Female, 1856–1924
VA 724, Chief Commissioner of Police
VPRS 1557, Letter Books, inc Memoranda and Reports, Bourke Street Police Department, 1853–1889
VPRS 937, Inwards registered correspondence, 1853–1894

Queensland State Archives, Runcorn
Wolston Park Hospital [formerly Goodna], A/45606, folio 126, 1885

Royal Melbourne Hospital Archives, Melbourne
Records of the Immigrants' Aid Society, 1870s–1900s
  Admissions, 1885–1982
  Daily Admission Book (Book 4: 1906–1916)
  The Genealogical Society of Victoria, Mount Royal Cumulative Index, 2007
  Immigrants' Aid Society Minute Books, 1869–1871; 1872–1875
  Medical Officers' Report Books, 1904–1919
  Statistical registers July 1878–March 1887

BIBLIOGRAPHY

State Library of Victoria, Melbourne
Annual Reports of the Immigrants' Aid Society's Home for Houseless and Destitute Persons 1860–1872; 1870–1901 (La Trobe Pamphlet Collections)

University of Melbourne Archives, Melbourne
Melbourne City Mission Records
  89/90 Annual Reports, Melbourne City Mission 1903–1936, 5/1
  89/90 City Mission Record 1900–1906, 14/1/1
  89/90 Loving Service in Our Community 1855–1962, Percival Dale 9/2
  89/90 Melbourne and Suburban City Mission Journal: Thomas Murray, Missionary, Hotham, 1877–1881, 15/13
  89/90 Melbourne City Mission Jubilee, 1906, Public Meeting 31 May, 7/1

Legislation
An Act for the Better Prevention of Vagrancy and Other Offences, 1852 (Victoria, Australia)
An Act to Make Provision for Certain Immigrants, 1855 (in Victoria, the Chinese Immigration Act)
Census of Victoria, 1881 (Australia)
Chinese Immigrants Act, 1881 (New Zealand)
Contagious Diseases Act, 1869 (UK)
Hospitals and Charitable Institutions Act, 1885 (New Zealand)
Imbecile Passengers Act, 1882 (New Zealand)
Immigration Restriction Act, 1899 (New Zealand)
Immigration (Restriction) Act, 1901 (Australia)
Lunacy Act, 1868 (New Zealand)
Lunatics Act, 1867 (Victoria, Australia)
Mental Defectives Act, 1911 (New Zealand)
Mental Deficiency Act, 1913 (UK)
Passengers Act, 1855 (UK)
Vagrant Act, 1866 (New Zealand)

Official publications
Balls-Headley, Dr Walter. *Royal Commission on Charitable Institutions, Synopsis, Minutes of Evidence and Appendix*. Melbourne: Robert S. Brain, Government Printer, 1892.
Bryce, Peter H. *Insanity in Immigrants*. Ottawa: Government Printing Bureau, 1910.
Forty-Seventh Annual Report of the Committee of the Melbourne City Mission for the Year Ending 20th of June 1903. In 89/90 Annual Reports, 1903–1936. Melbourne: Melbourne City Mission.
Greig, Dr James Saunders. *Report of the Royal Commission into Charitable Institutions, Victoria Parliamentary Papers*, 1870; 1871.
Greig, Dr James Saunders. *Royal Commission on Charitable Institutions, Synopsis, Minutes of Evidence and Appendix*. Melbourne, 1892.

BIBLIOGRAPHY

Report of Commission on the Costley Home, New Zealand, *Appendices to the Journal of the House of Representatives (AJHR)*, H-26, 1904.
Report of the Inspector-General of Hospitals and Charitable Aid in the Domi, AJHR, H-22, 1909.
Report of the Inspector of Asylums on the Hospitals for the Insane for the Year 1870. In *Victoria Parliamentary Papers*. Melbourne, 1871.
Report of the Inspector of Asylums on the Hospitals for the Insane for 1870. Melbourne: John Ferres, Government Printer, 1871.
Report of the Joint Committee on Lunatic Asylums, AJHR, H-10. Wellington, 1871.
Report of the Royal Commission on Asylums for the Insane and the Inebriate, Victoria Parliamentary Papers, 1886–1888. Melbourne: John Ferres, Government Printer, 1886.
Report of Sub-Committee of the IAS, Appointed on the 6th of June, 1873, to Examine into the Condition and Prospects of the Inmates – Male and Female – at Present Resident in the Immigrants' Home, Princes Bridge. Flinders Lane West: Mason, Firth, & McCutcheon, General Printers, 1873.
Reports on Lunatic Asylums in New Zealand. In *AJHR*, 1870.
Treadway, Walter L. *Mental Hygiene with Special Reference to the Migration of People*. Washington: Government Printing Office, 1925.
Twenty-first Annual Report of the Immigrants' Aid Society. Flinders Lane West: Mason, Firth & McCutcheon, General Printers, 1874.
Twenty-Seventh Annual Report of the Immigrants' Aid Society. Flinders Lane West: Mason, Firth, & McCutcheon, General Printers, 1880.

Newspapers and periodicals

Auckland Star
Australian Medical Journal
Illustrated Australian News
Illustrated Melbourne Post
Intercolonial Medical Congress of Australasia, 1887–1902
Intercolonial Medical Journal of Australasia, 1896–1903
Melbourne and Suburban City Mission Journal
New Zealand Graphic
New Zealand Herald
Transactions and Proceedings of the Royal Society of New Zealand, 1868–1961
Victorian Year Book

Published articles and books

Algar, Frederic. *A Description of the Province of Victoria: Australia*. London: Algar and Street, 1858.
Askew, John. *A Voyage to Australia and New Zealand Including a Visit to Adelaide, Melbourne, Sydney, Hunter's River, Newcastle, Maitland, and Auckland; With a Summary of the Progress and Discoveries Made in Each Colony From its Founding to the Present Time. By a Steerage Passenger*. London: Simpkin, Marshall and Co., 1857.

BIBLIOGRAPHY

Auckland Industrial and Mining Exhibition, Official Handbook and Catalogue. Auckland: Geddis and Blomfield, Observer Office, 1898.

Author, Unknown. *Auckland Illustrated: 53 Views of City and Suburbs.* Gold Medal Series. Auckland, Christchurch, Sydney and London: Fergusson, c. 1910.

Author, Unknown. *Auckland Industrial and Mining Exhibition, Official Handbook and Catalogue.* Auckland: Geddis and Blomfield, Observer Office, 1898.

Brett, Henry. *Brett's Colonists' Guide and Cyclopedia of Useful Knowledge.* Auckland: H. Brett, 1883.

Butler, Samuel. *A First Year in Canterbury Settlement, With Other Early Essays.* Edited by R. A. Streatfeild. London: A. C. Fifield, 1914.

Chisholm, Caroline. *Female Immigration Considered: In a Brief Account of the Sydney Immigrants' Home.* Sydney: James Tegg, 1842.

Clouston, T. S. *Clinical Lectures on Mental Diseases.* London: J. & A. Churchill, 1883.

Clouston, T. S. *The Hygiene of Mind.* 7th edn. London: Methuen & Co, 1918 [1906].

Cyclopedia of New Zealand [Auckland Provincial District], The. Christchurch: Cyclopedia Company Ltd, 1902.

Earley, Dr H. *Hints Upon Health, Addressed to Newly Arrived Immigrants.* Melbourne: B. Lucas, Collins Street, 1853.

Ellis, Ellen E. *Everything is Possible to Will.* London, 1882.

Fowler, Frank. *Southern Lights and Shadows.* Sydney: Sydney University Press, 1975 [1859].

Franklin, Miles. *My Brilliant Career.* Melbourne: William Blackwood & Sons, 1901.

Garran, Andrew (ed.). *Picturesque Atlas of Australasia.* Vol. 3. Sydney, Melbourne and London: Picturesque Atlas Publishing Company, 1980 [1886].

'Hopeful'. *'Taken in'; Being, a Sketch of New Zealand Life.* 2nd edn. London: W. H. Allen & Co., 1877; reprint 1974.

Howitt, William. *Land, Labour, and Gold, or, Two Years in Victoria with Visits to Sydney and Van Diemen's Land.* Sydney: Sydney University Press, 1972 [1855].

James, John Stanley. *The Vagabond Papers.* Edited by Michael Cannon. Abridged edn. Melbourne: Melbourne University Press, 1969.

Jarritt, Reverend William. *Hints to Immigrants Upon Colonial Life and Its Requirements.* Melbourne: Argus, Collins Street, 1853.

Kernot, M. J. *Reminiscences of the Carlton Refuge 1854 to 1919.* Carlton, Melbourne: Ford and Son, 1919.

Kerr, John Hunter [attrib.]. *Glimpses of Life in Victoria, by 'A Resident'.* Melbourne: Melbourne University Press, 1996 [1876].

MacGregor, Duncan. 'The problem of poverty in New Zealand', Part I. *New Zealand Magazine,* January 1876.

Manning, F. Norton. 'A contribution to the study of heredity'. *Australasian Medical Gazette,* 17 July (1885).

BIBLIOGRAPHY

Manning, F. Norton. *Ten Years at Gladesville*. Sydney: Thomas Richards, Government Printer, 1880.

McNab, Robert (ed.). *Historical Records of New Zealand*. Vol. 1. Wellington: Government Printer, 1908.

Mickle, William Julius. *General Paralysis of the Insane*. London: H. K. Lewis, 1886 [1880].

Moore, John Murray. *New Zealand for the Emigrant, Invalid, and Tourist*. London: Sampson Law, Marston, Searle and Rivington, 1890.

Morris, E. E. (ed.). *Cassell's Picturesque Australasia*. Vol. 3. Christchurch: Cadsonbury Publications, 1998 [1890].

Morris, E. E. (ed.). *Pictorial New Zealand*. London, Paris and Melbourne: Cassell & Company, 1895.

Mulgan, Alan. *Spur of Morning*. London: Whitcombe and Tombs, 1934.

Newman, A. K. 'Speculations on the physiological change obtaining in the English race when transplanted to New Zealand'. *Transactions and Proceedings of the Royal Society of New Zealand*, 30 September 1876.

Nicholls, Mary (ed.). *Traveller Under Concern: The Quaker Journals of Frederick Mackie on His Tour of the Australasian Colonies, 1852–1855*. Launceston: Foot and Playsted, 1973.

Philips, David and Susanne Davies (eds). *A Nation of Rogues? Crime, Law and Punishment in Colonial Australia*. Parkville: Melbourne University Press, 1994.

Pollard, N. W. *Homes in Victoria, or, the British Emigrant's Guide to Victoria, to Accompany Passage Warrants*. Vol. 1: Victorian Institutions and Establishments. Melbourne: Walker, May & Co., 1861.

Reeves, William Pember. *State Experiments in Australia and New Zealand*. Vol. 2. South Melbourne: Macmillan of Australia, 1969 [1902].

Rosenblum, Edward E. 'Premonitory symptoms of general paralysis of the insane'. *Intercolonial Medical Congress of Australasia*, Third Session. Sydney: W. M. Maclardy, Printer, 1892.

Ross, Chisholm. 'Race and insanity in New South Wales, 1878–1887'. *Transactions of the Intercolonial Medical Congress of Australasia* (1889).

Segar, H. W. 'Insanity: Some comparative statistics'. *Transactions*, 41 (Auckland: Auckland Institute 1908), pp. 221–30.

Singleton, John. *A Narrative of Incidents in the Eventful Life of a Physician*. Melbourne: M. L. Hutchinson, 1891.

Sommerville, Harold Archibald. *Auckland Hospital and Charitable Aid Board: A History of Its Buildings and Endowments*. Auckland: Whitcombe & Tombs, 1919.

Syder, C. Mingay *The Voice of Truth in Defence of Nature: And Opinions Antagonistic to Those of Dr Kilgour, Upon the Effect of the Climate of Australia Upon the European Constitution in Health and Disease*. Geelong: Heath and Cordell, 1855.

'Tempe'. *A Summer Holiday in Victoria and New Zealand, or, Leaves from a Tourist's Note Book*. Singleton: 'Argus' Steam Printing Works, 1882.

BIBLIOGRAPHY

Treadway, Walter L. *Mental Hygiene with Special Reference to the Migration of People*. Public Health Bulletin. Washington: Government Printing Office, 1925.

Trollope, Anthony. *Australia and New Zealand*. 2 vols. London: Dawsons of Pall Mall, 1873.

Twopeny, R. E. N. *Town Life in Australia*. Reprint. Sydney: Sydney University Press, 1973 [1883].

Vaile, E. Earle. *Some Interesting Occurrences in Early Auckland City and Province*. Christchurch, Auckland, Wellington: Whitcombe and Tombs Ltd, 1955.

Vogel, Sir Julius (ed.). *The Official Handbook of New Zealand: A Collection of Papers by Experienced Colonists on the Colony as a Whole, and on the Several Provinces*. London: Wyman & Sons, 1875.

Woods, W. J. *A Visit to Victoria*. London: Wyman and Sons, 1886.

Secondary material

Journal articles

Ahmad, Waqar I. U. and Hannah Bradby. 'Locating ethnicity and health: Exploring concepts and contexts'. *Sociology of Health and Illness*, 29:6 (2007), pp. 795–810.

Anderson, Warwick. 'The trespass speaks: White masculinity and colonial breakdown'. *American Historical Review*, 102:5 (1997), pp. 1343–70.

Anderson, Warwick. '"Where every prospect pleases and only man is vile": Laboratory medicine as colonial discourse'. *Critical Inquiry*, 18:3 (1992), pp. 506–29.

Andrews, Jonathan. 'Case notes, case histories, and the patient's experience of insanity at Gartnavel Royal Asylum, Glasgow, in the nineteenth century'. *Social History of Medicine*, 11:2 (1998), pp. 255–81.

Attwood, Bain. 'Tarra Bobby, a Brataualung man'. *Aboriginal History*, 11:1–2 (1987), pp. 41–57.

Bagnall, Kate. 'Rewriting the history of Chinese families in nineteenth-century Australia'. *Australian Historical Studies*, 42:1 (2011), pp. 62–77.

Ballantyne, Tony. 'Archives, empires and histories of colonialism'. *Archifacts* (April 2004), pp. 21–36.

Ballantyne, Tony. 'On place, space and mobility in nineteenth-century New Zealand'. *New Zealand Journal of History*, 45:1 (2011), pp. 50–70.

Barry, Lorelle and Catharine Coleborne. 'Insanity and ethnicity in New Zealand: Māori encounters with the Auckland Mental Hospital, 1860–1900'. *History of Psychiatry*, 22:3 (2011), pp. 285–301.

Bashford, Alison and Sarah Howard. 'Immigration and health: Law and regulation in Australia, 1901–1958'. *Health and History*, 6:1 (2004), pp. 97–112.

Bhavsar, Vishal and Dinesh Bhugra. 'Bethlem's Irish: Migration and distress in nineteenth-century London'. *History of Psychiatry*, 20:2 (2009), pp. 184–98.

BIBLIOGRAPHY

Boucher, Leigh. 'Masculinity gone mad: Settler colonialism, medical discourse and the white body in late nineteenth century Victoria'. *Lilith*, 13 (2004), pp. 51–67.

Brickell, Chris. 'Court records and the history of male homosexuality'. *Archifacts* (October 2008), pp. 25–44.

Brickell, Chris. 'Same-sex desire and the asylum: A colonial experience'. *New Zealand Journal of History*, 39:2 (2005), pp. 158–78.

Brooking, Tom, Dick Martin, David Thomson and Hamish James. 'The ties that bind: Persistence in a new world industrial suburb, 1902–22'. *Social History*, 24:1 (1999), pp. 55–73.

Burnham, John C. 'Psychotic delusions as a key to historical cultures: Tasmania, 1830–1940'. *Journal of Social History*, 13:3 (1980), pp. 368–83.

Chesser, Lucy. 'A woman who married three wives': Management of disruptive knowledge in the 1879 Australian case of Edward De Lacy Evans'. *Journal of Women's History*, 9:4 (1998), pp. 53–77.

Coleborne, Catharine. '"His brain was wrong, his mind astray": Families and the language of insanity in New South Wales, Queensland and New Zealand, 1880s–1910'. *Journal of Family History*, 31:1 (2006), pp. 45–65.

Coleborne, Catharine. 'Insanity, gender and empire: Women living a "loose kind of life" on the colonial institutional margins, 180–1910'. *Health and History*, 14:1 (2012), pp. 77–99.

Coleborne, Catharine. 'Pursuing families for maintenance payments to hospitals for the insane in Australia and New Zealand, 1860s–1914'. *Australian Historical Studies*, 40:3 (2009), pp. 308–22.

Coleborne, Catharine. 'Reading insanity's archive: Reflections from four archival sites'. *Provenance*, 9 (2010), pp. 29–42.

Coleborne, Catharine. 'Regulating "mobility" and masculinity through institutions in colonial Victoria, 1870s–1890s'. *Law Text Culture*, 15 (2011), pp. 45–71.

Coleborne, Catharine. 'White men and weak masculinity: Men in the public asylums in Victoria and New Zealand, 1860s–1900s'. *History of Psychiatry* (December 2014).

Comaroff, John L. 'Reflections on the colonial state, in South Africa and elsewhere: Factions, fragments, facts and fictions'. *Social Identities*, 4:3 (1998), pp. 321–61.

Cooper, Annabel. 'Poor men in the land of promises: Settler masculinity and the male breadwinner economy in late nineteenth-century New Zealand'. *Australian Historical Studies*, 39:2 (2008), pp. 245–61.

Cresswell, Tim. 'Embodiment, power and the politics of mobility: The case of female tramps and hobos'. *Transactions of the Institute of British Geographers*, 24:2 (1999), pp. 175–92.

Curry, Gerard. 'A bundle of vague diverse offences: The Vagrancy Laws with special reference to the New Zealand experience'. *Anglo-American Law Review*, 1 (1972), pp. 523–36.

Dawson, Maree. 'Clouston in the colonies? General paralysis of the insane at the Auckland Mental Hospital and beyond, 1868–1899'. Forthcoming.

BIBLIOGRAPHY

Dawson, Maree. 'Halting the "sad degenerationist parade": Medical concerns about heredity and racial degeneracy in New Zealand psychiatry, 1853-1899'. *Health and History*, 14:1 (2012), pp. 38-55.

Ernst, Waltraud. 'European madness and gender in nineteenth-century British India'. *Social History of Medicine*, 9:3 (1996), pp. 357-82.

Ernst, Waltraud. 'Idioms of madness and colonial boundaries: The case of the European and "Native" mentally ill in early nineteenth-century British India'. *Comparative Studies in Society and History*, 39:1 (1997), pp. 153-81.

Ernst, Waltraud. 'Madness and gender in nineteenth-century British India'. *Social History of Medicine*, 9:3 (1996), pp. 357-82.

Ewington, F. G. 'The treatment of lunatics, historically considered'. *Transactions and Proceedings of the Royal Society of New Zealand*, Vol. 27 (6 August 1894).

Fairburn, Miles. 'Vagrants, "folk devils" and nineteenth-century New Zealand as a bondless society'. *Australian Historical Studies*, 21:85 (1985), pp. 495-514.

Finnane, Mark. 'Asylums, families and the state'. *History Workshop Journal*, 20:1 (1985), pp. 134-48.

Gandevia, Bryan. 'Land, labour and gold: The medical problems of Australia in the nineteenth century'. *Medical Journal of Australia*, 47:1 (1960), pp. 753-62.

Garton, Stephen. 'Sound minds and healthy bodies: Re-considering eugenics in Australia, 1914-1940'. *Australian Historical Studies*, 26:103 (1994), pp. 163-81.

Goldberg, Ann. 'The limits of medicalization: Jewish lunatics and nineteenth-century Germany'. *History of Psychiatry*, 7 (1996), pp. 265-85.

Goodman, David. 'Reading gold-rush travellers' narratives'. *Australian Cultural History*, 10 (1991), pp. 99-112.

Hawk, Angela. 'Going "mad" in gold country: Migrant populations and the problem of containment in Pacific mining boom regions'. *Pacific Historical Review*, 80:1 (2011), pp. 64-96.

Jarvis, G. Eric. 'Changing psychiatric perception of African Americans with psychosis'. *European Journal of American Culture*, 27:3 (2008), pp. 227-52.

Jordanova, Ludmilla. 'The social construction of medical knowledge'. *Social History of Medicine*, 8:3 (1995), pp. 361-81.

Keller, Richard. 'Madness and colonization: Psychiatry in the British and French Empires, 1800-1962'. *Journal of Social History*, 35:2 (2001), pp. 295-326.

Kimber, Julie. 'Poor Laws: A historiography of vagrancy in Australia'. *History Compass*, 11:8 (2013), pp. 537-50.

Kirkby, Kenneth C. 'History of psychiatry in Australia, pre-1960'. *History of Psychiatry*, 10:38 (1999), pp. 191-204.

Knewstubb, Elspeth. '"Believes the devil has changed him": Religion and patient identity in Ashburn Hall, Dunedin, 1882-1910'. *Health and History*, 14:1 (2012), pp. 56-76.

Kolchin, Peter. 'Whiteness studies: The new history of race in America'. *Journal of American History*, 89:1 (2002), pp. 154-73.

Leckie, Jacqueline. 'The embodiment of gender and madness in colonial Fiji'. *Fijian Studies*, 3:2 (2005), pp. 311–36.
Le Couteur, Howard. 'Of intemperance, class and gender in colonial Queensland: A working-class woman's account of alcohol abuse'. *History Australia*, 8:3 (2011), pp. 139–57.
Lewis, Milton and Roy MacLeod. 'A workingman's paradise? Reflections on urban mortality in colonial Australia 1860–1900'. *Medical History*, 31 (1987), pp. 387–402.
Lovejoy, Valerie. 'Chinese in late nineteenth-century Bendigo: Their local and translocal lives in "this strangers' country"'. *Australian Historical Studies*, 42:1 (2011), pp. 45–61.
Manning, Corinne. 'Imprisoned in State care? Life inside Kew Cottages 1925–2008'. *Health and History*, 11:1 (2009), pp. 149–71.
McCarthy, Angela. 'A difficult voyage'. *History Scotland*, 10:4 (2010), pp. 26–31.
McCarthy, Angela. 'Ethnicity, migration and the lunatic asylum in early twentieth-century Auckland, New Zealand'. *Social History of Medicine*, 21:1 (2008), pp. 47–65.
Mein Smith, Philippa. 'Blood, birth, babies, bodies'. *Australian Feminist Studies*, 17:39 (2002), pp. 305–23.
O'Brien, Anne. 'Pauperism revisited'. *Australian Historical Studies*, 42:2 (2011), pp. 212–29.
Pietsch, Roland. 'Hearts of oak and jolly tars? Heroism and insanity in the Georgian Navy'. *Journal for Maritime Research*, 15:1 (2013), pp. 69–82.
Porter, Dorothy. 'The mission of social history of medicine: An historical view'. *Social History of Medicine*, 8:3 (1995), pp. 349–59.
Reeves, Keir. 'Tracking the dragon Down Under: Chinese cultural connections in gold rush Australia and Aotearoa, New Zealand'. *Graduate Journal of Asia-Pacific Studies*, 3:1 (2005), pp. 49–66.
Reeves, Keir and Tseen Khoo. 'Dragon tails: Re-interpreting Chinese Australian history'. *Dragon Tails: New Perspectives in Chinese Australian History*: A Special Issue of *Australian Historical Studies*, 42:1 (2011), pp. 4–9.
Roberts, Phillip. 'Determining the meaning behind historical disease terminology through an examination of patterns of terminology used in the mortality statistics of Victoria, 1853–1900'. *Health and History*, 10:1 (2008), pp. 63–87.
Rollison, David. 'Exploding England: The dialectics of mobility and settlement in early modern England'. *Social History*, 24:1 (1999), pp. 1–16.
Scott, Joan W. 'Gender: A useful category of historical analysis'. *American Historical Review*, 91:5 (1986), pp. 1053–75.
Sicherman, Barbara. 'The uses of a diagnosis: Doctors, patients, and neurasthenia'. *Journal of the History of Medicine*, 32:1 (1977), pp. 33–54.
Smith, Leonard D. 'Insanity and ethnicity: Jews in the mid-Victorian lunatic asylum'. *Jewish Culture and History*, 1:1 (1988), pp. 27–40.
Swain, Shurlee. 'The value of the vignette in the writing of welfare history'. *Australian Historical Studies*, 39:2 (2008), pp. 199–212.

BIBLIOGRAPHY

Swain, Shurlee. 'Writing the history of women and welfare'. *Australian Feminist Studies*, 22:52 (2007), pp. 43–7.
Swartz, Sally. 'The Black insane in the Cape, 1891–1920'. *Journal of Southern African Studies*, 21:3 (1995), pp. 399–415.
Swartz, Sally. 'Changing diagnoses in Valkenberg Asylum, Cape Colony, 1891–1920: A longitudinal view'. *History of Psychiatry*, 6:24 (1995), pp. 431–51.
Swartz, Sally. 'Colonial lunatic asylum archives: Challenges to historiography'. *Kronos*, 34:1 (2008), pp. 285–302.
Swartz, Sally. 'Lost lives: Gender, history and mental illness in the Cape, 1891–1910'. *Feminism and Psychology*, 9:2 (1999), pp. 152–8.
Swartz, Sally. 'The regulation of British colonial lunatic asylums and the origins of colonial psychiatry, 1860–1864'. *History of Psychology*, 13:2 (2010), pp. 160–77.
Tennant, Margaret. 'Elderly indigents and old men's homes, 1880–1920'. *New Zealand Journal of History*, 17:1 (1983), pp. 3–20.
Tosh, John. 'What should historians do with masculinity? Reflections on nineteenth-century Britain'. *History Workshop*, 38 (1994), pp. 179–202.
Twomey, Christina. 'Courting men: Mothers, magistrates and welfare in the Australian colonies'. *Women's History Review*, 8:2 (1999), pp. 231–46.
Wright, David. 'Getting out of the asylum: Understanding the confinement of the insane in the nineteenth century'. *Social History of Medicine*, 10:1 (1997), pp. 137–55.

Electronic journal articles

Field, Jacob and Amy Erickson. 'Prospects and preliminary work on female occupational structure in England from 1500 to the national census'. Occupations Project Paper (2009). The Cambridge Group for the History of Population and Social Structure, Department of Geography and Faculty of History, University of Cambridge, www.geog.cam.ac.uk/research/projects/occupations/categorisation, accessed 27 December 2013; 1 August 2014.
Rhook, Nadia. 'Listen to nodes of empire: Speech and whiteness in Victorian hawker's license courts'. *Journal of Colonialism and Colonial History*, 15:2 (2014). Project Muse, http://muse.jhu.edu.ezproxy.waikato.ac.nz/journals/journal_of_colonialism_and_colonial_history/v015/15.2.rhook.html, accessed 1 August 2014.
Shin, Ji-Hye. 'Immoral women, delusional men: Gender and racial differences among the U.S. immigrant insane, 1892–1930'. *Thinking Gender Papers* (2010), UCLA Center for the Study of Women. http://escholarship.ucop.edu/uc/item/5x7239zg, accessed 19 January 2015.
Smith, Daniel and John Protevi, 'Gilles Deleuze'. *The Stanford Encyclopedia of Philosophy* (Spring 2013 edition), Edward N. Zalta (ed.). http://plato.stanford.edu/archives/spr2013/entries/deleuze/, accessed 17 June 2014.
Swain, Shurlee. 'Immigrants Home'. In *eGold: Electronic Encyclopedia of Gold in Australia*. University of Melbourne and Heritage Victoria, www.egold.net.au/biogs/EG00090b.htm.

BIBLIOGRAPHY

Book chapters

Anderson, Warwick. 'Postcolonial histories of medicine'. In Huisman and Warner (eds), *Locating Medical History*.

Arnold, Rollo. 'The Australasian peoples and their world, 1888–1915'. In Keith Sinclair (ed.), *Tasman Relations*.

Bashford, Alison. 'Insanity and immigration restriction'. In Cox and Marland (eds), *Migration, Health and Ethnicity in the Modern World*.

Bashford, Alison. 'Medicine, gender, and empire'. In Levine (ed.), *Gender and Empire*.

Besley, Joanna and Mark Finnane. 'Remembering Goodna: Stories from a Queensland mental hospital'. In Coleborne and MacKinnon (eds), *Exhibiting Madness in Museums*.

Boucher, Leigh, Jane Carey and Katherine Ellinghaus. 'Historicising whiteness: Towards a new research agenda'. In Boucher, Carey and Ellinghaus (eds), *Historicising Whiteness*.

Brookes, Barbara. 'Men and madness in New Zealand, 1890–1916'. In Bryder and Dow (eds), *New Countries and Old Medicine*.

Brookes, Barbara. 'Pictures of people, pictures of places: Photography and the asylum'. In Coleborne and MacKinnon (eds), *Exhibiting Madness in Museums*.

Burton, Antoinette. 'Introduction: The unfinished business of colonial modernities'. In Burton (ed.), *Gender, Sexuality and Colonial Modernities*.

Carey, Jane and Claire McLisky. 'Introduction: Creating white Australia: New perspectives on race, whiteness and history'. In Carey and McLisky (eds), *Creating White Australia*.

Coleborne, Catharine. 'Disability in colonial institutional records: Bodily difference and the archive'. In Rembis, Nielsen and Kudlick (eds), *Oxford Handbook of Disability History*.

Coleborne, Catharine. 'Law's mobility: Vagrancy and imperial legality in the trans-Tasman colonial world'. In Pickles and Coleborne (eds), *New Zealand's Empire* (forthcoming).

Coleborne, Catharine. 'Legislating lunacy and the body of the female lunatic in 19th-century Victoria'. In Kirkby (ed.), *Sex, Power and Justice*.

Coleborne, Catharine. 'Locating ethnicity in the hospitals for the insane: Revisiting case books as sites of knowledge production about colonial identities in Victoria, Australia, 1873–1910'. In McCarthy and Coleborne (eds), *Migration, Ethnicity, and Mental Health*.

Coleborne, Catharine. 'Making "mad" populations in settler colonies: The work of law and medicine in the creation of the colonial asylum'. In Kirkby and Coleborne (eds), *Law, History, Colonialism*.

Coleborne, Catharine. 'Passage to the asylum: The role of the police in committals of the insane in Victoria, Australia, 1848–1900'. In Porter and Wright (eds), *The Confinement of the Insane*.

Coleborne, Catharine. '"She does up her hair fantastically": The production of femininity in patient case-books of the lunatic asylum in 1860s Victoria'. In Long, Gothard and Brash (eds), *Forging Identities*.

BIBLIOGRAPHY

Cox, Catherine, Hilary Marland and Sarah York. 'Itineraries and experiences of insanity: Irish migration and the management of mental illness in nineteenth-century Lancashire'. In Cox and Marland (eds), *Migration, Health and Ethnicity in the Modern World*.

Curthoys, Anna. 'White, British and European: Historicising identity in settler societies'. In Carey and McLisky (eds), *Creating White Australia*.

Daley, Caroline. 'A gendered domain: Leisure in Auckland, 1890–1940'. In Daley and Montgomerie (eds), *The Gendered Kiwi*.

Dalziel, Raewyn. 'Railways and relief centres (1870–1890)'. In Sinclair (ed.), *The Oxford Illustrated History of New Zealand*.

Daniels, Kay. 'Introduction'. In Daniels, Murnane and Picot (eds), *Women in Australia*.

Davies, Susanne. '"Ragged, dirty ... infamous and obscene": The "vagrant" in late-nineteenth-century Melbourne'. In Philips and Davies (eds), *A Nation of Rogues?*.

Deacon, Harriet. 'Insanity, institutions and society: The case of the Robben Island Lunatic Asylum, 1846–1910'. In Porter and Wright (eds), *The Confinement of the Insane*.

Edmonds, Penelope. 'The intimate, urbanising frontier: Native camps and settler colonialism's violent array of spaces around early Melbourne'. In Mar and Edmonds (eds), *Making Settler Colonial Space*.

Ernst, Waltraud. 'Out of sight and out of mind: Insanity in early nineteenth-century British India'. In Melling and Forsythe (eds), *Insanity, Institutions and Society*.

Evans, Raymond. 'The hidden colonists: Deviance and social control in colonial Queensland'. In Roe (ed.), *Social Policy in Australia*.

Finn, Edmund. 'How port Phillip was peopled'. In Weidenhofer (ed.), *Garryowen's Melbourne*.

Finnane, Mark. 'The ruly and the unruly: Isolation and inclusion in the management of the insane'. In Strange and Bashford (eds), *Isolation: Places and Practices of Exclusion*.

Ford, Ruth. 'Sexuality and "madness": Regulating women's gender "deviance" through the asylum, the Orange Asylum in the 1930s'. In Coleborne and MacKinnon (eds), *'Madness' in Australia*.

Fox, Charlie. 'Jumna Khan'. In Gothard (ed.), *Asian Orientations*.

Garton, Stephen. 'The dimensions of dementia'. In Burgmann and Lee (eds), *Constructing a Culture*.

Garton, Stephen. 'Eugenics in Australia and New Zealand: Laboratories of racial science'. In Bashford and Levine (eds), *The Oxford Handbook of the History of Eugenics*.

Garton, Stephen. 'On the defensive: Poststructuralism and Australian cultural history'. In Teo and White (eds), *Cultural History in Australia*.

Gibbons, Peter. 'The climate of opinion'. In Rice (ed.), *The Oxford History of New Zealand*.

Goldstein, Jan. 'Psychiatry'. In Porter and Bynum (eds), *Companion Encyclopedia of the History of Medicine*.

BIBLIOGRAPHY

Graham, Jeanine. 'Settler society'. In Rice (ed.), *The Oxford History of New Zealand*.

Gronemann, Claudia. 'A hybrid gaze from Delacroix to Djebar: Visual encounters and the construction of the female "other" in the colonial discourse of Maghreb'. In Fischer-Tiné and Gehrmann (eds), *Empires and Boundaries*.

Hacking, Ian. 'Making up people'. In Heller, Sosna and Wellbery (eds), *Reconstructing Individualism*.

Hall, Catherine. 'Of gender and empire: Reflections on the nineteenth century'. In Levine (ed.), *Gender and Empire*.

Hall, Di. 'Irishness, gender and household space in "An up-country township"'. In Proudfoot and Roch (eds), *(Dis)Placing Empire*.

Hamer, David. 'Centralization and nationalism (1891–1912)'. In Sinclair (ed.), *The Oxford Illustrated History of New Zealand*.

Hammerton, A. James. 'Gender and migration'. In Levine (ed.), *Gender and Empire*.

Hoult, Adrienne. 'Intellectual disability: The patient population of Tokanui, 1912–1935'. In Catharine Coleborne and the Waikato Mental Health History Group (eds), *Changing Times, Changing Places: From Tokanui Hospital to Mental Health Services in the Waikato, 1910–2012*. Hamilton: Half Court Press, 2012.

Kinealy, Christine. 'At home with the Empire: The example of Ireland'. In Hall and Rose (eds), *At Home with the Empire*.

Levine, Philippa. 'Sexuality and empire'. In Hall and Rose (eds), *At Home with the Empire*.

Levine, Philippa. 'Sexuality, gender and empire'. In Levine (ed.), *Gender and Empire*.

Labrum, Bronwyn. 'The boundaries of femininity: Madness and gender in New Zealand, 1870–1910'. In Chan, Chunn, and Menzies (eds), *Women, Madness and the Law*.

Lake, Marilyn. 'On being a white man, Australia, circa 1900'. In Teo and White (eds), *Cultural History in Australia*.

Leckie, Jacqueline. 'Unsettled minds: Gender and settling madness in Fiji'. In Mahone and Vaughan (eds), *Psychiatry and Empire*.

Lutz, Tom. 'Varieties of medical experience: Doctors and patients, psyche and soma in America'. In Gijswijt-Hofstra and Porter (eds), *Cultures of Neurasthenia*.

Macdonald, Charlotte. 'The "social evil": Prostitution and the passage of the Contagious Diseases Act (1869)'. In Brookes, Macdonald and Tennant (eds), *Women in History*.

Malcolm, Elizabeth. '"A most miserable looking object" – the Irish in English asylums, 1851–1901: Migration, poverty and prejudice'. In Belchem and Tenfelde (eds), *Irish and Polish Migration in Comparative Perspective*.

Malcolm, Elizabeth. 'Mental health and migration: The case of the Irish, 1850s–1990s'. In McCarthy and Coleborne (eds), *Migration, Ethnicity and Mental Health*.

BIBLIOGRAPHY

McCarthy, Angela. 'Migration and ethnic identities in the nineteenth century'. In Byrnes (ed.), *The New Oxford History of New Zealand*.

McCarthy, Angela. 'Migration and madness in New Zealand's asylums, 1863–1910'. In McCarthy and Coleborne (eds), *Migration, Ethnicity, and Mental Health*.

McCarthy, Angela and Catharine Coleborne. 'Introduction: Mental health, migration, and ethnicity'. In McCarthy and Coleborne (eds), *Migration, Ethnicity, and Mental Health*.

McDonald, Donald. 'Hospitals for the insane in the young colony'. In Pearn and O'Carrigan (eds), *Australia's Quest for Colonial Health*.

McDonald, Peter. 'Demography'. In Brown-May and Swain (eds), *The Encyclopedia of Melbourne*.

McKenzie, Kirsten. 'Opportunists and imposters in the British imperial world: The tale of John Dow, convict, and Edward, Viscount Lascelles'. In Deacon, Russell, and Woollacott (eds), *Transnational Lives*.

McLaren, Angus. 'Males, migrants and murder in British Columbia, 1900–1923'. In Iacovetta and Mitchinson (eds), *On the Case*.

McLennan, Nicole. 'Glimpses of unassisted English women arriving in Victoria, 1860–1900'. In Richards (ed.), *Visible Women*.

Megahey, Norman. 'More than a minor nuisance: Insanity in colonial Western Australia'. In Fox (ed.), *Historical Refractions*.

Mein Smith, Philippa. 'The Tasman world'. In Byrnes (ed.), *The New Oxford History of New Zealand*.

Melling, Joseph. 'Sex and sensibility in cultural history: The English governess and the lunatic asylum, 1845–1914'. In Andrews and Digby (eds), *Sex and Seclusion*.

Menzies, Robert and Ted Palys. 'Turbulent spirits: Aboriginal patients in the British Columbia psychiatric system, 1879–1950'. In Moran and Wright (eds), *Mental Health and Canadian Society*.

Michael, Pamela. 'Class, gender and insanity in nineteenth-century Wales'. In Andrews and Digby (eds), *Sex and Seclusion*.

Mitchinson, Wendy. 'Reasons for committal to a mid-nineteenth-century Ontario insane asylum: The case of Toronto'. In Mitchinson and McGinnis (eds), *Essays in the History of Canadian Medicine*.

Mongia, Radhika Viyas. 'Race, nationality, mobility: A history of the passport'. In Burton (ed.), *After the Imperial Turn*.

Olssen, Erik. 'Towards a new society'. In Rice (ed.), *The Oxford History of New Zealand*.

Porter, Roy. 'Nervousness, eighteenth and nineteenth century style: From luxury to labour'. In Gijswijt-Hofstra and Porter (eds), *Cultures of Neurasthenia*.

Probyn, Elspeth. 'The spacial imperative of subjectivity'. In Anderson, Domosh, Pile and Thrift (eds), *Handbook of Cultural Geography*.

Richards, Eric. 'Migrations: The career of British white Australia'. In Schreuder and Ward (eds), *Australia's Empire*.

Salesa, Damon. 'New Zealand's Pacific'. In Byrnes (ed.), *The New Oxford History of New Zealand*.

Sørensen, John Kousgård. 'Ingeborg Stuckenberg in New Zealand'. In Bender and Larsen (eds), *Danish Emigration to New Zealand*.
Springhall, John. 'Building character in the British boy: The attempt to extend Christian manliness to working-class adolescents, 1880–1914'. In Mangan and Walvin (eds), *Manliness and Morality*.
Starrett Hughes, John. 'The madness of separate spheres: Insanity and masculinity in Victorian Alabama'. In Carnes and Griffen (eds), *Meanings for Manhood*.
Stoler, Ann Laura. 'Colonial archives and the arts of governance: On the content in the form'. In Hamilton, Harris, Taylor, Pickover, Reid and Saleh (eds), *Refiguring the Archive*.
Suzuki, Akihito. 'Lunacy and labouring men: Narratives of male vulnerability in mid-Victorian London'. In Bivins and Pickstone (eds), *Medicine, Madness and Social History*.
Swain, Shurlee. 'The poor people of Melbourne'. In Davison, Dunstan and McConville (eds), *The Outcasts of Melbourne*.
Tabili, Laura. 'A homogeneous society? Britian's internal "others", 1800–present'. In Hall and Rose (eds), *At Home with the Empire*.
Thomson, Mathew. 'Neurasthenia in Britain: An overview'. In Gijswijt-Hofstra and Porter (eds), *Cultures of Neurasthenia*.
Tomes, Nancy. 'The Anglo-American asylum in historical perspective'. In Smith and Giggs (eds), *Location and Stigma*.
Walker, Pamela J. '"I live but not yet I for Christ liveth in me": Men and masculinity in the Salvation Army, 1865–90'. In Roper and Tosh (eds), *Manful Assertions*.
Wilson, Dean. '"Well-set-up men": Respectable masculinity and police organizational culture in Melbourne 1853–c.1920'. In Barrie and Broomhall (eds), *A History of Police and Masculinities*.
Woollacott, Angela. 'Whiteness and "the imperial turn"'. In Boucher, Carey and Ellinghaus (eds), *Historicising Whiteness*.
Wright, David. 'Delusions of gender?: Lay identification and clinical diagnosis of insanity in Victorian England". In Andrews and Digby (eds), *Sex and Seclusion*.

Books

Adam, Jack, Vivien Burgess and Dawn Ellis. *Rugged Determination: Historical Window on Swanson, 1854–2004*. Auckland: Swanson Residents and Ratepayers Association, 2004.
Allen, Judith A. *Sex and Secrets: Crimes Involving Australian Women Since 1880*. Melbourne and Oxford: Oxford University Press, 1990.
Anderson, Benedict. *Imagined Communities*. London and New York: Verso, 1983.
Anderson, Kay, Mona Domosh, Steve Pile and Nigel Thrift (eds). *Handbook of Cultural Geography*. London: Sage, 2003.
Anderson, Warwick. *Colonial Pathologies: American Tropical Medicine, Race, and Hygiene in the Philippines*. Durham, NC, and London: Duke University Press, 2006.
Andrews, Jonathan and Anne Digby (eds). *Sex and Seclusion, Class and*

BIBLIOGRAPHY

Custody: Perspectives on Gender and Class in the History of British and Irish Psychiatry. Clio Medica 73: The Wellcome Series in the History of Medicine. Amsterdam and New York: Rodopi, 2004.

Ashcroft, Bill, Gareth Griffiths and Helen Tiffin. *Post-Colonial Studies: The Key Concepts*. Abingdon and New York: Routledge, 2000.

Atkinson, Alan. *The Europeans in Australia. Volume 2 Democracy*. Melbourne and New York: Oxford University Press, 2004.

Attwood, Bain and S. G. Foster (eds). *Frontier Conflict: The Australian Experience*. Canberra: National Museum of Australia, 2003.

Ballantyne, Tony. *Orientalism and Race: Aryanism in the British Empire*. Basingstoke and New York: Palgrave, 2002.

Ballantyne, Tony. *Webs of Empire: Locating New Zealand's Colonial Past*. Wellington: Bridget Williams Books, 2012.

Ballantyne, Tony and Antoinette Burton (eds). *Bodies in Contact: Rethinking Colonial Encounters in World History*. Durham NC: Duke University Press, 2005.

Ballantyne, Tony and Antoinette Burton (eds). *Moving Subjects: Gender, Mobility, and Intimacy in an Age of Global Empire*. Chicago: University of Illinois Press, 2009.

Barrie, David G. and Susan Broomhall (eds). *A History of Police and Masculinities, 1700–2010*. Abingdon and New York: Routledge, 2012.

Bashford, Alison and Philippa Levine (eds). *The Oxford Handbook of the History of Eugenics*. Oxford and New York: Oxford University Press, 2010.

Beier, A. L. *Masterless Men: The Vagrancy Problem in England 1560–1640*. London and New York: Methuen, 1985.

Belchem, John and Klaus Tenfelde (eds). *Irish and Polish Migration in Comparative Perspective*. Essen: Klartext Verlag, 2003.

Belich, James. *Replenishing the Earth: The Settler Revolution and the Rise of the Anglo-World, 1783–1939*. Oxford and New York: Oxford University Press, 2009.

Bender, Henning and Birgit Larsen (eds). *Danish Emigration to New Zealand*. Translated by Karen Veien. Aalborg: Danes Worldwide Archives, 1990.

Benton, Lauren. *A Search for Sovereignty: Law and Geography in European Empires, 1400–1900*. Cambridge and New York Cambridge University Press, 2010.

Bivins, Roberta and John V. Pickstone (eds). *Medicine, Madness and Social History: Essays in Honour of Roy Porter*. Basingstoke: Palgrave Macmillan, 2007.

Bloomfield, G. T. *New Zealand: A Handbook of Historical Statistics*. Reference Publication in International Historical Statistics. Boston: G. K. Hall, 1984.

Bongiorno, Frank. *The Sex Lives of Australians: A History*. Collingwood: Black Inc., 2012.

Boucher, Leigh, Jane Carey and Katherine Ellinghaus (eds). *Historicising Whiteness: Transnational Perspectives on the Construction of an Identity*.

BIBLIOGRAPHY

Melbourne: RMIT Publishing, in association with the School of Historical Studies, University of Melbourne, 2007.

Bradbury, Bettina and Tamara Myers (eds). *Negotiating Identities in 19th and 20th Century Montreal*. Vancouver and Toronto: University of British Columbia Press, 2005.

Braslow, Joel. *Mental Ills and Bodily Cures: Psychiatric Treatment in the First Half of the Twentieth Century*. Berkeley, Los Angeles and London: University of California Press, 1997.

Brickell, Chris. *Manly Affections: The Photographs of Robert Gant, 1885–1915*. Dunedin: Genre Books, 2012.

Brookbanks, Warren (ed.). *Psychiatry and the Law: Clinical and Legal Issues*. Wellington: Brooker's Ltd, 1996.

Brookes, Barbara and Jane Thomson (eds). *'Unfortunate Folk': Essays on Mental Health Treatment 1863–1992*. Dunedin: Otago University Press, 2001.

Brookes, Barbara, Charlotte Macdonald and Margaret Tennant (eds). *Women in History: Essays on European Women in New Zealand*. Sydney: George Allen & Unwin, 1986.

Broome, Richard. *Aboriginal Australians: Black Responses to White Dominance 1788–2001*. 3rd edn. Crows Nest: Allen & Unwin, 2001.

Broome, Richard. *The Victorians Arriving*. Sydney: Fairfax, Syme and Weldon, 1984.

Brothers, C. R. D. *Early Victorian Psychiatry, 1835–1905*. Melbourne: A. C. Brooks, Government Printer [between 1957 and 1964].

Brown-May, Andrew. *Melbourne Street Life: The Itinerary of Our Days*. Melbourne: Australian Scholarly Press/Arcadia and Museum Victoria, 1998.

Brown-May, Andrew and Shurlee Swain (eds). *The Encyclopedia of Melbourne*. Cambridge, New York and Melbourne: Cambridge University Press, 2005.

Bryder, Linda and Derek A. Dow (eds). *New Countries and Old Medicine: Proceedings of an International Conference on the History of Medicine and Health*. Auckland: Pyramid Press, 1995.

Buckley, Ken and Ted Wheelwright. *No Paradise for Workers: Capitalism and the Common People in Australia, 1788–1914*. Oxford: Oxford University Press, 1988.

Burgmann, Verity and Jenny Lee (eds). *Constructing a Culture: A People's History of Australia Since 1788*. Ringwood: McPhee Gribble/Penguin, 1988.

Burns, Stanley B. *Seeing Insanity: Photography and the Depiction of Mental Illness*. Burns Archive Press, 2007.

Burton, Antoinette (ed.). *After the Imperial Turn: Thinking With and Through the Nation*. Durham, NC: Duke University Press, 2003.

Burton, Antoinette (ed.). *Gender, Sexuality and Colonial Modernities*. Routledge Research in Gender and History. London and New York: Routledge, 1999.

Bush, G. W. A. *Decently and in Order: The Government of the City of Auckland 1840–1971*. Auckland and London: Collins, 1971.

Byrne, Bridget. *White Lives: The Interplay of 'Race', Class and Gender in Everyday Life*. Abingdon and New York: Routledge, 2006.

BIBLIOGRAPHY

Byrnes, Giselle (ed.). *The New Oxford History of New Zealand*. Auckland and Melbourne: Oxford University Press, 2009.

Carnes, Mark C. and Clyde Griffen (eds). *Meanings for Manhood: Constructions of Masculinity in Victorian America*. Chicago and London: University of Chicago Press, 1990.

Cannon, Michael. *Australia in the Victorian Age*. 2 vols. Melbourne: Thomas Nelson, 1975.

Cannon, Michael. *Melbourne After the Gold Rush*. Main Ridge: Loch Haven Books, 1993.

Carey, Jane and Claire McLisky (eds). *Creating White Australia*. Sydney: Sydney University Press, 2009.

Chan, Wendy, Dorothy E. Chunn and Robert Menzies (eds). *Women, Madness and the Law: A Feminist Reader*. London, Portland, OR, and Coogee: GlassHouse Press, 2005.

Clarke, Patricia. *The Governesses: Letters from the Colonies 1862–1882*. Sydney, Wellington, London and Boston: Allen & Unwin, 1985.

Coleborne, Catharine. *Madness in the Family: Insanity and Institutions in the Australasian Colonial World, 1860–1914*. Basingstoke and New York: Palgrave Macmillan, 2010.

Coleborne, Catharine. *Reading 'Madness': Gender and Difference in the Colonial Asylum in Victoria, Australia, 1848–1888*. Perth: Network Books, Australian Public Intellectual Network, 2007.

Coleborne, Catharine and Dolly MacKinnon (eds). *Exhibiting Madness in Museums: Remembering Psychiatry through Collections and Display*. Routledge Research in Museum Studies. New York and London: Routledge, 2011.

Coleborne, Catharine and Dolly MacKinnon (eds). *'Madness' in Australia: Histories, Heritage and the Asylum*. UQP Australian Studies. St Lucia: University of Queensland Press, 2003.

Cooper, Frederick and Ann Laura Stoler (eds). *Tensions of Empire: Colonial Cultures in a Bourgeois World*. Berkeley and Los Angeles: University of California Press, 1997.

Cox, Catherine. *Negotiating Insanity in the Southeast of Ireland, 1820–1900*. Manchester and New York: Manchester University Press, 2012.

Cox, Catherine and Hilary Marland (eds). *Migration, Health and Ethnicity in the Modern World*. Science, Technology and Medicine in Modern History. Basingstoke and New York: Palgrave Macmillan, 2013.

Cronin, Kathryn. *Colonial Casualties: Chinese in Early Victoria*. Melbourne: Melbourne University Press, 1983.

Crowther, M. Anne and Marguerite W. Dupree. *Medical Lives in the Age of Surgical Revolution*. Cambridge Studies in Population, Economy and Society in Past Time 43. Cambridge and New York: Cambridge University Press, 2007.

Dale, Colonel Percival. *Loving Service in Our Community, 1855–1962: Being the Story of the Work of the Melbourne City Mission*. 89/90, Percival Dale, 9/2. Carlton: Melbourne City Mission [c. 1963].

BIBLIOGRAPHY

Daley, Caroline and Deborah Montgomerie (eds). *The Gendered Kiwi*. Auckland: Auckland University Press, 1999.

Damousi, Joy. *Depraved and Disorderly: Female Convicts, Sexuality and Gender in Colonial Australia*. Cambridge and Melbourne: Cambridge University Press, 1997.

Daniels, Kay, Mary Murnane and Anne Picot (eds). *Women in Australia: An Annotated Guide to Records*. Vol. 1. Canberra: Australian Government Publishing Service, 1977.

Davison, Graeme. *The Rise and Fall of Marvellous Melbourne, 1880–1895*. Melbourne: Australian National University, 1969.

Davison, Graeme and Shirley Constantine (eds). *Out of Work Again: The Autobiographical Narrative of Thomas Dobeson, 1885–1891*. Monash Publications in History 6. Melbourne: Monash University, 1990.

Davison, Graeme, David Dunstan and Chris McConville (eds). *The Outcasts of Melbourne: Essays in Social History*. Sydney, London and Boston: Allen & Unwin, 1985.

Davison, Graeme, J. W. McCarty and Ailsa McLeary (eds). *Australians 1888*. Broadway: Fairfax, Syme & Weldon, 1987.

Day, David. *Claiming a Continent: A New History of Australia*. Sydney: HarperCollins, 2001 [1996].

Deacon, Desley, Penny Russell and Angela Woollacott (eds). *Transnational Lives: Biographies of Global Modernity, 1700–Present*. Palgrave Macmillan Transnational History Series. Basingstoke and New York: Palgrave Macmillan, 2010.

Dingle, Tony. *The Victorians Settling*. Melbourne: Fairfax, Syme and Weldon, 1984.

Dixson, Miriam. *The Imaginary Australian: Anglo-Celts and Identity, 1788 to the Present*. Sydney: University of New South Wales Press, 1999.

Driver, Felix and David Gilbert (eds). *Imperial Cities: Landscape, Display and Identity*. Studies in Imperialism. Manchester: Manchester University Press, 2003.

Duncan, James S. *In the Shadows of the Tropics: Climate, Race and Biopower in Nineteenth Century Ceylon*. Re-Materialsing Cultural Geography. Aldershot and Burlington: Ashgate, 2007.

Edmonds, Penelope. *Urbanizing Frontiers: Indigenous Peoples and Settlers in Nineteenth-Century Pacific Rim Cities*. Vancouver and Toronto: University of British Columbia Press, 2010.

Ehrhardt, Penny with Ann Beaglehole. *Women and Welfare Work, 1893–1993*. Wellington: Department of Social Welfare/Historical Branch, 1993.

Ernst, Waltraud and Thomas Mueller (eds). *Transnational Psychiatries: Social and Cultural Histories of Psychiatry in Comparative Perspective c. 1800–2000*. Newcastle upon Tyne: Cambridge Scholars Publishing, 2010.

Fairburn, Miles. *The Ideal Society and Its Enemies: The Foundations of Modern New Zealand Society, 1850–1900*. Auckland: Auckland University Press, 1989.

BIBLIOGRAPHY

Fairburn, Miles. *Nearly Out of Heart and Hope: The Puzzle of a Colonial Labourer's Diary.* Auckland: Auckland University Press, 1995.

Finch, Lynette. *The Classing Gaze: Sexuality, Class and Surveillance.* Sydney: Allen & Unwin, 1993.

Finlay, Henry. *To Have But Not to Hold: A History of Attitudes to Marriage and Divorce in Australia 1858–1975.* Annandale: Federation Press, 2005.

Fischer-Tiné, Harald and Susanne Gehrmann (eds). *Empires and Boundaries: Rethinking Race, Class, and Gender in Colonial Settings.* Routledge Studies in Cultural History. New York and London: Routledge, 2009.

Flannery, Tim (ed.). *The Birth of Melbourne.* Melbourne: Text Publishing, 2002.

Fox, Charlie (ed.). *Historical Refractions.* Studies in Western Australian History 14. Crawley: University of Western Australia, 1993.

Frances, Raelene. *The Politics of Work: Gender and Labour in Victoria, 1880–1939.* Cambridge, New York and Melbourne: Cambridge University Press, 1993.

Fraser, Lyndon and Katie Pickles (eds). *Shifting Centres: Women and Migration in New Zealand History.* Dunedin: University of Otago Press, 2002.

Freeman, Mark and Gillian Nelson (eds). *Vicarious Vagrants: Incognito Social Explorers and the Homeless in England, 1860–1910.* Lambertville: True Bill Press, 2008.

Garton, Stephen. *Medicine and Madness: A Social History of Insanity in New South Wales, 1880–1940.* Sydney: New South Wales University Press, 1988.

Garton, Stephen. *Out of Luck: Poor Australians and Social Welfare.* The Australian Experience. Sydney: Allen & Unwin, 1990.

Ghosh, Durba and Dane Kennedy (eds). *Decentring Empire: Britain, India and the Transcolonial World.* New Perspectives in South Asian History. Hyderabad: Orient Longman, 2006.

Gijswijt-Hofstra, Marijke and Roy Porter (eds). *Cultures of Neurasthenia: From Beard to the First World War.* Clio Medica 63: The Wellcome Series in the History of Medicine. Amsterdam and New York: Rodopi, 2001.

Gilbert, Helen and Anna Johnston (eds). *In Transit: Travel, Text, Empire.* New York: Peter Lang, 2002.

Goodman, David. *Gold Seeking: Victoria and California in the 1850s.* Sydney: Allen & Unwin, 1994.

Gothard, Jan (ed.). *Asian Orientations: Studies in Western Australian History.* Studies in Western Australian History. Crawley: University of Western Australia, 1995.

Gothard, Jan. *Blue China: Single Female Migration to Colonial Australia.* Melbourne: Melbourne University Press, 2001.

Hacking, Ian. *The Taming of Chance.* Ideas in Context. Cambridge: Cambridge University Press, 1990.

Hall, Catherine. *Civilising Subjects: Metropole and Colony in the English Imagination 1830–1867.* Chicago: University of Chicago Press; Cambridge: Polity, 2002.

BIBLIOGRAPHY

Hall, Catherine. *White, Male and Middle Class: Explorations in Feminism and History*. Cambridge: Polity, 1992.

Hall, Catherine and Sonya O. Rose (eds). *At Home with the Empire: Metropolitan Culture and the Imperial World*. Cambridge: Cambridge University Press, 2006.

Hamilton, Carolyn, Verne Harris, Jane Taylor, Michele Pickover, Graeme Reid and Razia Saleh (eds). *Refiguring the Archive*. Dordrecht, Boston and London: Kluwer Academic Publishers, 2002.

Heller, Thomas C., Morton Sosna and David E. Wellbery (eds), with Arnold I. Davidson, Ann Swidler and Ian Watt. *Reconstructing Individualism: Autonomy, Individuality, and the Self in Western Thought*. Stanford: Stanford University Press, 1986.

Hodgson, Terence. *The Heart of Colonial Auckland, 1865–1910*. Auckland: Random Century, 1992.

Howell, Philip. *Geographies of Regulation: Policing Prostitution in Nineteenth-Century Britain and the Empire*. Edited by Alan Baker, Richard Dennis and Deryck Holdsworth. Cambridge Studies in Historical Geography 43. Cambridge: Cambridge University Press, 2009.

Huisman, Frank and John Harley Warner (eds). *Locating Medical History: The Stories and Their Meanings*. Baltimore and London: Johns Hopkins University Press, 2004.

Iacovetta, Franca and Wendy Mitchinson (eds). *On the Case: Explorations in Social History*. Toronto, Buffalo and London: University of Toronto Press, 1998.

Jackson, Lynette A. *Surfacing Up: Psychiatry and Social Order in Colonial Zimbabwe, 1908–1968*. Cornell Studies in the History of Psychiatry. Ithaca: Cornell University Press, 2005.

Jackson, Will. *Madness and Marginality: The Lives of Kenya's White Insane*. Studies in Imperialism. Manchester and New York: Manchester University Press, 2013.

Kennedy, Richard. *Charity Warfare: The Charity Organisation Society in Colonial Melbourne*. Melbourne: Hyland House, 1985.

Kingston, Beverley. *My Wife, My Daughter, and Poor Mary Ann: Women and Work in Australia*. Melbourne: Thomas Nelson, 1975.

Kingston, Beverley. *The Oxford History of Australia, Volume 3: 1860–1900, Glad Confident Morning*. Melbourne, Oxford and Auckland: Oxford University Press, 1988.

Kirkby, Diane. *Barmaids: A History of Women's Work in Pubs*. Cambridge, New York and Melbourne: Cambridge University Press, 1997.

Kirkby, Diane (ed.). *Sex, Power and Justice: Historical Perspectives on Law in Australia*. Melbourne: Oxford University Press, 1995.

Kirkby, Diane and Catharine Coleborne (eds). *Law, History, Colonialism: The Reach of Empire*. Studies in Imperialism. Manchester: Manchester University Press, 2001.

Lake, Marilyn and Henry Reynolds. *Drawing the Global Colour Line: White Men's Countries and the International Challenge of Racial Equality*.

Critical Perspectives on Empire. Cambridge and New York: Cambridge University Press, 2008.
Lambert, David and Alan Lester (eds). *Colonial Lives across the British Empire: Imperial Careering in the Long Nineteenth Century*. Cambridge and New York: Cambridge University Press, 2006.
Lawrence, Dianne. *Genteel Women: Empire and Domestic Material Culture, 1840–1910*. Studies in Imperialism. Manchester: Manchester University Press, 2012.
Levine, Philippa (ed.). *Gender and Empire*. Oxford History of the British Empire. Oxford: Oxford University Press, 2004.
Levine, Philippa. *Prostitution, Race and Politics: Policing Venereal Disease in the British Empire*. New York and London: Routledge, 2003.
Lewis, Milton James. *Managing Madness: Psychiatry and Society in Australia, 1788–1980*. Canberra: Australian Government Publishing Service, 1988.
Long, Jane, Jan Gothard and Helen Brash (eds). *Forging Identities: Bodies, Gender and Feminist History*. Nedlands: University of Western Australia Press, 1997.
Lucas, Gavin. *An Archaeology of Colonial Identity: Power and Material Culture in the Dwars Valley, South Africa*. Contributions to Global Historical Archaeology. New York: Springer, 2006.
Mahone, Sloan and Megan Vaughan (eds). *Psychiatry and Empire*. Cambridge Imperial and Post-Colonial Studies. Basingstoke and New York: Palgrave Macmillan, 2007.
Main, William. *Auckland Through a Victorian Lens*. Wellington: Millwood Press, 1977.
Mangan, J. A. and James Walvin (eds). *Manliness and Morality: Middle-Class Masculinity in Britain and America, 1800–1940*. Manchester: Manchester University Press, 1987.
Mar, Tracey Banivanua and Penelope Edmonds (eds). *Making Settler Colonial Space: Perspectives on Race, Place and Identity*. Basingstoke: Palgrave Macmillan, 2010.
Marland, Hilary. *Dangerous Motherhood: Insanity and Childbirth in Victorian Britain*. Basingstoke and New York: Palgrave Macmillan, 2004.
Matlock, Jann. *Scenes of Seduction: Prostitution, Hysteria, and Reading Difference in Nineteenth-Century France*. New York: Columbia University Press, 1994.
McCalman, Janet. *Struggletown: Public and Private Life in Richmond, 1900–1965*. Carlton: Melbourne University Press: 1985.
McCarthy, Angela. *Scottishness and Irishness in New Zealand since 1840*. Studies in Imperialism. Manchester: Manchester University Press, 2011.
McCarthy, Angela and Catharine Coleborne (eds). *Migration, Ethnicity, and Mental Health: International Perspectives, 1840–2010*. Routledge Studies in Cultural History. New York and Abingdon: Routledge, 2012.
McClintock, Anne. *Imperial Leather: Race, Gender and Sexuality in the Colonial Contest*. New York and London: Routledge, 1995.

BIBLIOGRAPHY

McClure, Margaret. *Saving the City: The History of the Order of the Good Shepherd and the Community of the Holy Name in Auckland, 1894–2000*. Auckland: Hostel Advisory Group/David Ling, 2002.

Melling, Joseph and Bill Forsythe (eds). *Insanity, Institutions and Society, 1800–1914: A Social History of Madness in Comparative Perspective*. Studies in the Social History of Medicine. Abingdon and New York: Routledge, 1999.

Millen, Julia. *Colonial Tears and Sweat: The Working Class in Nineteenth-Century New Zealand*. Wellington: Reed, 1984.

Mills, James H. *Madness, Cannabis and Colonialism: The 'Native-Only' Lunatic Asylums of British India, 1857–1900*. London and New York: Macmillan and St Martin's, 2000.

Mills, James H. and Satadru Sen (eds). *Confronting the Body: The Politics of Physicality in Colonial and Post-Colonial India*. Anthem South Asian Studies. London: Anthem Press, 2003.

Mitchinson, Wendy and Janice Dickin McGinnis (eds). *Essays in the History of Canadian Medicine*. Toronto: McClelland and Stewart, 1988.

Mohanram, Radhika. *Imperial White: Race, Diaspora, and the British Empire*. Minneapolis: University of Minnesota Press, 2007.

Monk, Lee-Ann. *Attending Madness: At Work in the Australian Colonial Asylum*. Clio Medica 84: The Wellcome Series in the History of Medicine. Amsterdam and New York: Rodopi, 2008.

Moran, James E. and David Wright (eds). *Mental Health and Canadian Society: Historical Perspectives*. Studies in the History of Medicine, Health and Society. Montreal: McGill-Queen's University Press, 2008.

Otzen, Roslyn. *Dr John Singleton, 1808–1891: Christian, Doctor, Philanthropist*. Melbourne: Melbourne Citymission, 2008.

Parle, Julie. *States of Mind: Searching for Mental Health in Natal and Zululand, 1868–1918*. Scottsville: University of KwaZulu-Natal Press, 2007.

Pearn, John and Catherine O'Carrigan (eds). *Australia's Quest for Colonial Health: Some Influences on Early Health and Medicine in Australia*. Brisbane: Department of Child Health, 1983.

Phillips, Jock. *A Man's Country? The Image of the Pakeha Male: A History*. Revised ed. Auckland: Penguin, 1996 [1987].

Phillips, Roderick. *Divorce in New Zealand: A Social History*. Auckland: Oxford University Press, 1981.

Picard, Liza. *Victorian London: The Life of a City 1840–1870*. New York: St Martin's Press, 2005.

Pick, Daniel. *Faces of Degeneration: A European Disorder, c. 1848 – c. 1918*. Ideas in Context. Cambridge: Cambridge University Press, 1989.

Pickles, Katie and Catharine Coleborne (eds). *New Zealand's Empire*. Studies in Imperialism. Manchester: Manchester University Press (forthcoming).

Porter, Roy and W. F. Bynum (eds). *Companion Encyclopedia of the History of Medicine*. Routledge Companion Encyclopedias. London and New York: Routledge, 1993.

BIBLIOGRAPHY

Porter, Roy and David Wright (eds). *The Confinement of the Insane: International Perspectives, 1800–1965*. Cambridge and New York: Cambridge University Press, 2003.

Povinelli, Elizabeth A. *The Empire of Love: Toward a Theory of Intimacy, Genealogy, and Carnality*. Durham, NC: Duke University Press, 2006.

Proudfoot, Lindsay J. and Dianne P. Hall. *Imperial Spaces: Placing the Irish and Scots in Colonial Australia*. Studies in Imperialism. Manchester: Manchester University Press, 2011.

Proudfoot, Lindsay J. and Michael M. Roche (eds). *(Dis)Placing Empire: Renegotiating British Colonial Geographies*. Heritage, Culture and Identity. Aldershot and Burlington: Ashgate, 2005.

Reaume, Geoffrey. *Remembrance of Patients Past: Patient Life at the Toronto Hospital for the Insane, 1870–1940*. Don Mills: Oxford University Press Canada, 2000.

Rembis, Michael A., Kim Nielsen and Catherine Kudlick (eds). *Oxford Handbook of Disability History*. Oxford: Oxford University Press (forthcoming).

Rice, Geoffrey W. (ed.). *The Oxford History of New Zealand*. 2nd edn. Oxford: Oxford University Press, 1992.

Richards, Eric (ed.). *Poor Australian Immigrants in the Nineteenth Century*. Visible Immigrants: Two. Canberra: Australian National University, 1991.

Richards, Eric (ed.). *Visible Women: Female Immigrants in Colonial Australia*. Visible Immigrants: Four. Canberra: Australian National University, 1995.

Richards, Thomas. *The Imperial Archive: Knowledge and the Fantasy of Empire*. London and New York: Verso, 1993.

Robinson-Tomsett, Emma. *Women, Travel and Identity: Journeys by Rail and Sea, 1870–1940*. Gender in History. Manchester and New York: Manchester University Press, 2013.

Roe, Jill (ed.). *Social Policy in Australia: Some Perspectives 1901–1975*. Melbourne: Cassell, 1976.

Roper, Michael and John Tosh (eds). *Manful Assertions: Masculinities in Britain since 1800*. London and New York: Routledge, 1991.

Rose, Lionel. *'Rogues and Vagabonds': Vagrant Underworld in Britain 1815–1985*. London and New York: Routledge, 1988.

Russell, Lynette (ed.). *Colonial Frontiers: Indigenous-European Encounters in Settler Societies*. Studies in Imperialism. Manchester: Manchester University Press, 2001.

Russell, Penny. *A Wish of Distinction: Colonial Gentility and Femininity*. Melbourne: Melbourne University Press, 1994.

Russell, Penny (ed.). *For Richer, For Poorer: Early Colonial Marriages*. Melbourne: Melbourne University Press, 1994.

Salmon, J. H. M. *A History of Gold-Mining in New Zealand*. Wellington: Government Printer, 1963.

Schreuder, Deryck M. and Stuart Ward (eds). *Australia's Empire*. The Oxford History of the British Empire Companion Series. Oxford and New York: Oxford University Press, 2008.

BIBLIOGRAPHY

Shapiro, Ann-Louise. *Breaking the Codes: Female Criminality in Fin-de-Siècle Paris*. Stanford: Stanford University Press, 1996.

Showalter, Elaine. *The Female Malady: Women, Madness and English Culture, 1830–1980*. Michigan: Panthecn Books, 1985.

Sinclair, Keith (ed.). *The Oxford Illustrated History of New Zealand*. Oxford Illustrated Histories. Auckland and Oxford: Oxford University Press, 1990.

Sinclair, Keith (ed.). *Tasman Relations: New Zealand and Australia, 1788–1988*. Auckland: Auckland University Press, 1987.

Sinha, Mrinalini. *Colonial Masculinity: The 'Manly Englishman' and the 'Effeminate Bengali' in the Late Nineteenth Century*. Studies in Imperialism. Manchester: Manchester University Press, 1995.

Smith, Christopher J. and John A. Giggs (eds). *Location and Stigma: Contemporary Perspectives on Mental Health and Mental Health Care*. Boston: Unwin Hyman, 1988.

Stasiulis, Daiva and Nira Yuval-Davis (eds). *Unsettling Settler Societies: Articulations of Gender, Race, Ethnicity and Class*. Sage Series on Race and Ethnic Relations. London and Thousand Oaks: Sage, 1995.

Stedman Jones, Gareth. *Outcast London: A Study in the Relationship Between Classes in Victorian Society*. Oxford: Clarendon Press, 1971.

Steel, Frances. *Oceania under Steam: Sea Transport and the Cultures of Colonialism, c. 1870–1914*. Studies in Imperialism. Manchester and New York: Manchester University Press, 2011.

Stoler, Ann Laura. *Along the Archival Grain: Epistemic Anxieties and Colonial Common Sense*. Princeton and Woodstock UK: Princeton University Press, 2009.

Stoler, Ann Laura (ed.). *Haunted by Empire: Geographies of Intimacy in North American History*. Durham, NC: Duke University Press, 2006.

Stoler, Ann Laura. *Race and the Education of Desire: Foucault's History of Sexuality and the Colonial Order of Things*. Durham, NC, and London: Duke University Press, 1995.

Stone, Deborah. A., *The Disabled State*. Philadelphia: Temple University Press, 1984.

Stone, R. C. J. *Makers of Fortune: A Colonial Business Community and Its Fall*. Auckland: Auckland University Press, 1973.

Strahan, Lynne. *Out of the Silence: A Study of a Religious Community for Women: The Community of the Holy Name*. Melbourne: Oxford University Press, 1988.

Strange, Carolyn and Alison Bashford (eds). *Isolation: Places and Practices of Exclusion*. Routledge Studies in Modern History. London and New York: Routledge, 2003.

Sutphen, Mary P. and Bridie Andrews (eds). *Medicine and Colonial Identity*. Routledge Studies in the Social History of Medicine. London and New York: Routledge, 2003.

Swain, Shurlee. *Separate Spaces: Mapping the Melbourne of the Single Mother*. Melbourne: University of Melbourne, 1996.

BIBLIOGRAPHY

Swain, Shurlee with Renate Howe. *Single Mothers and Their Children: Disposal, Punishment and Survival in Australia.* Cambridge, New York, and Melbourne: Cambridge University Press, 1995.

Te Awekotuku, Ngahuia with Linda Waimarie Nikora. *Mau Moko: The World of Māori Tattoo.* North Shore: Penguin Viking, 2007.

Teo, Hsu-Ming and Richard White (eds). *Cultural History in Australia.* Sydney: University of New South Wales Press, 2003.

Tennant, Margaret. *The Fabric of Welfare: Voluntary Organisations, Government and Welfare in New Zealand, 1840–2005.* Wellington: Bridget Williams Books, 2007.

Tennant, Margaret. *Paupers and Providers: Charitable Aid in New Zealand.* Wellington: Allen & Unwin/Historical Branch, 1990.

Thomson, Rosemarie Garland, *Extraordinary Bodies: Figuring Physical Disability in American Culture and Literature.* New York: Columbia University Press, 1997.

Twomey, Christina. *Deserted and Destitute: Motherhood, Wife Desertion and Colonial Welfare.* Melbourne: Australian Scholarly Publishing, 2002.

Uhl, Jean. *Mount Royal Hospital: A Social History.* Parkville: Mount Royal Hospital, 1981.

Vamplew, Wray. *Australians: Historical Statistics.* Australians: A Historical Library 9. Melbourne: Fairfax, Syme and Weldon, 1987.

Vaughan, Megan. *Curing Their Ills: Colonial Power and African Illness.* Stanford: Stanford University Press, 1991.

Veracini, Lorenzo. *Settler Colonialism: A Theoretical Overview.* Basingstoke and New York: Palgrave Macmillan, 2010.

Warsh, Cheryl Krasnick. *Moments of Unreason: The Practice of Canadian Psychiatry and the Homewood Retreat, 1883–1923.* Montreal and Kingston: McGill-Queen's University Press, 1989.

Waterhouse, Catherine. *Going Forward in Faith: A History of the Melbourne Citymission.* Fitzroy: Melbourne Citymission, 1999.

Wear, Andrew (ed.). *Medicine in Society: Historical Essays.* Cambridge, New York and Melbourne: Cambridge University Press, 1992.

Weaver, John C. *A Sadly Troubled History: The Meanings of Suicide in the Modern Age.* McGill-Queen's/Associated Medical Services Studies in the History of Medicine, Health, and Society. Montreal and Kingston: McGill-Queen's University Press, 2009.

Weidenhofer, Maggie (ed.). *Gariyowen's Melbourne: A selection from the Chronicles of Early Melbourne, 1835 to 1852.* Melbourne: Thomas Nelson, 1967.

Wevers, Lydia. *Country of Writing: Travel Writing and New Zealand 1809–1900.* Auckland: Auckland University Press, 2002.

Wevers, Lydia. *Reading on the Farm: Victorian Fiction and the Colonial World.* Wellington: Victoria University Press, 2010.

White, Richard. *Inventing Australia.* The Australian Experience 3. St Leonard's: Allen & Unwin, 1981.

BIBLIOGRAPHY

Wilson, Dean. *The Beat: Policing a Victorian City*. Melbourne: Circa, 2006.
Wolfe, Patrick. *Settler Colonialism and the Transformation of Anthropology: The Politics and Poetics of an Ethnographic Event*. Writing Past Colonialism. London and New York: Cassell, 1999.
Wolff, Kurt H. *The Sociology of Georg Simmel*. New York: Free Press, 1950.

Unpublished theses

Brown, Hayley. 'Loosening the Marriage Bond: Divorce in New Zealand, c.1890s–c.1950s'. Ph.D. thesis, Victoria University of Wellington, 2011.
Elphick, Judith. 'Auckland 1870–74: A Social Portrait'. Masters thesis, University of Auckland, 1974.
Dawson, Maree. 'National Fitness or Failure? Heredity, Vice and Racial Decline in New Zealand Psychiatry: A Case Study of the Auckland Mental Hospital, 1868–99'. Ph.D. thesis, University of Waikato, 2013.
Hoult, Adrienne. 'Institutional Responses to Mental Deficiency in New Zealand, 1911–1935: Tokanui Mental Hospital'. Masters thesis, University of Waikato, 2007.
Murray, Caitlin. 'Settling the Mind: Psychiatry and the Colonial Project in Australia'. Ph.D. thesis, University of Melbourne, 2012.
Mutch, Margaret. 'Aspects of the Social and Economic History of Auckland, 1890–1896'. Masters thesis, University of Auckland, 1968.
Reeves, Carol Anne. 'Insanity and Nervous Diseases amongst Jewish Immigrants to the East End of London, 1880–1920'. Ph.D. thesis, University of London, 2001.
Robson, Belinda. 'The Construction and Experience of Female Mental Illness in Melbourne, 1906–1909'. Honours thesis. University of Melbourne, 1988.
Spooner, Emma. 'Digging for the Families of the "Mad": Locating the Family in the Auckland Asylum Archives, 1870–1911'. Masters thesis, University of Waikato, 2006.
Spooner, Emma. '"The mind is thoroughly unhinged": Reading the Auckland Asylum Archive, New Zealand, 1900–1910'. Honours dissertation, University of Waikato, 2004.
Twomey, Christina. '"Without Natural Protectors": Histories of Deserted and Destitute Colonial Women in Victoria 1850–1865'. Ph.D. thesis, University of Melbourne, 1995.
Wilson, Dean. 'Community Violence in Auckland, 1850–1875'. Masters thesis, University of Auckland, 1993.

Unpublished papers

Coleman, Jenny. 'Reframing benevolence: From palliative charity to social reform in early 1870s Auckland'. Unpublished paper presented at the Australasian Welfare History Workshop, Massey University, Palmerston North, and University of Waikato, Hamilton, 15–16 November 2011.
Marland, Hilary and Catherine Cox. 'Emaciated and exhausted: Irish minds and bodies in nineteenth-century Lancashire asylums'. EAHM Body and Mind Conference, Utrecht, September 2011.

BIBLIOGRAPHY

Wright, Katie. 'The arrival of therapeutic culture in Australia: Modern life, masculinity and the problem of "nerves"'. TASA Conference 2006 (The Australian Sociological Association), University of Western Australia and Murdoch University, 4–7 December 2006.

Internet sources

'1881 Victorian Census'. Revisiting Kew: Sources Historic Explanations, 1 August 2012. http://rbkr.wordpress.com/2012/08/01/1881-victorian-census-11/, accessed 4 August 2014.

Appendices to the Journals of the House of Representatives. AtoJsOnline. National Library of New Zealand/Te Puna Mātauranga o Aotearoa. http://atojs.natlib. govt.nz/cgi-bin/atojs, accessed 1 August 2014.

'Calling Australia Home'. Jewish Museum of Australia in Melbourne. www.jewishmuseum.com.au/exhibitions/permanent-exhibitions, accessed 18 November 2013.

eMelbourne: The City Past and Present. Encyclopedia of Melbourne online, University of Melbourne. www.egold.net.au/biogs/EG00090b.htm, accessed 1 August 2011.

'Hauhauism'. By Bernard John Foster. Te Ara: The Encyclopedia of New Zealand. www.teara.govt.nz/en/1966/hauhauism, accessed 20 June 2013.

Historical Census and Colonial Data Archive (HCCDA). Victorian Censuses 1865–1901. http://hccda.ada.edu.au/, accessed 4 August 2014.

'Immigration Chronology: Selected Events 1840–2008'. New Zealand Parliamentary Research Library. www.parliament.nz/en-nz/parl-support/research-papers/00PLSocRP08011/immigration-chronology-selected-events-1840-2008, accessed 1 August 2014.

'The Occupational Structure of Britain 1379–1911'. The Cambridge Group for the History of Population and Social Structure. Department of Geography and Faculty of History, University of Cambridge. www.geog.cam.ac.uk/research/ centres/campop/occupations/, accessed 27 December 2013; 1 August 2014.

Police Gazettes, Factsheet. National Archives of New Zealand. http://archives.govt.nz/ sites/default/files/Police_Gazettes.pdf, accessed 18 June 2013.

INDEX

Aboriginal missions 102
   Coranderrk 102
   Lake Condah 102
Aboriginal peoples 6, 20, 24, 30, 31, 43n1, 74, 88, 101–2, 171–4, 175
   and dispossession 74–5
Aboriginal protection 74
addiction 121, 170
admission 51–2, 58, 68, 86, 88, 99, 101, 106, 107, 109n8, 126, 127, 131, 143, 148, 179, 183, 187
   and Chinese 176
   and family 88, 168
   and Māori 168
   and police 88
   and readmission 88
alcoholism 38, 92, 116, 120, 123, 130
   see also drinking
Anderson, Warwick 9, 133
Andrews, Bridie 8
Andrews, Jonathan 90
Anglo-settler 'revolution' 5
anti-semitism 96
Argus 63
Arnold, Rollo 25
Ashburn Hall (New Zealand) 42
Askew, John 35
assemblages 5, 77, 88, 179, 183
asylums 3, 10, 15n12, 37–9, 41, 52, 53, 58, 61, 68, 96
   Annual Reports 68, 89, 97
   populations 54, 88, 91
      'colonial born' 14, 30, 37, 54–5, 87, 93, 94, 165, 174, 176, 177
      'foreign born' 12, 41, 53–5, 72, 87, 93
   public 69, 86,
   segregation 87
Atkinson, Alan 6
Auckland City Mission 69
Australian Medical Journal 176

Balls-Headley, Dr Walter 55
Batman, John 24
Belich, James 5

benevolence 57, 61, 70
benevolent homes (Victoria) 62, 64
bereavement 92
Besley, Joanna 187
birthrate 140, 174
boarding houses 57, 66, 121, 141
boarding-out 39
bodies 2, 4, 7, 12, 29, 37, 64, 87, 105–7, 117–18, 122, 140, 142, 144, 152–3, 156, 184, 187
Braslow, Joel 13
Brickell, Chris 128–9
Britain 2, 12, 25, 29, 30, 33 52, 56, 58, 60, 66, 97, 115, 122, 123, 126, 142, 143, 145, 147, 177, 178
British Columbia (Canada) 130
Brookes, Barbara 86, 107, 187
Butler, Samuel 28, 120

Calcutta 41
California 32
Cannon, Michael 52–3
Canterbury (New Zealand) 28, 120
Canvas Town 34–5, 57, 61
case note records 3
   conventions of 84, 89–91
   language 107
   and classification 107, 142, 168
Census reports 26, 93, 97, 146, 169
Central Board for Aborigines 31
   see also Aboriginal Protection
charitable institutions 52–5, 61, 69–70, 71–3
   see also welfare
children 58, 62, 63, 64, 127, 129, 130, 143, 146, 151, 158, 175
   neglected 68–9
   and mortality 153
Chisholm, Caroline 152–3
China 30, 93, 98, 171
Chinatown 1
Chinese 6, 14, 20, 28, 37, 57, 74, 81n92, 87–8, 97, 104, 117, 165–6, 167–71, 173, 175, 177, 178, 185, 186

[218]

INDEX

Clarke, Patricia 146
class 2, 3, 6, 8, 9, 10, 13, 26, 27–31, 33, 36, 38, 40, 55, 58–60, 62, 63, 65, 68, 76–7, 86–7, 91, 96, 98, 99, 103, 114–15, 118–19, 121–2, 124, 128, 130, 133, 141–3, 145–7, 150, 156, 157, 184, 186, 188
Clouston, Thomas 37
Colombo 41
colonial medicine 14
  and discourse 6, 142
colonisers 4, 9
commerce 20, 33
Commercial Bay (Auckland) 24
communication 25, 170
convicts 100
Coromandel (New Zealand) 21
Costley, Edward 70
Costley Home for the Aged Poor (Auckland) 3, 51, 53–4, 70–4, 75, 77n12
Cox, James 131

Dale, Colonel Percival 58
database 3, 13, 56, 85, 92, 93, 95, 99, 104, 105, 109n8, 110n25
Dawson, Maree 125
death 38, 53, 72, 88, 105, 125, 126, 153, 172, 175
degeneracy 1, 37, 161n70
delinquency 63, 152
delusions 1, 40, 41, 51 75, 83n144, 93, 94, 102–5, 114, 116, 119, 124, 125, 127, 129, 130, 144–5, 153–4, 156, 170–1, 175
demography 12
deserted wives 27, 53, 58, 63, 141
diagnoses 87–8, 104–5, 107, 116, 120, 124–7, 136n48, 140, 150–2
  General Paralysis of the Insane (GPI) 37, 164, 68, 73, 104, 116, 125–7, 148, 153, 168–9, 183
  hysteria 123, 130, 139, 153
  puerperal insanity 104, 140, 146, 154–5, 164, 174
  sunstroke 116, 118–19, 124, 187
Dick, Dr Thomas 68
disguises 103
Dixson, Miriam 7
Dobeson, Thomas 119–20

domesticity 98, 130, 140
  language of 129
Donegal 64
drinking 36, 38, 46n77, 120, 128, 148, 150
  see also alcoholism
Dunedin 32–3, 42, 86

Earley, Dr H. 34, 60
Edmonds, Penelope 5, 186
England 21, 29, 30, 37, 41, 42, 55, 69, 84, 93, 96, 97, 114, 119, 127
Ernst, Waltraud 9
ethnicity 3, 6, 7–10, 13, 14, 18n57, 26, 29, 76, 87, 91, 93, 94, 116, 118, 120, 122, 126, 128, 133, 140, 142–4, 164–5, 168–9, 175–6, 188
  Afghan 128, 170
  Anglo-Celtic 7, 88
  Danish 39, 73
  Irish 7, 9, 12, 20, 29, 32, 33, 37, 41, 64, 87–8, 93–4, 97, 103, 120, 126, 131, 143, 144, 147, 156–7, 177
  Jewish 32, 36, 37, 95–7,143
  non-white 8–9, 13, 14, 27, 28, 33, 65, 101, 122, 133, 142, 158, 165, 175, 178–9, 186–7
  Scottish 7, 33, 88,
  and accents 56, 93, 144
  and heterogeneity 28
  and language 56, 93, 144, 171, 173
  see also Chinese; Māori
European empire 4
excitement 20–1, 60, 66, 119
extra-institutional care 39

factory 25, 37, 145–6, 148–9
families 10, 26, 27, 29, 32, 38, 39, 41, 57, 58, 61, 66, 71, 92, 99 104, 117, 127, 133, 139, 141, 145, 151, 153, 155, 158, 166, 168, 174, 177
  and violence 124
Female Middle Class Emigration Society 146
female refuge 69
feminist 12, 14, 29, 130, 142, 156
Finnane, Mark 187
Foucault, Michel 184

[219]

INDEX

Franklin, Miles 147
friendship 122, 129
frontier 11, 23, 28, 30
fugitive 27

Galton, Francis 37
gambling 36
Garton, Stephen 121, 187
gender 2, 3, 4, 6, 7–10, 13–14, 26–7, 29, 38, 51, 56, 65, 74–5, 76–7, 86–7, 91, 92, 101, 105, 108, 117, 133, 139, 165, 172, 174, 183, 184–6
  femininity 139–58
  masculinity 114–33
  norms 104
  relations 116, 186
  and identity 101, 129–30, 187–8
  and labour 97–9, 122
  and sexuality 127
geography 12, 22, 97
Glasgow 40, 51, 124
gold mining 30, 122, 168
Goldberg, Ann 96
goldrush 20–1, 24, 25, 27, 28, 30, 52, 58, 100, 118, 122, 141
Goodman, David 101, 103
governmentality 5, 86
Grace, Dr M. 41
Graham, Jeanine 25
Greig, Dr James Saunders 54–5
grief 40, 92, 114, 130, 165
  see also death; bereavement

Hall, Catherine 86, 164, 183, 188
Hawk, Angela 100
Hay, Dr Frank 177
health 8, 12, 14, 21, 27, 34, 36, 43, 52, 56, 60, 61, 64, 69, 74–6, 91, 118, 131, 140, 142, 144, 150, 153, 155, 156, 164, 166–7, 176, 187
heredity 1, 10, 119, 152, 155, 173, 178
Hodges, C. P. 169
homosexuality 31, 127, 128
Howitt, William 28, 34, 61, 119–21
hybridity 176–7, 188

identity formation 7, 12, 149, 183, 188

Illustrated Australian News 35, 58, 62
Illustrated Melbourne Post 117
Immigrant's Aid Society (Melbourne) 3, 34, 53–4, 57, 59–60, 62–3, 68, 74, 131, 151
immigration advice booklets 53
Immigration Agent 31
Immigration Officer 55
imperial pension 71
'imperial turn' 4, 179, 183
Industrial Schools 152
Intercolonial Medical Congress of Australasia 3, 126, 176
Intercolonial Medical Journal of Australasia 130
Ireland 29, 30, 42, 51, 55, 93, 98, 127, 144
isolation 3, 6, 39, 60–1, 188

James, John Stanley 59
Jarritt, Rev William 34, 60
Joint Committee on Lunatic Asylums (New Zealand) 41

Kernot, M. J. 65
Kerr, John Hunter 27, 35
Kilkenny District Asylum 41
King, Frederic Truby 128
King, John (Inspector of Asylums) 31, 39

Labrum, Bronwyn 141, 187
Ladies' Benevolent Society (Auckland) 69
Ladies' City Mission (Melbourne) 57
  see also Melbourne City Missions
Lake, Marilyn 132
Lancashire 37
legislation 13, 90, 100, 133, 179
  An Act for the Better Protection of Vagrancy and Other Offences (Victoria, 1852) 100
  Contagious Diseases 156
  Hospitals and Charitable Institutions Act (New Zealand, 1885) 71
  Imbecile Passengers Act (New Zealand, 1882) 166
  Immigration (Restriction) Act (Australia 1901) 166

[220]

INDEX

Lunacy Act (New Zealand, 1868) 89
Lunatics Act (Victoria, 1867) 89
Mental Defectives Act (New Zealand, 1911) 178
Mental Deficiency Act (UK, 1913) 178
Passengers Act (UK, 1855) 166
Vagrant Act (New Zealand, 1866) 100
Levine, Philippa 156
literacy 123, 148
Liverpool 37
lodging houses 57
London 32, 36, 56, 62, 63, 103, 145–6
lunatics 6, 31, 38, 69, 70, 71, 88, 89, 174
lying-in hospital 52

MacGregor, Duncan 55, 70, 78n28,
Mackie, Frederick 57, 79n41
Malcolm, Elizabeth 97, 143, 18n48
Manchester 131, 145
manhood 27, 120, 122, 134n10
Manning, Frederic Norton 61, 125, 126
Māori 21, 75, 106, 171, 173
March, J. Edwin 55
marital status 76, 86, 91, 92, 98, 105, 129, 142, 145, 175, 185
marriage 27–9, 127, 141, 145–6, 154
McCarthy, Angela 7, 17, 18n57, 44n22, 49n152, 93, 109n1, 180n12
McClure, Margaret 73
McCreery, J. V. 174
McKenzie, Kirsten 103
McLaren, Angus 130
medical journals 3, 155
medical officer 34, 59, 62, 64, 68, 73, 126, 167
medical superintendents 66, 119
Megahey, Norman 112n53, 168
Melbourne City Mission 38, 52, 57–8, 68
  see also Ladies City Mission
Melbourne Gaol 53
Melbourne Hospital 53, 155
Melling, Joseph 147
menopause 154–5

mental
  defective 139, 151
  defects 61, 68, 151–2

health 3, 23, 39–41, 53, 54, 60, 68, 75, 118, 120, 145, 153–4, 165–7, 174, 177
hygiene 14, 165–6, 176
influences 70
Menzies, Bob 172
Mickle, William Julius 37
migration networks 28
  see also immigration
migration patterns 5–6, 51
military medical personnel 4
Mission to the Street and Lanes (Auckland) 58, 73–4
missionaries 57–8, 74
mobility 6, 11–12, 14, 17n46, 20–3, 25–34, 36–37, 40–3, 44n20, 51, 77, 100–1, 108, 119, 122, 131, 156–7, 185–7
Monk, Lee-Ann 71
Moore, John Murray 21, 26, 36, 69, 77n18
morality 56, 156
mortality 35, 60
Moss, Mr and Mrs 73
Mulgan, Alan 33
Murray, Caitlin 174

narratives 2, 27, 32, 77, 84–5, 90, 108, 183
New South Wales 10, 30, 61, 120, 187
New Zealand Magazine 55
Newton, Reverend Isaac 120
nomads 22
North Island (New Zealand) 6, 20–1, 38, 69, 122–3, 171–2
Northland (New Zealand) 21, 172

occupations 97–9, 116–17, 121, 123–4, 140, 145, 149, 169, 172
  banker 30
  barmaid 98, 148–9
  bootmaker 149
  bushmen 61
  domestic servant 87, 98, 144–5, 147, 154
  factory hand 145, 149

[221]

INDEX

occupations (*cont.*)
 gardener 51, 169
 governess 98–9, 139, 146–8
 gum digger 21, 71, 98, 103, 123, 172–3
 labourer 84, 87, 93, 98, 99–100, 119, 121–3, 131, 133, 150, 169, 183, 187
 miner 30, 46n75, 61, 87, 93, 98, 100, 103, 118, 168–9, 187
 pub-keeper 30
 sealer 24
 seamstress 99, 149
 servant 30, 87, 98, 144–8, 154
 settler's daughter 149
 settler's wife 150
 soldier 31
 storekeeper 30, 123
 tailoress 149
 teacher 98–9, 123, 145, 147–8, 153
official statistics 91,177
old age 39, 68, 92, 124, 173
Old Age Pension 25, 71
Old Colonists Association Home 62
Old Men's Refuge (Auckland) 69
opium 1, 28, 58, 121, 175
Otago 25, 32, 80, 78n28, 97
outdoor relief 52–3, 62
 see also welfare

Pacific islands 26
Paimārire Church 97, 173
Paley, Dr Edward 38–9, 54
Palys, Ted 172
parenthood 129
paupers 31, 52, 55, 101
pension 25, 71, 99
pensioner 99
Philson, Dr Thomas 69
photographs 86, 107
photography 106
Point Britomart 24
police 1, 28, 30–2, 64, 71, 84–5, 88, 100, 102–6, 114, 121, 127, 132, 146, 148, 154, 157, 168, 170–3, 175, 183
 Irish constabulary 103
 London Metropolitan 103
Police Gazettes 102–3
policing 14, 32, 56, 58, 103
Pollard, N. W. 61, 114

population 2–6, 8–9, 11–14, 20–2, 24–6, 29–30, 32–9, 52–5, 58, 60, 65, 68, 74, 76
Port Phillip 24, 30, 56, 143
poverty 3, 12, 20, 31, 37, 39, 48n131, 52, 54–5, 57–8, 60, 63, 68, 70, 74, 92, 100, 117, 120–1, 144, 158, 171, 178
pregnancy 141, 146, 154, 156
prison (Mount Eden, Auckland) 101
prisoners 6, 101
professions 36, 71, 96, 114, 149
 see also occupations
prostitution 4, 28, 69, 100, 156, 170
provincial surgeon 69

Queen Street (Auckland) 23, 33
Queensland 10, 120, 187

race 1, 2, 6, 8–10, 13–14, 29, 37, 41–2, 86–8, 133, 142–3, 156, 164, 167, 174–7, 186
 and psychopathology
religion 76, 87, 169, 173, 188
religious affiliations 96
 Anglican 32, 69, 73–4
 Catholic 1, 32, 64, 69, 87, 94–5, 131, 144, 146
 Christian 32, 57, 94–5, 97, 115, 117, 134n16, 144, 173
 Church of Scotland 32, 94
 Hauhauism 95, 97, 173
 Lutheran 94–5, 144
 Presbyterian 32, 94–5
 Wesleyan 32, 79n39, 94–5, 171
religious charity 57, 61
Report of the Commission on the Costley Home (1904) 73
Rhook, Nadia 170
Rosenblum, Dr Edward E. 126
Ross, Dr Chisholm 176–7
Royal Commission into Charitable Institutions (Victoria, 1871) 54
Royal Commission on Charitable Institutions (Victoria, 1890) 55
Royal Commission on Employees in Factories and Shops (Victoria 1882–84) 148
Royal Society of New Zealand 3
rural community 61, 63

[222]

INDEX

Sailors' Homes 58, 70
Salvation Army Maternity Home (Melbourne) 64
Scotland 29–30, 40, 55, 93, 97, 127
Seacliff Asylum 42
Segar, Dr H.W. 177
settler jurisdictions 24
settling 2, 8, 12, 20, 28–9, 34, 54, 101–2, 186
sexual health 56
sexuality 4, 10, 13, 31, 91–2, 116, 125–9, 140–2, 151–2, 154, 156, 170, 188
  heterosexuality 127
  homosexuality 31, 127–8
  masturbation 128, 153
  see also gender
shipping records 39
shipping trade 26
Showalter, Elaine 186
sickness 52, 62, 120
Singleton, Dr John 38, 66, 68, 158
Sinha, Mrinalini 165
Skae, Dr Frederick 52
skin 106–7, 120–1
slum 32–3, 36, 74, 121
Smith, Leonard 96
'social identity' 7–8, 10–1, 13–14, 86, 115, 165, 176, 184, 186, 188
social institutions 1–7, 12
social policy 25
sojourners 22, 26
South Australian 10
South Island 10, 21, 69, 97, 120, 152, 187
street urchins 31
Staffordshire Asylum 41
Steel, Frances 26
Stoler, Ann Laura 85
strangers 12, 26, 34, 56–7, 60, 66, 78n36
Stuckenberg, Ingeborg 39, 73
subjectivity 7
suburbs 33, 35, 57, 96
suicide 39–40, 42, 61, 68, 73, 158, 164, 170
Sunbury Asylum 40, 131, 176
Sutphen, Mary P. 8
Suzuki, Akihito 98
Swain, Shurlee 76
Syder, Mingay 142

syphilis 37, 40, 68, 117, 125–6, 148, 156
Syria 94

Tasman world 29
tattoos 102, 106
Tennant, Margaret 52, 71, 99
Thames (New Zealand) 21, 25
Tosh, John 115, 127
towns 21, 34–6, 38–9, 122, 147, 155, 169
tramp 101–2, 131
Transactions and Proceedings of the New Zealand Institute 3
transcolonial 5, 186
transfers 53, 68, 109n6
  institutional 75, 88
  transience 26, 34, 43n14, 74, 118
  see also vagrancy
transnational 4, 108, 183
transport 25, 33
travel writing 27, 53, 75
traveller 3–4, 20, 22, 26–7, 29, 35, 75, 101–2, 123, 132
Treadway, Walter L. 167
trial leave 88, 105, 170
Trollope, Anthony 20–1, 28, 34, 37, 75, 164
tropics 56, 118

Uhl, Jean 55, 65
United States Treasury Department 167
urban 1–2, 5–6, 8, 20–2, 29, 31–2, 35–8, 42, 54, 58, 63, 66, 69, 73–4, 100, 103, 118, 121–4, 126, 149, 156, 167–8, 170, 186

vagrancy 28, 58, 66, 100–3, 121, 131, 144, 157
  see also transience
vagrant 31, 33, 65, 71, 97–8, 100–1, 106, 131–2, 139–40, 156–7, 184, 186
Victorian Parliament 54
vital statistics 36, 48n128
voluntary contributions 57, 71
voluntary sector 52

Wales 30, 55, 93
wanderer 27, 102, 163n98

INDEX

welfare 1–5, 14, 27, 39, 53–4, 61, 65, 69–71, 74–6, 78n28, 139, 151, 157–8, 181n22
  assistance 6, 52, 70–1, 118
  dependants 139
  institutions 2–5, 12, 14, 42–3, 52–4, 57, 73, 75–6, 85, 101, 103, 109n6, 183
  organisations 52
  orphanages 69
  rescue work 57, 74
West Coast (New Zealand) 40
Western Australia 10, 101, 168
whiteness 9–10, 13, 88, 116, 132–3, 140, 164–5, 174, 187, 188
widowers 92
widows 58, 63, 92, 141, 155
Wilson, Dean 101
womanhood 13
women 2, 5, 8–9, 12–13, 27–8, 30, 32, 35, 51, 54–65, 68–9, 71, 73–6, 84, 87, 91–5, 97–106, 116–17, 120, 123, 125, 128–30, 133, 139–63, 164, 169–74, 177, 184, 186–7
  classes of 63, 141–2
  English 9, 145
  'fallen' 158
  genteel 141
  Irish 120, 143–4, 156
  respectable 157
Woods, W. J. 114
work 9, 11, 21, 25, 27, 29, 31, 34, 37, 41, 47n99, 52–4, 58, 60–2, 64, 66, 68–9, 74, 86, 91, 93, 96–9, 102, 114–15, 117–19, 121–3, 129–31, 133, 139, 141–2, 144–53, 156, 158, 160n43, 167, 169, 172–3, 175, 179, 186
  seasonal 34, 61
  see also occupations
workhouses 48n131, 53
working man's paradise 60

Zox, Ephraim 176

EU authorised representative for GPSR:
Easy Access System Europe, Mustamäe tee 50,
10621 Tallinn, Estonia
gpsr.requests@easproject.com

www.ingramcontent.com/pod-product-compliance
Ingram Content Group UK Ltd.
Pitfield, Milton Keynes, MK11 3LW, UK
UKHW041914140426
5217IPUK00002B/36